Natural Fertility

THE COMPLETE GUIDE TO AVOIDING OR ACHIEVING CONCEPTION

REVISED EDITION

FRANCESCA NAISH

SALLY MILNER PUBLISHING
MILNER HEALTHY LIVING GUIDE

First published in 1991 by
Sally Milner Publishing Pty Ltd
P O Box 2104
Bowral NSW 2576
Australia

Reprinted 1993, 1994, 1996, 2000

© Francesca Naish, 1991
This edition published in 2000 by
Sally Milner Publishing Pty Ltd

Design by Anna Warren, Warren Ventures P/L
Diagrams by Bookserve
Illustrations by Jacqueline Bateman
Printed and bound in Australia by Australian Print Group

National Library of Australia
Cataloguing-in-Publication data:

Naish, Francesca.
    Natural fertility.

    3rd ed.
    Includes index.
    ISBN 1 86351 268 3.

    1. Fertility, Human. 2. Conception. 3. Infertility. 4. Contraception. I. Title.
    (Series : Milner health series).

613.94

Cover painting:
Arnold Shore 1897–1964 Australian
Bella Donna, 1931
Oil on canvas on hardboard
76.5 x 64.2 cm
Purchased 1957
Reproduced with permission of the National Gallery of Victoria

Disclaimer

The information provided in this book is intended for general information and guidance only and should not be used as a substitute for consulting a qualified health practitioner. Neither the author nor the publisher accept liability or responsibility for any person or entity with respect to any loss, damage or injury caused or alleged to be caused directly or indirectly by the information contained in this book.

Dedication

For my mother — whose work of art was her children.

Acknowledgements

First, my thanks must go to all those who have researched and written on the topics discussed in this book before me, without whom I and many other women would be less healthy and happy.

Thanks go to Drs Evelyn and John Billings, two Australians whose work pioneered the use of the mucus method, to Dr Eugen Jonas, the Czechoslovakian whose work discovering and using the lunar cycle added another dimension to fertility management, and to Denis Stewart and Raymond Khoury, who greatly increased my love and knowledge of herbal medicine.

Next, my thanks go to my friends and colleagues (past and present) at the Village Healing and Growth Centre — which grew from my practice and helped my practice to grow, and which has now evolved into the Jocelyn Centre for Natural Fertility Management and Holistic Medicine — for their enormous contribution to my understanding and treatment of fertility, and for providing me with a second home and family.

Further thanks go to my dear friend Jacqueline Bateman for her wonderful pictures, to my illustrator, Judy Pownall, whose graphic skill enlivens these pages, to Anna Warren, for designing the book so attractively, to my editors, Lynn Humphries, for her painstaking care with the text of the first edition, and to Sandra Goldbloom Zurbo for her work on the changes to this edition, to my patient and supportive Australian publishers, Sally Milner and Margaret Bowman, Ian Webster and Libby Renney for their support for this new updated edition, and to my dear friend Valerie, who opened up her new home to me as a writer's retreat and kept me cheerful through the stresses of creativity.

Last, great thanks and love to my family for their continued good humour as more and more of my energy went into completing this book, which I could never even have begun if it weren't for the experiences of all my patients. It is they who have provided me with a wealth of material over the last 25 years of practice, on which to develop my understanding of fertility. My gratitude to womankind, everywhere.

A Note on the Author

Francesca Naish DCH, MATMS, MANTA, MNHAA, is an accredited herbalist, naturopath and hypnotherapist who is the director of a unique natural and holistic health care fertility clinic in Sydney, where she lives with her family. Her practical and humorous approach comes from 25 years of experience in practice, using the methods described in this book, both for herself and her clients. Over 10 000 women and their partners have consulted her and her associates during this time to find answers to their contraception, infertility and reproductive health problems, and to plan their ideal babies.

Francesca works at the Jocelyn Centre for Natural Fertility Management and Holistic Medicine, at which a diverse team of practitioners from both medical and natural health backgrounds offers a wide range of holistic therapies, and from which a national and international network of Natural Fertility Management counsellors are trained and supported. Francesca pioneered the use of the lunar cycle in combination with other timing techniques, and has created a unique blend of approaches to fertility management. As well as the programs offered through the clinic and through the network of trained counsellors, many women and couples are helped through the postal conception and contraception services.

She appears often on radio and television, talking on her speciality subjects of natural birth control, infertility, preconception health care and reproductive health. She writes extensively for natural health magazines, has been the subject of interviews and articles in the press, lectured at all the natural health training colleges in Sydney and to countless interested groups and conventions. She has previously published *The Lunar Cycle*, a book which explores the personal lunar phase cycle and its relationship to fertility, first published *Natural Fertility* in Australia in 1993, since when it has enjoyed best-seller status, as has her third book, *The Natural Way to Better Babies*, co-authored with Janette Roberts and published by Random House (also published as *Healthy Parents, Better Babies* in the USA by The Crossing Press and in the UK by Gill and Macmillan). This has been followed by two more books co-authored with Janette, *The Natural Way to a Better Pregnancy* and *The Natural Way to a Better Birth and Bonding*, both published by Doubleday, with two more in the pipeline on breastfeeding and miscarriage.

Having grown up in England, been educated at Godolphin School, Salisbury, and at Sussex University where she studied mathematics, Francesca went on to work with computers, manage a health food shop, and work in both theatre and circus as a mime–clown–comedienne. She extended this work to become involved with children in schools, open spaces and institutions, but on arriving in Australia in her late twenties, gave up the theatre in favour of concentrating on her interests in natural health and women. She then changed the emphasis of the natural birth control methods that she had employed for contraception and planned her family.

To join her two stepchildren came her first child, conceived on Friday the thirteenth and born a few weeks early on April Fool's Day! Her second consciously conceived child followed 6 years later.

Francesca's inspirations, apart from her work, are her family, music, literature and the countryside. Although a self-confessed workaholic, she has ambitions to one day spend less time at the former and more with the latter!

Contents

Introduction

All the ideas and information in this book have arisen from my experiences in managing my own fertility, and helping my patients to avoid or achieve conception, and retain or regain reproductive health. I'm sure that I've learnt as much from them over the past 25 years as (I hope) they have from me. Because my practice is a unique blend of techniques and remedies for fertility management, I felt there might be a need to spread the word.

Nearly all women have problems with their fertility at some point in their lives, and have a constant need to manage it. Either they have too much of it when they don't want to conceive, or too little when they do. In between, their hormones can plague them with a host of physical and emotional problems, and on top of that, the devices and drugs used to correct all of these difficulties simply create more.

In this book I have tried to give guidelines to help you manage your fertility, overcome all these 'women's problems' so you can take your rightful place in the world, be able to function in good health at all times, and have your children when and if you want them — rejoicing in your womanhood, not falling prey to it.

I firmly believe in women's right to this information about their bodies and their inherent good sense and ability to use it to make informed choices and enhance their lives.

It is my hope that the information in this book will help you to

- make clear and informed choices about the 'orthodox' and natural alternatives open to you

- understand and cooperate with your fertility cycles (rather than attempting to override or manipulate them), through observing body signs such as cervical mucus and basal body temperature, and combining this knowledge with your personal biorhythmic lunar cycle

- use these methods to avoid or achieve conception

- combine natural fertility awareness with other contraception techniques

- conceive consciously and in good health

- plan for the conception of your ideal baby

- overcome fertility problems (men, too) and achieve reproductive and hormonal health.

In other words, that the information will help you to learn to manage your fertility from puberty to menopause, and teach you how to adapt to the different needs of the different times in your life.

Effective, natural contraception and hormonal and reproductive health are the best possible foundations for conceiving in consciousness and good health when — and if — the time comes for you to have your children. Preparation for pregnancy well before conception has been shown to result overwhelmingly in healthier, brighter, more beautiful and well-adjusted babies.

Although many of the methods in this book, such as mucus, temperature and rhythm methods, have been written about fairly extensively, as far as I'm aware there is little that discusses their use in conjunction with the lunar cycle, which I have found in my practice to give the extra edge to success.

Objections to the use of the lunar cycle have often arisen from the fact that it is sometimes called 'astrological' birth control. In fact, it is not really astrological, as it only deals with a monthly repeating cycle and the relationship between only two heavenly bodies — the sun and the moon. In some ways, then, the name 'astrological' birth control as applied to this method is a misnomer, which may alienate those who might otherwise be prepared to consider the moon's role in influencing fertility.

The lunar cycle itself is not based on traditional astrological philosophy, but on empirically proven fact. In Chapter 7 I have tried to give some idea of how we might come to a proper scientific understanding of the effect of this cycle. In my first book, *The Lunar Cycle*, I look at these ideas more fully, but am only too aware of the areas in which we have no answers. Further research is needed, and we hope to get a preliminary study on the effects of this cycle happening in the near future.

Orthodox medicine has also often objected to the use of natural fertility awareness techniques. These objections are based on many medical practitioners' doubts as to whether women can successfully manage their own reproductive affairs. Most of these practitioners are men. My experience of women has been that they are overjoyed to have a more interactive role to play in their fertility management — especially one that poses no threat to their physical or psychological health — and show great sensitivity and responsibility. So, of course, do an increasing number of medical practitioners, both male and female, and I must apologise here if any of my remarks offend them.

My apologies, too, to any male readers of this book, who have been given such a small slice of attention and to whom the book is not directly addressed. My use of the female pronoun is not meant to be exclusive, and I heartily welcome any interest shown in fertility management by the male sex. It's just that most of the people concerned with fertility are women, so I've written the book (mostly) for them. Male fertility is linear rather than cyclic, which means that there is less to write about!

It's this cyclic quality of women that this book celebrates. We are about change and renewal; by learning to tune in to our personal rhythms and those of the planet we live on, we can learn to adapt our lifestyles to accommodate our cyclical natures. Hormonal and reproductive health can never be achieved through suppression, so much of the information in this book is to encourage you to balance your hormonal health, not juggle it. Healthy lifestyle is essential for healthy bodies. I'm sure it's not natural for so many women to have so many problems, rather, a result of depleted and depleting lifestyles and environments.

The incidence of common disorders of the reproductive system (both female and male) seems to be increasing, although with the lack of records on this still-taboo subject, it's difficult to be sure. Much of this book is dedicated to help you reach full reproductive and hormonal health, and there is plenty of advice on self-help methods.

However, this information is intended as a general guide: any treatment of individual physical disorders should be supervised by a competent health practitioner. Although the ideas in this book have worked for large numbers of women, they do rely on informed use to be effective. Responsibility lies with the user to remain aware, and not to abuse the methods. No guarantee of their success can be made in individual cases, although it is with confidence that I present them to you here, with my best wishes for:

Confident contraception, conscious conception, functional fertility, hormonal health and a good, healthy preparation for pregnancy.

Children are precious, may all yours be healthy
and come when they are welcome.

CHAPTER 1

The Natural Approach

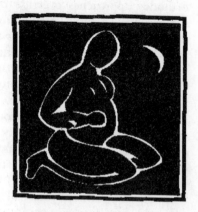

If there is one area of our lives where the natural approach is appropriate, it is surely that of fertility. After all, Mother Nature *is* fertility! She is reproduction. All other concerns bow to this one, the continuation of the species (us!).

Now, it could certainly be argued that one of the biggest threats to our survival comes from overpopulation—not having too many children is as important for the human race as having enough. This is where we can look to Mother Nature for guidance.

In her desire to have us reproduce, Nature has given us all unmistakable and wonderful signs of fertility.

This book is about how to recognise these signs, and use them for the appropriate purpose: to prevent or achieve conception.

It is fair to say that if you cooperated fully with natural cycles, you would conceive more often than not. As you read through these pages, it will become obvious that Mother Nature and your body are in a (benign) conspiracy to aid and abet the process of conception.

However, through learning about and understanding the changes in your body, as well as the forces that affect it, you can come to a point of control through response rather than through ignorance, suppression and manipulation. And, along the way, you will reap the benefits to your mental, emotional and physical health, your relationships and many other aspects of your well-being.

Countless women—and their partners—have felt the benefits of these methods and experienced the transformation they bring to their lives. This book aims to help you to do the same.

Body awareness

Tuning in or turning off? These are basically the choices when it comes to fertility management.

In the orthodox medical approach to treatment of infertility, drugs and surgery take over. As far as contraception is concerned, all the available orthodox approaches override or manipulate natural body functions in some way in a futile attempt to repress them. The difference with the methods outlined in this book is that here, the emphasis is on encouraging you into further involvement with, and understanding of, your reproductive functions, rather than on attempting to conceal them.

Knowledge is power. The more you understand what you are doing, and why, the more control you have.

Natural methods of fertility control return power to the individual. They enable you to deal with fertility in a manner appropriate to each set of circumstances instead of having to rely on the second-hand, poorly explained and partial answers that encourage dependence on devices, chemicals and specialists.

In *Natural Fertility*, you will embark on an amazing and wonderful adventure of discovery into your own body and be given the chance to learn the hows and whys of it all so that you can make your body work for you and not in spite of you. *You will learn how to give your body back to yourself and feel so much better for it.*

Sex and reproduction

Part of the understanding that comes from this journey of discovery is that sex and reproduction are aspects of the same process. Sex and sexuality are the tools of reproduction.

You don't have to make the quantum leap to supposing that sexual expression is 'wrong' if it's not carried out for the express purpose of creating another human being, but you can come to understand that denial of this basic truth can harm your efforts towards self-awareness and the greater harmony of mind and body.

Freeing the sexual energy

When the contraceptive pill (the Pill) came along, there was a lot of talk of 'sexual freedom', of women being 'freed' from the burden of unwanted pregnancies. Little did we know then that we were adding to our burdens. Not only has the contraceptive pill turned out to be a big problem for the physical and psychological health of many women who take it, but it has also brought us a new bondage — uncaring relationships.

The Pill brought with it the expectation that women should be sexually available at all times. Women felt obliged to provide, regardless of health hazards, while men were encouraged to be takers and to ignore any responsibility to prevent conception. These are hardly the ingredients for caring and responsible relationships; more the stuff of alienation, chauvinism and resentment, even leading to sexual turn-off rather than turn-on.

Some women are so bitter about the risks they feel obliged to take with their health that problems with their sexuality, including frigidity, can result.

Let us redefine sexual freedom to mean the capacity to give ourselves sexually in love and in trust, in tune with natural cycles and in the full knowledge that we are in no way endangering our health for the sake of our relationships.

Joyful and uninhibited sexual expression is both beneficial to and desirable for a fully rounded life. With Natural Fertility Management methods, this can truly be achieved by those of you who do not want to conceive in the times when you know yourself to be infertile.

Cooperation of the sexes

Far from laying the responsibility for contraception or conception firmly on the woman's shoulders, to be borne alone, along with whatever health hazards may accompany it, let us bring the whole issue out in the open and encourage a full and frank discussion and the sharing of information and responsibility.

Natural methods offer the male partner a chance to contribute to the processes of achieving or preventing conception in more ways than just depositing the seed. A cooperative partner is a big help for a woman using these methods, and most relationships flourish as a result of adopting them. But these methods can also be used by women on their own. The single or uninvolved woman can feel highly confident in her ability to control and understand her fertility whether or not she has a participating partner. *It can be each woman's decision to share the responsibility or not, as she sees fit.*

Reliability

Many women, health-conscious in all other aspects of their lives, take their contraceptive pill along with their vitamins and minerals, in the mistaken belief that natural methods of contraception are not a safe alternative.

Although the many myths about huge Catholic families conceived on the Rhythm Method have some basis in fact, many people do not realise that natural methods have been updated: these days they are well-researched and precise. Despite being dissatisfied with their current contraceptive method, these women have left the subject of natural methods unexplored, as have many of their sisters who are suffering from infertility, and have looked to the hi-tech approaches for the answers to their problems. *Natural methods of contraception, when used correctly, are between 97 and 99 per cent effective.*

This rate of effectiveness is as good as that for any other method of contraception, except, perhaps, the combination Pill, but not the Mini-pill.

Of course, the methods have to be used correctly. Even the use of the Pill can be abused or not understood — I once knew a woman who took her entire month's supply at the beginning of each cycle.

Easy to apply

Another incorrect assumption about natural methods of contraception is that they are difficult to implement. Nothing could be further from the truth. Over and over again, the statistics show that women, however simple or uneducated, can easily be taught how to recognise signs of fertility and be given the guidelines on what measures to take, according to what outcome they desire.

Although it may seem that there is a great deal of information to absorb in this book, the methods are really learnt through application, with *most women feeling confident of their command of them within a few cycles.* Your fertility becomes another part of your self-awareness, in the same way as you are aware of whether or not you have a cold, and the methods of identification become an easy part of your daily routine, requiring little time or effort.

Commitment and motivation, along with a healthy curiosity about your own body, are really all that are required if you are willing to give your energy to this approach. The learning period requires the most time and attention, but once the methods have become a part of your daily routine, confidence, and the subsequent relief from anxiety, quickly become established in nearly all cases.

Regularity is not essential

Another reason why some women feel that these methods are not for them is because they have irregular cycles.

Fertility can be recognised whether it is present every other week or only once in a blue moon. In fact, *these methods are applicable at all stages of a woman's fertile life, from puberty to the onset of menopause* (often a confusing and chaotic time, when this information can be invaluable), *and can be used either to avoid conception or to help achieve it.* Understanding the effect that different circumstances have on your body is part of the process, and it allows greater efficiency in the application of the methods.

So, if you want to interfere with your body functions as little as possible and, at the same time, retain control over your fertility, or if you merely have a problem finding a suitable and reliable method of birth control, then you will be pleased to learn that there is a real and effective natural solution.

Individual approaches

One of the things this book will try to do is give you information, not rules. The trouble with rules is that, although they are, of course, sometimes necessary, they do not always educate. When conditions change, guidelines may be missing and this can result in confusion.

If you truly understand the principles on which these methods are based, there should be no circumstance which lies outside their effective application and you will be able to confidently meet the demands of any new situation.

There are different answers for different times, and different strokes for different folks. So, while there are not always set formulae for each situation, there is help, guidance and information that should give each person the resources and confidence to meet each new circumstance with an appropriate response.

There are several ways to identify fertility. Some are more effective than others and some more appropriate in a given situation. Most women work out a combination that best suits them, flexibility being the most successful approach. In this way, if one method is invalidated by circumstance, another can be substituted.

I recommend that you become familiar with, and adept at, each of the approaches outlined in *Natural Fertility*. Then, when you fully understand what you are doing, you can make informed choices.

You might even make an informed choice to use chemical or mechanical means of contraception to meet the perceived needs of a certain phase in your life. *As long as you know you have options, and what the consequences of your actions are, then the choices are yours alone.*

Too often, women and girls blindly follow the advice of a less-than-thorough medical practitioner and end up choosing a program of fertility control that is not appropriate simply because they have no other information and, therefore, no option.

Overkill versus minimalism

Fertility is an issue for most women for most of their lives, which makes it too significant a matter for ill-informed decisions. The consequences are considerable, continuous and sometimes irreversible.

The Pill, though its history is comparatively short, is taken in greater quantities than any other prescribed drug in history. There may be long-term and generational effects that we have yet to discover.

Although fertility is a full-time concern for most women, *there are only a few days each month when it is actually possible to conceive.* Therefore, orthodox methods that protect against conception 100 per cent of the time represent overkill, which is, by definition, unnecessary.

Natural methods are minimalist in their approach, identifying the fertile days so that choices only have to be made a small proportion of the time — so much more streamlined. Some of the other problems associated with orthodox methods will be explored in greater depth in the next chapter.

The natural advantage

Let us summarise the advantages of natural methods of fertility management. Then, if you're convinced, you can continue reading this book to find out how to make them work for you.

SELF-SUFFICIENCY

With natural methods, there is no reliance on manufactured goods or specialist knowledge. The resources are right there in your own body, which means that these methods can be used effectively in any circumstances, including having an irregular cycle, during breastfeeding, when trying to conceive, and during the approach to menopause (see Chapter 11, 'Times of Change').

You could go bush and remain able to control your fertility; you could survive medical and pharmaceutical breakdowns or strikes; you could travel to uncharted lands or indulge in other exotic escapades — you will still remain confident and in control.

NO SIDE-EFFECTS

As natural methods involve no intrusive techniques, there can be no side-effects. With these methods you learn to cooperate with your body, not abuse it. All other methods have side-effects to some extent. We will explore these more fully in Chapter 2.

SELF-KNOWLEDGE

The mastering of natural methods will reward both your curiosity and the harmonious interaction of your body and mind. Observation of the changes that take place during a cycle can often lead to other discoveries about your body and health, as well as informing you of when you are fertile. You will become much more sensitive to, and less at the mercy of, changes in energy and emotional states, in levels of sensuality and sexual desire and other cyclical changes, both physical and mental. Patterns that emerge are fascinating and usually bring to full consciousness a hitherto vague awareness of changes, making sense of previously unexplained phenomena.

Increased self-knowledge can bring a whole new dimension of awareness to sexual activity. Sexual blocks are often the result of ignorance and fear. Self-knowledge can defuse these situations, allowing a woman to feel more comfortable in her body, and less threatened by another's intimacy. And, of course, *knowledge is power*.

LOW COST

Although it is best to get some professional guidance while learning these methods through the first few cycles, once the system is an established part of your day-to-day life, there are no further expenses — no prescription fees or costs for services, no bills for treatment and checkups. Natural Fertility Management is a *truly maintenance-free method*.

SHARED RESPONSIBILITY

The adoption of natural methods represents a chance for couples to work together with mutual consideration and respect, to take common responsibility for what is, after all, a common concern. And all this without loss of control for the woman. She need feel no threat from using these methods, and no resentment at having to abuse her body for the sake of the relationship: a truly liberating experience for all concerned.

WOMAN–CONTROLLED CONTRACEPTION

It is not necessary to have a cooperative partner, or, indeed, a stable relationship to use these methods. Many women wonder why they take the Pill in periods of sexual inactivity: the reason is usually 'just in case'. Natural Fertility Management methods offer a chance for a woman to feel confident that she can have effective control over her fertility whenever she has the need.

Barrier methods (condom, female condom, diaphragm and cap) are available and can be used *if necessary and if desired*, when abstinence is inappropriate. Diaphragms (or Dutch caps, as they are sometimes called) offer a chance for the woman to stay discreet and in control. Condoms offer the male partner a chance to contribute — and the woman a chance to find out if he's willing to do so (see Chapter 9, 'Sexual Expression in Fertile Times').

HAVING CHILDREN WHEN THEY'RE WANTED

Information about fertility can be used to achieve conception, as well as to avoid it. The identification techniques remain the same; the uses to which they are put can vary. Some couples use this information to achieve conscious conception (see Chapter 13, 'Conscious Conception'). Natural Fertility Management gives you a chance to prepare for conception and then achieve it in full awareness. Many pregnancies are accidental, the parents becoming reconciled to them at a later date. Others are wished for but not acknowledged until several weeks into the pregnancy.

On so few occasions in our lives do we have the chance to welcome in another being — in this way we can do so in confidence and with joy, benefiting both your pregnancy and your child.

Some couples have fertility problems, an increasing difficulty these days as a result of the stress of modern lives, poor health, environmental hazards and pollution, and exacerbated by contraceptive programs and sexually transmitted disease.

Low levels of fertility (see Chapter 13 again) can be helped enormously by pinpointing the most fertile time in a woman's cycle and properly preparing for it. So, the same information that was used for contraception can be reversed in its application.

No other method of birth control can make this claim. In fact, most of them are more likely to contribute to fertility problems.

NO OVERKILL

Natural contraception methods allow you to guard against pregnancy only when it is a possibility. Orthodox methods of birth control are employed continuously, despite the fact that *you are fertile only for a few days each cycle.*

This means that the rest of the time you are free to make pure, unprotected love, confident that it will not result in an unwanted pregnancy.

NO DANGER TO FUTURE PREGNANCIES OR FERTILITY
Many contraception methods pose a threat to a child conceived while they are being employed. Conception is a possibility, albeit slight, with all methods of contraception — there is no such thing as 100 per cent contraception.

In Chapter 2, 'The Unnatural Approach', we shall look at how a pregnancy can be affected by the contraception method used at the time of conception.

One thing can be certain with natural methods of contraception: the only complication can be a *normal* pregnancy (given that all other possible mutagens are absent), and the chances of this occurring are about as low as with any other method.

MORALLY AND ETHICALLY IMPECCABLE
There can be no objections to these methods on moral, religious or ethical grounds, unless barrier methods are used at fertile times, and this is a matter of individual choice.

Some other methods of birth control (such as the intrauterine device — IUD) may involve the abortion of a fertilised egg, a fact of which the user may be unaware. Many religions prohibit contraception methods that interfere with the process of conception. Natural methods are perfectly acceptable on all these grounds.

Hi-tech, *in vitro* fertility treatments, which are becoming more and more unnatural in their approaches, often use sperm and eggs from donors and may involve experimentation on, and storage of, fertilised eggs. These methods and experiments are giving rise to many ethical and religious concerns.

The extent of medical alienation from the natural process of reproduction is illustrated by one recent suggestion, taken seriously by at least some of the medical establishment, that, as an alternative to using surrogate mothers, newly-dead women (*neo morts*) could be kept alive on life-support systems and used as incubators for babies. The intent behind this extraordinarily insensitive plan is to overcome legal objections to surrogacy, as the law, so far, only applies to live women.

For anyone who believes in the importance of the psychological, physical and spiritual environments at the time of conception, these artificial methods present additional problems. Whether or not these problems are worth enduring in the quest for a child is a matter for individual decision, but many couples would feel a lot easier in their consciences if natural methods were explored fully as a first option.

RELIABILITY

Despite the findings of a recent survey in the USA showing that fewer than half the physicians whom women consult about reproductive issues discuss natural methods, and that the physicians seriously underestimate the effectiveness of these methods, the truth is far more reassuring.

Statistics show us between 97 and 99 per cent successful results for natural methods of contraception (when used correctly). The only method which has a (very slightly) higher rate is the combination Pill. The Mini-pill, more often prescribed these days, does not.

Natural methods also enjoy a higher success rate than the hi-tech procedures used in dealing with infertility, and are much less stressful and expensive.

Natural methods are no longer the hit-and-miss affair of old. They have been updated, and are precise and reliable. So, here's wishing you confident contraception and conscious conception.

CHAPTER 2

The Unnatural Approach

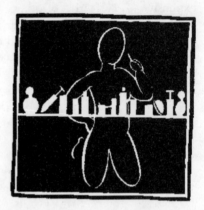

There is a long history of regarding the menstrual cycle and its effects as a curse. Indeed, it is traditionally seen as woman's punishment for Eve's 'sins'. Throughout the ages, we have examples of women being considered unclean at the time of their menstruation, being forbidden access to social activities, having a taboo placed on their preparation of food and, most particularly, on their participation in sexual activity. As late as the end of the nineteenth century, it was believed that the touch of a menstruating woman could turn a ham rancid.

In some patriarchal societies, there was a belief that menstruating women were dangerous and could infect people and objects with which they came into contact. In some cases, this even went as far as a fear of death.

Blessed or cursed?

It has been suggested that if we go back further than the nineteenth century, we may find that these fears originated in the recognition that, at the time of menstruation, a woman is in touch with magical or psychic powers, a connection made much of by the Yaqui Indian sorcerer Don Juan in books by Carlos Casteneda, and with roots in many cultural and religious traditions. (Interestingly, the Old English derivative of the word *blessing* is *blestian*, which means 'bleeding'.) Such contact means the woman needs to psychologically withdraw at this time, and requires solitude.

There is a decrease in the external senses of sight, smell, hearing and colour discrimination at menstruation, with a corresponding increase in the body's internal senses, such as thinking, feeling and memory.

The Sabbath had its origin in the Sabbatu, the menstruation of the Babylonian goddess Ishtar, which took place at full moon, and at which time no work was done, no cooked food was eaten and no journeys undertaken. *Sa-bat* means 'heart rest', the day of rest that the moon takes when it is full, neither increasing nor decreasing in size.

The fulfilment of psychic and physical needs, the rest taken from normal duties at this time of menstruation — by goddesses and women alike — is something we are completely out of touch with today. Although many cultures have respected these needs, even to the extent of providing a menstruation hut or a women-only bathhouse for retreat, most modern women in the Western world are presumptuous enough to consider themselves removed from 'primitive' natural cycles, and attempt to keep their activities at consistent levels without recognition of their influences.

We can see here one possible cause of the widespread suffering of premenstrual syndrome (PMS) and other menstrual distress these days, which could, perhaps, be partially interpreted as the result of women being out of touch with their cyclical nature and needs — physical, psychological and psychic.

The old ways of acknowledging women's cycles were religious and firmly embedded in social customs. Today, we have to fulfil these needs individually. The modern woman's chance to tune in to her physical self and her cycles involves personal exploration, observation and understanding of her sexuality and reproductive functions.

Unfortunately, the society in which we live does not encourage such attitudes. The menstrual cycle is seen by men as a nuisance, a reason why women are unreliable in the workforce and as something of an embarrassment, to be acknowledged as little as possible. Many women also see it this way, as an inconvenience and a destructive force in their lives.

As a result, our contraception methods reflect these attitudes. They are largely attempts to disguise and suppress the natural cycle. The total obliteration of cyclical change was found to have deeply disturbing effects on women, which is why there is a 'pretend' period on the Pill, a sop to women's cyclical nature.

Unfortunately, this negative approach has all sorts of problems attached to it, which we shall now discuss.

The Pill
There are basically two types of contraceptive pill, each one working in slightly different ways.

THE COMBINATION/SEQUENTIAL/TRIPHASIC PILL

This medication contains oestrogen and progesterone. It acts by

◆ *sterilisation* — inhibiting ovarian activity

◆ *abortion* — altering the womb's lining to prevent implantation

◆ *contraception* — making the mucus in the cervix hostile to sperm.

THE MINI-PILL

This medication contains *only* progesterone; it contains no oestrogen. It does not necessarily inhibit ovulation, relying instead on the second and third actions described above.

As notorious as the Pill is, millions of women still use it. Medicine acknowledges that there are many women for whom the Pill is contra-indicated. These include women with a personal or family history of the following medical conditions.

> Diabetes
>
> Blood clots
>
> Heart or kidney disease
>
> Epilepsy
>
> Known or suspected pregnancy
>
> Unusual vaginal bleeding
>
> Angina pectoris (pains in the heart)
>
> Stroke
>
> High blood pressure
>
> High cholesterol and triglycerides
>
> Very irregular menstrual cycles or late menarche (onset of first menstruation)
>
> Known or suspected cancer of the breast, liver or reproductive organs
>
> Breast nodules or fibrocystic disease of the breast
>
> Multiple sclerosis
>
> Tuberculosis
>
> Sickle-cell anaemia
>
> Large, swollen and tender varicose veins
>
> Cigarette smoking
>
> Obesity
>
> Migraines or recurrent headaches
>
> Fibroid tumours of the uterus
>
> Diseases triggered by pregnancy, for example, jaundice, herpes, chloasma

Gallbladder disease or gallstones

Liver tumours, disorders or damage

Recurrent or active hepatitis

Crohn's disease

Malabsorption syndrome

Depression

Also, women who are currently breastfeeding, women over 35 (especially if they smoke or suffer from poor circulation), and adolescents who have been menstruating for less than 2 years This is not a complete list, and, too often, little case-taking is done by busy medical practitioners. Unfortunately, many of these at-risk women end up taking the Pill on the recommendation of their physician. Perhaps if they had access to some of the following information, they would have made a different choice.

In the USA, detailed warnings of possible side effects (which fill two foolscap pages) are compulsory with each prescription for the Pill.

The Pill has been in use for less than 40 years which means that long-term and generational effects are still to be fully explored. However, here are some of the proven side-effects noted so far.

MINOR SIDE-EFFECTS

Weight gain

Appetite changes

Skin discolouration (chloasma)

Migraines

Fungal infections and tinea

Vaginal discharges, including a much greater tendency to vaginal thrush (candida, or yeast infestation)

Systemic candida infection

Genital warts

Urinary tract infections

Nausea

Allergic reactions, such as incidence of rhinitis, hay fever, asthma, skin rashes

Eye disorders, such as double vision, swelling of optic nerve, contact-lens intolerance, corneal inflammation

Secretions from the breasts

Lumpy or tender breasts

Disturbances in liver function

Dizziness and neurological problems

Breakthrough bleeding

Decreased immune response

Fluid retention (oedema) and bloating

Eczema

Acne

Mouth ulcers

Cervical erosions

Hair loss (alopecia)

Facial and body hair growth

Varicose veins

Psychological and emotional disorders, often labelled depression, including mood swings or loss of libido (sex drive), jokingly referred to as the way the Pill works. (Suicide is much more common among Pill users than those using other forms of contraception.)

If you suffer from even some of these effects to any great degree, you may wonder why they are called minor — it's because they are not life-threatening. However, they are certainly quality-of-life threatening.

A 10-year research program undertaken by the California Walnut Creek Drug Study of hospital admissions reports significantly increased inflammatory diseases in women under 40 who have taken, or currently take, the Pill. These inflammatory conditions include respiratory, digestive, urogenital and musculoskeletal disorders.

Many women coming off the Pill report a much greater feeling of well-being, both physical and psychological, although the feelings are often unrelated to specific conditions and only fully realised as the effects of the Pill wear off.

MAJOR SIDE-EFFECTS

Significantly increased chance of suffering a stroke (risk increasing with age and duration of Pill usage)

Two to eight-fold increased risk of blood clots (thrombosis)

Three to six-fold increase in risk of heart attacks (according to age)

Increased chance of hardening of the arteries, circulatory disease and high blood pressure

Disturbances to blood-sugar metabolism (possibly contributing to diabetes or hypoglycaemia)

Increased risk of gallbladder disease (gallstones) Liver tumours (increasing with duration of Pill usage)

Significantly increased risk of ectopic pregnancy

Possible link with cancer of the endometrium (lining of the

womb), cervix, ovaries, liver and lungs

Significantly higher risk of developing breast cancer

Strong probability of more rapid development of pre-
existing cancers and progression to cancer of abnormal cells

Osteoporosis

Possible arrest of bone growth in adolescent girls

The probability of incidence of all of these effects is disputed, and some have only been noted (so far) as resulting from the high-dosage Pill that is now less commonly prescribed, though studies show that the third generation pills now in use have increased the risk of thrombosis. Long-term statistics inevitably include a period when the higher doses were commonplace. For each set of statistics showing negative results, there seems to be a corresponding set denying them.

All the health-conscious person can conclude is that there is sufficient evidence to cast grave doubts on the safety of taking contraceptive pills.

This also seems to be the view of the British Government's Committee on the Safety of Medicines, which was sufficiently startled by statistics from Oxford University showing a significant link with higher rates of breast cancer, to write to every doctor in the UK advising them of the study and suggest that they seriously consider alternative forms of contraception for their patients.

Taking the Pill causes deficiencies in a large number of nutrients, as it affects vitamin metabolism, and this, of course, contributes to our list of side-effects.

VITAMIN AND MINERAL DEFICIENCIES EXPERIENCED BY PILL TAKERS

Vitamin A (retinol) — Various studies have shown disruption to vitamin A levels in the blood. Some show increases in retinol levels, which may simply mean less of the vitamin is stored in the liver, and others show a marked reduction in beta-carotene (the precursor to vitamin A). The implications are not yet clear. Eyesight changes can result from a deficiency in vitamin A, as this vitamin is needed for the normal, healthy functioning of the eyes. Increased susceptibility to infections, dry and scaly skin, lack of appetite and vigour, defective teeth and gums, heavy menstrual bleeding, cervical problems and retarded growth are also reported in the case of a deficiency. Vitamin A is also an important antioxidant and anticancer vitamin, and better taken as mixed carotenoids (or, if unavailable, betacarotene) to avoid toxicity.

Vitamin B1 (thiamin) — There is a probability that Pill takers are deficient in this vitamin. Side-effects include fatigue, weakness, insomnia, vague aches and pains, weight loss, depression, irritability, lack of initiative, constipation, oversensitivity to noise, loss of appetite or sugar cravings and circulatory problems.

Vitamin B2 (riboflavin) — Requirements of the body are raised by use of the Pill, leading to deficiencies. Side-effects include gum and mouth infections, dizziness, depression, eye irritation, skin problems and dandruff.

Vitamin B6 (Pyridoxin) — Depletion varies from marginal to severe. Side-effects include nausea, low stress tolerance, lethargy, anxiety, depression, weakness, nervousness, emotional flare-ups, fatigue, insomnia, mild paranoia, skin eruptions, loss of muscular control, eye problems, herpes infection and oedema (fluid retention). Vitamin B6 is needed to help convert tryptophan to serotonin (a brain compound that affects pain response, eating patterns, moods, sleep patterns, psychological drive and sexual desire), to normalise sugar metabolism, to help prevent blood clots forming and to keep homocysteine levels under control (see Vitamin B9, folic acid).

Vitamin B9 (folic acid) — Levels are significantly reduced on the Pill. The most severe problem resulting from this is if conception occurs during Pill use, or in the immediate period following, when the body is still recovering. Since folic acid is required by the body to facilitate cell division, a process that starts immediately after conception, if this nutrient is deficient, there is a much higher risk of abnormal synthesis of DNA and congenital abnormalities, including neural tube defects, spina bifida, deformed limbs and mongolism. Deficiency can also lead to damage to the wall of the small intestine, anaemia and raised homocysteine levels, which have been associated with cardiovascular disease, various gynaecological conditions and repeated miscarriage. Homocysteine can be kept to healthy levels if folic acid and vitamins B6 and B12 are in adequate supply. Raised levels of this amino acid may be the pathway whereby deficiencies of these nutrients can lead to neural tube defects, such as spina bifida.

Vitamin B12 (cobalamin) — Levels in the blood are lowered in Pill users, especially vegetarians. Resulting effects include anaemia, sore tongue, weight loss, depression and raised homocysteine levels (see Vitamin B9, folic acid).

Vitamin C (ascorbic acid) — The breakdown of vitamin C is increased by the Pill; levels can be reduced by up to 30 per cent. This is worsened by smoking, stress, high pollution levels, infections and some medications. The effectiveness of vitamin C supplementation may also be reduced. This can result in bruising, bleeding gums, 'spider' veins, heavy menstrual bleeding, eye problems, loss of appetite, muscular weakness, anaemia, fatigue and lowered immune response.

This vitamin is also necessary for the production of the sex hormones, something your body will have to start doing for itself when you come off the Pill. A deficiency can make it even harder for your body to resume normal production.

The lack of the bioflavonoids that naturally occur with vitamin C can exacerbate many of these symptoms.

Ironically, if vitamin C is taken in high doses (more than 2 grams daily) it can interfere with the effectiveness of the Pill. This is because it increases the potency of chemical hormones, so when the dosage is reduced, your body can misinterpret this as a reduction in hormone levels and ovulation can occur.

Vitamin E (mixed tocopherols or, if unavailable, alpha tocopherol) — There is an increased need for vitamin E as a result of oestrogen levels being higher when you are taking the Pill (this vitamin helps to normalise oestrogen levels). Effects of insufficient vitamin E include anaemia, muscle degeneration, subsequent low fertility, changes in the menstrual cycle and hot flushes. It is also needed to help offset the greater risk of blood-clot formation and possible carcinogenic effect of the oestrogen, as is selenium, which plays a part in vitamin E absorption. Selenium levels are also decreased by the Pill.

Vitamin K (menadione) — Higher levels may lead to blood-clot formation. Other factors involved in blood clotting are also increased in Pill users.

Iron — Less iron may be lost due to lighter periods.

Calcium — Absorption is improved. Though this may seem like an advantage, it can further imbalance overall nutritional status..

Magnesium — Levels of this important mineral are reduced in those taking the Pill. Deficiency can cause a variety of premenstrual symptoms, lumpy breasts, muscle cramps, anxiety, sleeplessness, chocolate or sugar cravings and cardiovascular problems.

Copper — Absorption is increased, raising the body's need for vitamin C, disrupting the zinc:copper balance and leading to insomnia, depression, migraine, hair loss and the possibility of high blood pressure and clotting tendencies.

Zinc — Levels are significantly lowered by the Pill. This can lead to diabetes, sugar cravings, loss of appetite, poor resistance to infection, skin infections, lowered fertility and many other problems. This mineral is crucial for normal growth, cell division and tissue repair. Zinc is very important during pregnancy, as it is involved in over 200 enzyme systems in the body, and is crucial for the development of brain function and a competent immune system, another reason to avoid conceiving while on, or soon after using, the Pill. Long-term Pill users can find it difficult to rebuild their zinc status to an adequate level.

Prostaglandins — Levels of certain prostaglandins are lowered on the Pill. These prostaglandins are normally made from essential fatty acids, using zinc as a catalyst. They decrease tendencies to clot formation.

Blood lipids — Low and very low density lipids, cholesterol and triglycerides (the villains) are increased on the Pill, raising the chances of heart disease.

Serum proteins — All are altered by the Pill.

SUGGESTED SUPPLEMENTATION LEVELS IF ON THE PILL (AND FOR SEVERAL MONTHS AFTER WITHDRAWAL)

Mixed carotenoids or betacarotene — 6 mg

Vitamin B-complex — 50 mg each of B_1, B_2, B_3, B_5, B_6, 400 mcg B_{12} and folic acid

Vitamin C — 1000–3000 mg (with bioflavonoids)

Vitamin E — 200–400 iu (except if you have high blood pressure)

Magnesium — 100–200 mg

Zinc — 50 mg

Manganese — 10 mg

Essential fatty acids (evening primrose and fish oils) — 500–1000 mg 3 x d

Garlic (2–5000 mg) and lecithin are also useful to help reduce the raised level of blood fats

Check calcium and iron levels, and remember that the best source of nutrients is your diet. Eating wisely will help recovery. (See Chapter 12, 'Natural Remedies for Hormonal and Reproductive Health' and Chapter 13, 'Conscious Conception', for more details on food sources and the effects of food on reproductive and foetal health.)

It is extremely important to stop taking the Pill and replenish nutrients for at least 6 months before attempting conception, as the egg needs to mature for almost 3 months in a nutrient-rich environment.

Once a woman decides to stop taking the Pill, whether to start a family or for any other reason, she may find she is suffering from the most ironic, and perhaps distressing, side-effect of all.

TEMPORARY, OR EVEN PERMANENT, STERILITY

Sometimes the body has difficulty responding after ovulation and mucus production are no longer suppressed, as there is a resulting hormonal imbalance and the cycle does not recommence satisfactorily. This results in a lack of

◆ menstruation

◆ ovulation

◆ normal endometrial function, or

◆ sufficient mucus reduction.

There may also be other associated problems, such as irregularity and increased incidence of PMS or dysmenorrhoea, which may last several years.

Women who previously had long cycles, whose cycles were irregular, or who began menstruating late (after age 15), and women who are lightweight, are more likely to be affected by post-Pill amenorrhoea or hormonal imbalance. Happily, natural remedies are very effective in most cases (see Chapter 12, 'Natural Remedies for Hormonal and Reproductive Health').

PROBLEM PREGNANCIES

Of course, even the Pill is not 100 per cent effective. In fact, no method is, except total abstinence. Nowadays, pills are prescribed in lower dosage and many women are on the progesterone-only, or Mini-pill. To be effective, these pills have to be taken with great regularity and at the same time each day; the user success rate is, therefore, lower. There is also a problem of lowered effectiveness if some antibiotics (including penicillin and tetracycline) are taken at the same time as the Pill, as they speed up the elimination of the synthetic hormones.

This means that more pregnancies are started while the mother is on the Pill, a situation which may continue into the first few months of the pregnancy, conception not being obvious. This severely alters the climate in which the foetus grows.

Deficiencies of folic acid, for example, have been linked to a greatly increased chance of giving birth to a child with spina bifida and limb defects. The incidence of Down syndrome has been linked to deficiencies in a number of nutrients, including selenium, folic acid and zinc. An increase in heart defects has also been associated with conceptions taking place while the mother is on the Pill, and other defects, such as limb deformities, have been linked with ingested oestrogens and progesterone.

There is also a much higher incidence of stillbirths, miscarriages and congenital abnormalities in children conceived within a month of coming off the Pill. Women who have, at any stage, taken the Pill, have a 4.3 per cent increased chance of having offspring with congenital abnormalities. It seems highly likely that nutrient deficiencies and imbalances may be a major contributing factor to the greater incidences of abnormalities and problem pregnancies experienced by these mothers. There may also be an increased chance of gestational diabetes in these women (the Pill has a proven link with diabetes and blood-sugar metabolism disturbances), and of hypertension and toxaemia (because the Pill tends to increase blood pressure).

Another possible problem has emerged in recent studies. It appears that a woman's immune system, her sense of smell and her body odour are intimately connected. Under natural conditions, women and men are attracted to someone who smells unlike them, thus ensuring an extended immune response gene pool for their child. Unfortunately, when taking the oral contraceptive pill (OCP), this natural imperative becomes confused, and women are likely to chose partners who smell similar to themselves.

This creates two problems. First, there are likely to be increased chances of infertility, miscarriage and health problems in the offspring, and second, when the woman goes off the Pill in order to conceive, her olfactory responses return to normal so she may stop being sexually attracted to her mate! Perhaps this could be part of the reason (along with the nutrient deficiencies) for the increased level of infertility in women who have previously used oral contraceptives.

The Mini-pill, or progesterone-only pill, which does not suppress ovulation but causes changes in the endometrium and the cervical mucus (see Chapter 4, 'Cervical Mucus Changes'), also interferes with the passage of the egg through the fallopian tubes. This may result in a greater likelihood of any pregnancies being ectopic or implanting in the fallopian tubes, a highly dangerous and potentially fatal condition. (As the Mini-pill must be taken at exactly the same time each day, pregnancies are more likely to occur.)

The residue of the Pill can take up to 6 months to be eliminated from the system. This is, therefore, the minimum amount of time that should elapse between coming off the Pill and conceiving. Luckily, the process of elimination can be sped up and guaranteed by using natural therapies such as herbal medicine, homoeopathy or acupuncture, along with good diet and nutritional supplementation (See Chapter 11, 'Times of Change', and Chapter 12, 'Natural Remedies for Hormonal and Reproductive Health').

The Mini-pill is also often prescribed for lactating mothers, despite the fact that this pill has been shown to severely deplete the nutrients available for the child in the mother's milk, as well as providing the baby with an overdose of synthetic hormones. Synthetic progesterone is known to act on the hypothalamus, an important brain centre, and may masculinise a female infant and contribute to neonatal jaundice.

The one effect that the Pill has on all users (this is, in fact, its modus operandi) is that it keeps the body in a continuous state of preparation for the (non-existent) developing foetus. In other words, it simulates a state of pregnancy for those anxious to avoid the real thing.

Many women feel that they don't want to live out their lives in this altered state, regardless of whether they suffer side-effects or not.

The IUD

IUD is the acronym for **intrau**terine **d**evice (a device in the womb).

For those women who don't want to take chemical contraception into their body orally, the next option is usually mechanical contraception via the vagina.

No one is certain how an IUD works, but it is largely, if not wholly, to do with the irritation and inflammation it causes in the uterus. This means that the fertilised egg cannot implant in the wall of the womb.

If intercourse occurs at the fertile time and there are no other problems with fertility, then the egg is fertilised most months. If an IUD is present, an abortion occurs because *the IUD is an abortifacient, not a contraceptive*, a fact that is little known, even by users, and can give rise to great moral or religious distress on its discovery.

Different types of IUD in common use

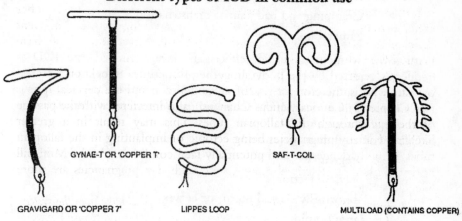

GYNAE-T OR 'COPPER T'

SAF-T-COIL

GRAVIGARD OR 'COPPER 7'

LIPPES LOOP

MULTILOAD (CONTAINS COPPER)

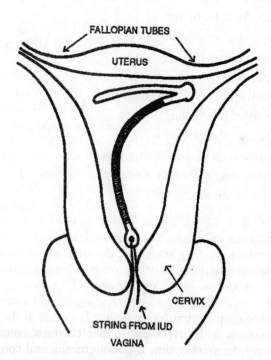

FALLOPIAN TUBES

UTERUS

CERVIX

STRING FROM IUD

VAGINA

A 'Copper 7' or Gravigard IUD in the Uterus

The inflammation and irritation caused by the IUD also give rise to the so-called minor side-effects.

MINOR SIDE-EFFECTS

Heavy bleeding

Possible hormonal changes

Dysplasia

Cramping and bad pain at menstruation

Mineral imbalances

With some women, these side-effects are severe. Indeed, the IUD is frequently rejected by the body altogether, sometimes unbeknown to the woman, who is, therefore, at risk of unwanted conception.

No woman with a history of dysmenorrhoea (period pain, heavy bleeding and so forth) should ever use an IUD.

Other contra-indications include:

pregnancy

pelvic infection

abnormally shaped uterus or cervix

large fibroids

multiple partners

cervical or uterine cancer

irregular cycles

previous uterine surgery

previous ectopic pregnancy

abnormal bleeding

heart-valve disease

anaemia / blood-clotting defect

high risk of sexually transmitted diseases (STDs)

autoimmune disease

immune deficiency

Since most IUDs are made of copper, and high levels of this mineral reduce the availability of zinc in the body, zinc deficiencies, which affect the skin and the reproductive and immune systems particularly adversely, may be a problem for those women using an IUD. Copper also causes melanaldehyde, which is known to be carcinogenic and mutagenic, to form in the cervical mucus.

A newer version of the IUD, called the IUS (intrauterine system), is impregnated with hormones, thus increasing the risks involved to include those associated with chemical contraception.

Of course, if you feel that your health is dependent on the free flow of energy through your body (the model of health on which traditional Chinese and Oriental medicine is based, for example the meridians of acupuncture), then you will be dubious about living with a constantly inflamed and irritated organ in your body.

MAJOR SIDE-EFFECTS

Pelvic inflammatory disease (PID) — This is the most common of the major side-effects, being a five-fold greater risk in women under 30. The perforated endometrium is susceptible to these infections that arise in the pelvic cavity, involving the uterus or the fallopian tubes, and sometimes spreading to the ovaries. It is believed that the bacteria responsible may climb up the cord that hangs from the sterile uterus into the non-sterile vagina, infecting the womb and tubes. *Unfortunately, these infections are often well-progressed before detected, and resultant scarring can cause adhesions, which may block the fallopian tubes and result in infertility.*

Surgery can sometimes correct this, but the outlook is not good. If the infection is severe, a hysterectomy (removal of the uterus) may be advised, and may even be necessary. It is, however, the most frequently performed, unnecessary operation in the Western world. If the ovaries are also removed, this can result in an unnaturally early menopause, the symptoms of which are usually treated with synthetic oestrogen.

You will be particularly susceptible to PID if you are exposed to STDs or have a copper IUD, which may cause chronic uterine inflammation and diminish immunity through the action of the copper.

Cervical damage — Insertion of the IUD, especially in women who have not yet had children, often results in tearing of the cervix, leading to later miscarriages as a result of an 'incompetent cervix'. There is also evidence showing a higher rate of cervical cell abnormalities and a greater risk of cervical cancer.

Uterine perforation — IUDs can become lodged in the uterus and may perforate it, leading to intestinal obstruction or severe bleeding, especially if the device contains copper. Removal is difficult, so much so that it could result in the need for a hysterectomy. It can also be life-threatening.

Failure due to diabetes — Diabetic women have a 37 per cent failure rate with copper IUDs as a result of their excessive metabolic production of sulphur and chlorides. These accumulate on the device, negating its effect. The resultant pregnancy could be problematic.

Problem pregnancies — There are also dangers to any pregnancies initiated while an IUD is in place. They have been known to lodge in the embryo (luckily, not too many cases are known to have occurred). More commonly, they cause the fertilised egg to attach in the fallopian tube (or, very occasionally, in the ovaries), instead of the womb, which is too inflamed. These ectopic pregnancies (which are nine times more likely to occur in women who use the IUD, amounting to 5–10 per cent of their pregnancies), are highly dangerous and sometimes fatal, requiring immediate surgery. The affected tube usually has to be removed, and there is a 50–60 per cent chance of resulting infertility. If you have been using a copper device, then your copper levels may be high, resulting in zinc deficiency, not good news for conception or pregnancy (see 'The Pill' above).

Miscarriage — There will be a 50 per cent chance of a miscarriage occurring if the IUD cannot be removed. This can only be done by a doctor pulling on the string, which may or may not be successful. The miscarriage rate for women using any other form of contraception is 17 per cent.

Septic abortion — A conception that occurs in the presence of an IUD is much more likely to result in a septic abortion in the fourth or fifth month of pregnancy.

Premature birth or bleeding — If the IUD remains in place during a pregnancy, there will be a slightly increased risk of a premature birth or bleeding later in the pregnancy. Removal of the IUD during pregnancy can, however, be hazardous for the child, and infectious complications are likely.

Uterine cancer — Increased risk for IUD users.

Anaemia and lowered immunity — From iron and zinc loss, and elevated copper.

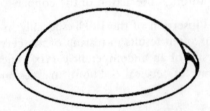

A Diaphragm made of a soft rubber dome with a rubber covered spring

Barrier methods

There are no major side-effects with barrier methods (diaphragm, condom, female condom and cap). As a result, these devices are becoming much more popular. One other reason for this is that the condom helps to protect against STDs. However, there are some minor side-effects.

MINOR SIDE-EFFECTS

Allergies — Some women and men are allergic to an ingredient in the rubber device and may develop a skin irritation. The allergy may be to the rubber itself, or to a chemical used as a lubricant or spermicide which may be used in combination with the device (or, in the case of condoms, impregnated in it).

Different manufacturers use different types of rubber and chemicals in their brands, so the allergy may be avoided by changing brands (see 'Spermicides', below), or by using a diaphragm or condom made from polyurethane (plastic).

Embarrassment — There can be embarrassment surrounding the use of barrier methods, especially with condoms (also with their purchase, particularly with women). However, if diaphragms are inserted in advance of any sexual activity, this problem can be avoided. Some women find the whole process of inserting the diaphragm messy and inconvenient; their sexual desire is somewhat reduced after chasing a slippery diaphragm around the bathroom for half an hour! Yet insertion is quite easy to learn and one can soon become accustomed to it.

Lack of spontaneity and tactile experience — Condoms and diaphragms, if not inserted in advance, can interrupt the spontaneity of sexual response. Some people find the obvious presence of barrier devices a sexual turn-off. Condoms particularly can reduce the tactile experience considerably, especially for the male partner, giving rise to the saying, 'Having sex with a condom is like having a shower in a raincoat.'

ADVANTAGES

The advantages of barrier methods are not only that they have few side-effects and protect against disease (condoms) and cervical dysplasia (diaphragms), but also that they can be used in conjunction with fertility identification techniques. This means that they only need to be used for a few days each cycle, which significantly reduces the nuisance factor. Their effectiveness is also increased as they are usually used more carefully, occasional use being nowhere near as negative an experience as continual use.

Their other advantage, even if they are used for all sexual encounters, is for those with sporadic sex lives, that is those who have long periods of sexual inactivity and need no protection at these times.

Spermicides

Spermicides are usually used in conjunction with a condom or diaphragm. They could be the main source of any allergic reaction.

There is also some concern that the spermicide might cause congenital abnormalities by damaging, instead of killing, the sperm on their way to fertilise the eggs. Luckily, this is fairly improbable, as defective sperm are unlikely to be the winners in this highly competitive race. There is, however, evidence that they can affect the embryo adversely, causing deformities if used into the early months of pregnancy; this is particularly likely if there is a mercury component in the spermicide. This evidence has been used successfully in American courts of law to sue for compensation.

Tubal ligation (female sterilisation)

This operation involves blocking, burning or severing the fallopian tubes so that the eggs, once released, cannot reach the womb. In the USA, as well as in some other countries, it may also involve a hysterectomy. This is a major operation and has much higher risks, including death.

Female Sterilization (Tubal Ligation)

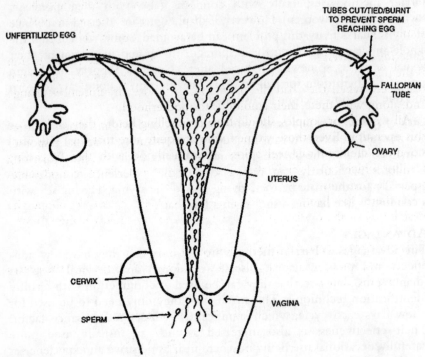

RISKS

Dysmenorrhoea — There is a greater risk of heavier periods after sterilisation (especially if you were previously on the Pill, or gave birth by caesarean section), and of pelvic infection and ectopic pregnancies. Blood supply to the uterus (if the uterus has not already been removed) is disturbed and may result in the need for a hysterectomy. This in turn can lead to premature menopause, depression, loss of libido and painful intercourse. PMT is often increased and cycles may become irregular, especially if there has been any damage to the ovaries.

Reversibility — Reversibility is not guaranteed. Attempts are not often successful if the tubes have been burnt or there has been significant damage. Its success may depend on the method of ligation used. However, unbeknown to the woman, the tubes occasionally grow back together again by themselves, and a pregnancy can result. Failure rate of sterilisation due to this effect is estimated at between 0.5 per cent and 7 per cent and there is a 10–20 per cent chance of this pregnancy being ectopic.

Surgical procedures — Of course, any operation that is done under a general anaesthetic (and nearly all sterilisations are) carries risks and can be fatal. There is also some risk of damage to a nearby organ, such as the bladder or bowel, or a blood vessel near the tubes. If there is significant tissue damage to the ovary or its blood supply, premature menopause can result. With a laparoscopy, a tiny incision is made, a tube is inserted and the abdomen inflated with nitrous oxide gas, then a tiny lens is inserted through the incision and photographs the condition of the reproductive system. Explosions have resulted from this process, as have cardiac failures.

Emotional distress — Perhaps the most upsetting side-effect of sterilisation is the distress felt by some women who were not clear enough about their real needs when they had the operation, or whose circumstances change and, along with these, their ambitions to motherhood.

All women, or couples, should have counselling before they embark on this operation. Even those women who are quite sure that they will want no more children can feel a loss of womanhood with their departing fertility, which can severely affect their sexuality and self-esteem, although sexual response, as such, is not usually affected.

If there has been any disagreement between a couple about the desirability of the operation, marital conflict and breakdown often occur.

Vasectomy (male sterilisation)
In this operation, the vas deferens are cut and tied to prevent the sperm reaching the semen.

Male Sterilization (Vasectomy)

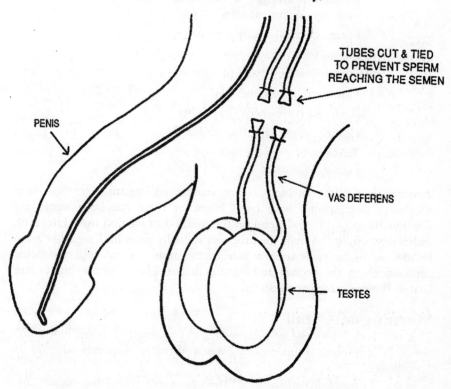

TUBES CUT & TIED
TO PREVENT SPERM
REACHING THE SEMEN

PENIS

VAS DEFERENS

TESTES

Cardiovascular disease, thyroid and joint disorders, prostatic, testicular and lung cancer, prostatitis and epididymitis, diabetes and changes in bone marrow are some of the many problems now being recognised as side-effects of this operation. However, the most commonly experienced problem the man has is, like the woman, emotional distress.

Vasectomy is not necessarily reversible. Even if the vas deferens are rejoined, there is often too much scar tissue, or the body has developed sperm antibodies. In some animal tests, these antibodies have been associated with hardening of the arteries. The success rate for reversal depends on the time that has elapsed since the operation. If it has been within 3 years, the success rate is 75 per cent. This declines after 8 years to 50 per cent, and 30 per cent after 15 years.

Termination (abortion)

The effects of termination are numerous. Although the decision to have an abortion is every woman's right, she must also be aware that it is not without consequences.

> Increase in infection
>
> Endometriosis
>
> Future ectopic pregnancies
>
> Future miscarriages in the fourth to sixth months of subsequent pregnancies
>
> Future cervical incompetence
>
> Future foetal death
>
> Future low birth-weight
>
> Future premature delivery
>
> Reduced reproductive capability
>
> Complications to future children
>
> Trauma
>
> Depression
>
> Guilt
>
> Grief
>
> Suppressed remorse

Deaths do occur with terminations, the a result of ensuing infections, perforations to the womb and haemorrhages. The risks are higher the further the pregnancy is advanced.

Morning-after pill

This is a very high dose of oestrogen and progesterone taken within 72 hours of unprotected intercourse, when there is a, perceived risk of conception.

There is a possibility of failure (0.16–5 per cent), with a subsequent risk of ectopic pregnancy, or abnormalities known as VACTERL:

V — vertebral

A — anal

C — cardiac

T — tracheo-oesophageal

R — renal

L — limb

If the morning-after pill works, the huge dose of hormones may well disrupt your subsequent cycles, and may also cause nausea and vomiting, or, more seriously (although, luckily, less likely), thrombosis or embolus.

Contraceptive injections

Depo-Provera, a synthetic progesterone that is injected every 3 months, prevents pregnancy by altering the normal growth of the endometrium. Depo-Provera is thought to interfere with normal interaction between the hypothalamus and pituitary glands, and the ovaries. Common side-effects of use include nausea, bloating, acne, breast tenderness, weight gain and mood changes. They may be related to the effects of androgenising (that is, the increase in male hormone).

It can cause a progressive decline in bleeding each cycle and if used for more than 2 years can lead to total menstrual cessation (amenorrhoea), which can last for months, years or forever. It can also lead to heavy and unpredictable bleeding. There is evidence that it takes longer to conceive after ceasing to use Depo-Provera (up to 1 year is common) than it does when stopping the Pill.

Problems in resultant pregnancies can involve congenital malformation of children and inadequate breast milk. Headaches, abdominal bloating and discomfort, breast tenderness, weight gain, depression, loss of libido and pain in the limbs are among the 'minor' side-effects, and many women become disturbed at the loss of cyclic activity. Long-term use can result in loss of bone density.

Vaginal ring

This is another way of absorbing chemical hormones, with side-effects similar to those from the Mini-pill. The vaginal ring commonly causes irregular bleeding.

Skin implants

Yet another method of administering synthetic progesterone, this time via time-release rods inserted under the skin of the arm and lasting for 5 years. Increased and unpredictable bleeding, a high rate of ectopic pregnancy, excess weight gain, mood changes, breast tenderness, acne, hair loss, migraine, blurred vision, rashes or pain around the implant and subsequent delays in the return of fertility are all possible associated problems. If scar tissue forms around the site of insertion, the rods can be difficult to remove, though at least removal of the chemical is possible, unlike when injections have been used.

The male Pill

Development of this form of chemical contraception has been delayed because of the perceived side-effects, such as a reduction in testosterone levels and sex drive, and an increase in acne, weight gain, heart disease and prostate cancer. It is tempting to say 'What's good for the goose is good for the gander', but of course the truth is, both sexes are better off without these problems.

Informed use of artificial methods

Don't despair if you feel that there is a real need for you to use one of these artificial contraception approaches. Certainly, there are times in many women's lives when they may choose to do so for any number of reasons. Most often, problems arise when neither the woman nor her physician is careful enough to check personal and family history, or to monitor the ongoing use of these methods. Of course, the most careful checking cannot eliminate all the risks, but forewarned is forearmed.

It is important to make an informed choice and not to follow blindly the advice of a less-than-thorough medical practitioner, as is unfortunately too often the case.

Natural methods are not suitable for all women all of the time, and can only be used by those who are motivated to do so. However, they do represent a real choice in that *it is possible for any woman, in any circumstances, to use natural methods if she so desires.*

CHAPTER 3

Bodies — An Introduction to Female and Male Anatomy and the Menstrual Cycle

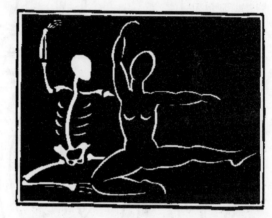

Through using natural methods of fertility management, you will become much more familiar with the workings of your body. Here is an introduction to those bits of you down there and how they work and play.

The man

Most men are fertile from puberty until approximately 70 years of age (older for some), every day of their lives. Men have no hormonal cycle to explore, although there can be variations in the levels of male fertility (see Chapter 7, 'The Lunar Cycle', and Chapter 13, 'Conscious Conception'). However, although there is not usually the need for the man to familiarise himself with his reproductive system in the cause of contraception, maybe you'd like to know anyway!

A man's hormonal and reproductive systems are controlled — as are a woman's — by the **pituitary gland**. This hangs like a little brown bag from the base of the brain and sends messages via the male hormones, called **androgens**, to various parts of the body, giving instructions on what to do next.

This gland starts to become more active around **puberty**, at which time it begins to be stimulated by the **hypothalamus** (a specialised part of the brain which controls body functions, and to which it is attached). This oft-maligned period of around 4 years, which starts between 8 and 12 years of age, is when a boy's body begins to change.

◆ 31

Male Pelvic and Reproductive Organs

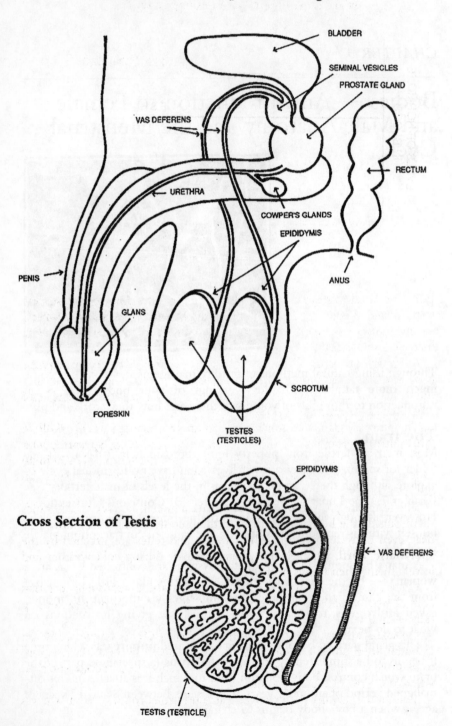

BLADDER

SEMINAL VESICLES

PROSTATE GLAND

VAS DEFERENS

RECTUM

URETHRA

COWPER'S GLANDS

EPIDIDYMIS

PENIS

ANUS

GLANS

SCROTUM

FORESKIN

TESTES
(TESTICLES)

EPIDIDYMIS

Cross Section of Testis

VAS DEFERENS

TESTIS (TESTICLE)

Male Hormone Levels during a month

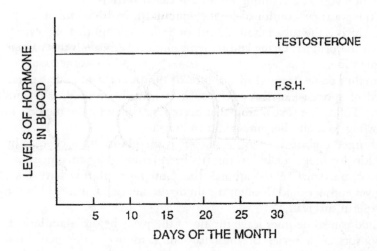

Body and facial hair grows, as does the penis, the testes drop, the voice starts to break and deepen, muscles develop, body shape changes, and wet dreams — involuntary nocturnal emissions of semen — start to occur, along with increased sexual desire.

All these events are the result of the production of **testosterone**, the male sex hormone, produced by the **testes** or testicles in response to a message from the pituitary gland and carried via the **interstitial cell stimulating hormone** (ICHS).

The pituitary gland also sends the testes another message, via the **follicle stimulating hormone** (FSH), to start them producing **sperm** (about 50~000 a minute). Each of these sperm is about 0.00423 cm (1/600 inch) in length. This means that it would take 25 million of them to cover this full stop.

The testes are protected by the **scrotum**, a pouch of tissue which holds them outside the body cavity to keep them cool. Sperm are destroyed by heat, even body temperature. The scrotum and testes are attached by the **spermatic cord**, which brings them in closer during cold weather and lowers them when things heat up!

Once the sperm are produced, they travel to the **epididymis**, the tiny coils of which are from 4–6 metres (13–20 feet) long, where they develop fully — and wait.

On sexual arousal, they travel through the **vas deferens**, a pair of 50 cm (20 inch) long tubes. The vas deferens go through a series of contractions to help the sperm, which cannot swim yet, to reach the **seminal vesicles**, where the seminal fluid is produced.

This fluid nourishes the sperm and, together, they continue along the vas deferens to the **prostate gland**. This small, roundish gland produces another nourishing fluid which increases sperm motility (their ability to propel themselves). The resulting mixture is called **semen**.

Now the journey continues to the **ejaculatory duct** and into the **urethra**, which is the tube (about 20 cm, or 8 inches, long) that also carries urine from the bladder. Urine and semen cannot pass through this passage at the same time.

The urethra passes through the centre of the **penis**, a muscular organ composed of sponge-like tissue. Unless it is sexually aroused, the penis hangs limp. Following sexual arousal, it becomes swollen by the increase in blood flowing to it and becomes rigid and erect.

The enlarged end of the penis is known as the **glans** and is covered by the **foreskin** (or prepuce), unless this has been removed by circumcision.

All this time, since sexual arousal, the **Cowper's glands** have been secreting yet another fluid through the urethra to neutralise urine, all in the cause of sperm survival.

This fluid can sometimes leave the tip of the penis before **ejaculation**, which consists of a series of muscular contractions in the penis and reproductive system that pump out the semen (containing up to 400~000 million sperm).

This is called **orgasm** and is generally regarded as the best bit of all!

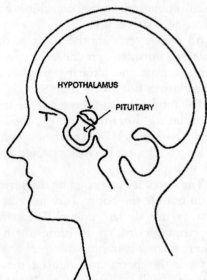

Hypothalamus and Pituitary Glands

The woman

A woman's reproductive system is far more complicated, which is why this book is devoted to helping her understand it. A woman's fertility is cyclic in nature and goes through constant change. These changes will be looked at in the next section; here we look at the bits that are involved in getting it all to work.

Female Pelvic & Reproductive Organs

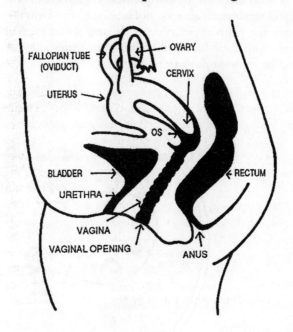

Cross section of Female Reproductive Organs

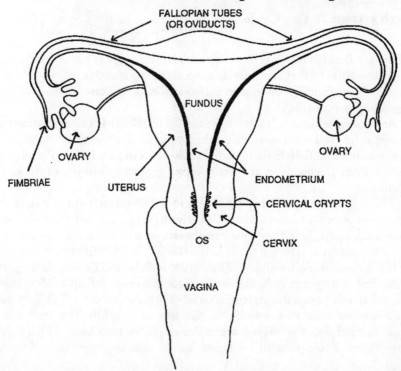

The woman's hormonal and reproductive systems are controlled and initiated, as with the man, by the **pituitary gland**. This lies at the base of the brain and sends messages, via hormones, to the **ovaries**.

These are the primary female sex organs, about the size and shape of prunes, and contain, at birth, all of the (immature) eggs, or **ova**, that will mature and be released during the woman's fertile life.

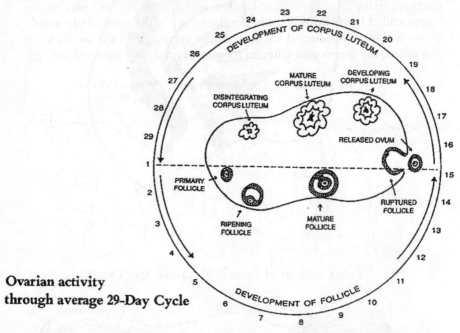

Ovarian activity through average 29-Day Cycle

There are about 300 000 cells which are potential eggs at puberty, although only about 400 of them actually develop. Each egg is about the size of a full stop and is surrounded by its own balloon called a **follicle**, which holds the egg in a protective fluid.

At the fertile time in each menstrual cycle, which is called **ovulation**, an egg is released from its follicle, which appears as a blister on the surface of the ovary. The follicle then changes into the **corpus luteum** (Latin for 'yellow body'), which acts as a temporary gland and produces a new set of hormones.

The egg is then collected by the nearest **fallopian tube**, or oviduct. These are about 10 cm (4 inches) in length, very thin and muscular, and have tendrils on their ends called **fimbriae**, which sweep the egg up into the tube and let it wait for the sperm to arrive and fertilise it.

If it is not fertilised within 8–24 hours, it will die and be absorbed by the body. But if a sperm (which can live much longer, for up to 3–6 days) reaches it and penetrates it, it will travel down the tube for 5–7 days and then implant itself in the lining of the **uterus** (womb). The uterus is a muscular, hollow, pear-shaped organ 7.5 cm (3 inches) long, which holds only about 1 teaspoonful of liquid in its non-pregnant state. During pregnancy, it houses the developing foetus (child), eventually stretching up to 500 times its normal size, then contracting at childbirth to push the baby out.

The lining of the womb is called the **endometrium**, and it goes through changes each cycle to prepare for this possibility. If a fertilised egg does not implant in it, it will be shed, along with blood, during **menstruation**. The blood and uterine lining leave the top part of the uterus, called the **fundus**, via the **cervix**, which is the neck of the womb. There is a small opening at the base of the cervix called the **os**, which is also where the sperm gain entry to the uterus on their journey to the egg.

Changes in the Endometrium at Menstruation

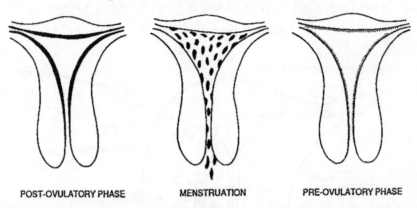

POST-OVULATORY PHASE   MENSTRUATION   PRE-OVULATORY PHASE

Though anatomically an extension of the uterine muscle, the cervix is an organ in its own right. It contains glands that produce protective mucus in the cervical crypts and goes through other changes during the menstrual cycle, such as rising and opening around the time of ovulation to allow the sperm easier passage.

During childbirth, the cervix dilates to allow the baby passage down into the **vagina** or birth canal, which is about 10–15 cm (4–6 inches) long, and muscular.

The vagina expands during sexual arousal when it becomes engorged with blood and secretes a lubricating fluid. It also does both these things during birth. It contracts (along with the uterine muscles) during **orgasm**, which some women don't experience as readily or as often as most men, but which, most of them would agree, is still the best bit.

Orgasm in the woman has been a controversial issue in that it has been categorised as being either 'vaginal' or 'clitoral', according to whether the sexual stimulation is applied vaginally (through penetration) or to the **clitoris**, which is a small organ above the vaginal opening made of the same tissue as the penis. The clitoris also becomes filled with blood, and firm and erect, during arousal.

The clitoris contains many nerve endings and is placed in such a position that it is (usually) stimulated during intercourse. It is protected by the

prepuce, the hood of the clitoris, which is where the inner vaginal lips, the **labia minora**, meet.

The labia minora are the soft folds of skin that protect the **vaginal opening**. together with the outer lips, the **labia majora**. The labia majora are fatter than the labia minora, have some hair covering and contain oil-producing glands.

The external genitalia are collectively called the **vulva**. This is separated from the **anus** by the **perineum**. The vulva also contains the **urethral meatus**, the urinary opening, which is just above the vaginal opening.

Above all this is the **mons pubis**, or **mons veneris** (Mount of Venus), which is the fatty pad that covers the pubic bone and is itself covered by pubic hair. This is one of the changes that take place at **puberty**, which occurs between 8 and 13 years of age, and lasts for about 4 years.

External Female Genitalia

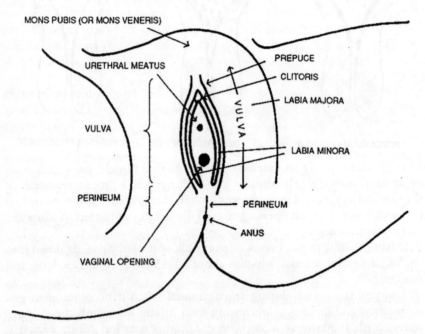

Other changes are the growth of the mammary glands, or **breasts**, the overall changes in shape and distribution of fat in the body, giving 'womanly' contours, the growth of body hair (underarm and pubic) and finally, the first bleeding at **menarche**, which is the onset of menstruation. The first egg may not be released for up to another couple of years.

After this time the girl will be fertile (although it may take 6–8 years for her reproductive system to fully mature), all going well, until the supply of eggs runs out at **menopause**. During this fertile period of her life she will experience, hopefully with some regularity (except when she is pregnant or breastfeeding), her menstrual cycle.

THE MENSTRUAL CYCLE

The menstrual cycle is the name given to the periodic changes that occur in a woman's body as a result of the activity of the endocrine glands and their secretion of hormones. The cycle is generally the length of a lunar (not calendar) month; the implications and origins of this are looked at more fully in Chapter 7, 'The Lunar Cycle'.

Individual women, for one reason or another, may have cycles that vary from much shorter to much longer than the norm. This may also vary within each single woman's experience, which may be of a very short cycle (say, 21 days) under some circumstances, and a rather long cycle (say, 36 days) at other times.

The length of the cycle is measured from the first day of bleeding (spotting doesn't count), which is called Day 1, to the first day of bleeding of the next menstrual period.

Mostly, the variation falls in the first half of the cycle, called the **follicular phase** (or pre-ovulatory phase), which lies between menstruation and ovulation, and not in the second half of the cycle, the **luteal phase** (or post-ovulatory phase), which is generally about 14 days long, give or take a couple of days. This stability of the second half of the cycle is the basis of the Rhythm Method (to be discussed in Chapter 6, 'Rhythm Method Calculations').

The first half of the cycle can be shortened or lengthened, or, in other words, ovulation can be precipitated or delayed. Delay, leading to longer cycles, is a more common experience and may be caused by any number of factors, including *stress, travel, ill health, drugs* (prescription or otherwise), *excessive exercise, weight changes, diet changes, fasting* or any other abnormal activity. This is because of the effect these events or activities have on the complex interaction of hormones from the pituitary gland and the ovaries.

The sequence is as follows.

As menstruation begins, the pituitary gland sends a message to the ovaries via the **follicle stimulating hormone** (FSH), which it releases in response to a signal from the **hypothalamus**. This is a specialised part of the base of the brain, which is concerned with the control of body functions. It, in its turn, contains a specialised portion called the **menstrual clock**, which is responsible for the periodic time of the menstrual cycle.

The hypothalamus and the pituitary gland are responsive to increased levels of light, such as that of the full moon, so it is no accident that our cycles are generally monthly.

When the FSH reaches the ovary, it stimulates the follicles to ripen several eggs and, as this process occurs, the ovaries release one of the major female sex hormones, which is called **oestrogen**.

Oestrogen is responsible for all sorts of effects, such as the development of 'womanly' characteristics at puberty, when the body changes its shape and distribution of fat, and for the earlier maturation of bones (which is why girls don't grow as tall as boys).

As levels of this hormone change during the menstrual cycle, it causes the following things to occur.

◆ The cervix softens and rises, and its opening, the os, widens, thus facilitating the passage of the sperm.

◆ The **mucus** produced in the cervical crypts changes in quantity and quality and become 'fertile' (see Chapter 4, 'Cervical Mucus Changes'), thus ensuring the life of the sperm (up to 3–6 days) and helps to channel them up into the uterus.

◆ The endometrium (lining of the womb) thickens and prepares to receive the fertilised egg (if there is one).

◆ The pituitary gland releases a sudden surge of **luteinising hormone** (LH) which causes the release of the ripest egg from its follicle at **ovulation**, leaving a crater on the surface of the ovary called the **corpus luteum**.

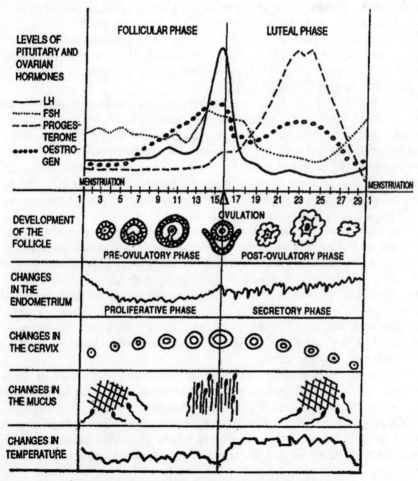

Female Hormone Levels during a Monthly Cycle

This now continues the release of oestrogen, but in reduced amounts. As the quantity of this hormone decreases, the cervix lowers, hardens and closes, and the mucus becomes 'infertile' and hostile to sperm.

However, this tiny and temporary endocrine gland starts secreting in greater quantity the second major female sex hormone, **progesterone**, which also has its specific effects. It causes

◆ the body-at-rest temperature to rise (see Chapter 5, 'Basal Body Temperature Changes')

◆ the cervical mucus to lessen and thicken

◆ the lining of the womb to thicken even more, so that within 5–7 days it is quite ready for the egg, fully supplied with blood and nutrients

◆ the ovary to cease releasing eggs.

If pregnancy does occur, the levels of progesterone continue to rise until the birth, when they fall precipitously.

If pregnancy doesn't occur, then the corpus luteum shrivels and leaves a tiny scar on the surface of the ovary. Its production of hormones having ceased, the uterine lining breaks down and, accompanied by blood, leaves the womb in the menstrual flow, or **menstruation**.

The lifespan of the corpus luteum is about 12–16 days, and it doesn't vary much, either from woman to woman, or cycle to cycle. So, *ovulation is nearly always about 2 weeks before the next period* and not, as used to be thought, 2 weeks after the last.

This all starts somewhere between 9 and 16 years of age, at **menarche**, and will continue, month after month — unless there is a problem, or a baby — until the supply of eggs runs out, usually somewhere between 45 and 55 years of age, at **menopause**.

CHAPTER 4

Cervical Mucus Changes

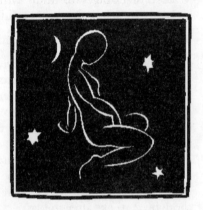

Now that you know how your body parts fit together, it is time to learn how to cooperate with it.

As the female body goes through all the changes of the menstrual cycle described in the last chapter, certain symptoms of these changes become externally apparent and are able to be used to identify a fertile state.

You can learn to distinguish these marvellous and unmistakable signs that your body gives you and use this information to avoid or achieve conception, depending on your choice, for the whole of your fertile life.

Assessing fertility

The fertile times in the menstrual cycle need to be assessed by each woman individually from cycle to cycle, as timing can be affected by

◆ stress

◆ drug-taking (prescription or otherwise)

◆ travel

◆ ill-health

◆ perimenopause

◆ diet and weight changes

◆ fasting

◆ or any other major change in circumstance.

The likely effects of these factors will vary from woman to woman and will, of course, be much more accurately assessed as you become more familiar with your cycle.

There are basically two ways of telling when the fertile time around ovulation occurs. One way is to use records of previous cycles to calculate the likely course of the next. This is called the *Rhythm Method*. The other is to observe changes in body symptoms such as the cervical mucus and body-at-rest temperature that occur at different stages of the cycle. Depending on which body symptoms are observed, this can be called the *Sympto-thermal Method*, which uses a mixture of all symptoms, including temperature, the *Ovulation Method*, which uses the cervical mucus observations only, the *Billings Method*, which is another name for the ovulation method, named in tribute to Dr Evelyn Billings and her husband, Dr John Billings, two Australian doctors who originally developed the method, or the *Temperature Method*, which uses the basal (or body-at-rest) temperature readings only.

Any of the methods can come under the umbrella terms of *Natural Family Planning* or *Natural Birth Control* (which implies strict abstinence at fertile times), or *Natural Fertility Awareness* (which doesn't, because it allows for the use of barrier methods).

These terms could also imply the observance of the Lunar (or Lunar Phase) Cycle (see Chapter 7, 'The Lunar Cycle'), which is sometimes called *Astrological Birth Control*. I prefer the term *Natural Fertility Management*, which embraces all of the above and more, as this approach includes natural and holistic remedies to correct fertility problems and optimise reproductive health.

Of the two ways of identifying ovulation and its approach — by calculation or observation of body symptoms — observation has three obvious advantages.

◆ Observation is more accurate than calculation.

◆ As a consequence, observation requires less abstinence (or protection) if conception is not required.

◆ Observation encourages involvement in, and awareness of, the reproductive functions, which leads to even greater accuracy.

The best course of action is to rely on the sympto-thermal observations whenever possible, and to use rhythm calculations as back-up, fail-safe, and as a warning of when ovulation is likely to be due.

Advantages of the mucus method

Of all of the ways available to a woman (and her partner) for assessing fertility on the ovulation cycle, observation of the changes in the cervical mucus is the most reliable and important because it is

◆ adaptable to times of change (see Chapter 11)

◆ easily learnt by almost all women

◆ applicable under nearly all conditions

◆ requires no technology or apparatus

◆ effective (usually assessed at 98.5 per cent reliable).

A World Health Organization survey in five countries (including undeveloped Third World societies) showed that 95 per cent of women were able to return an interpretable chart of the changes in their cervical mucus by the end of the first cycle.

All that is required is a healthy and curious attitude towards your body and its functions, and the motivation and determination to persevere in your monitoring of its cyclical changes.

The only limiting factor for the use of this method (apart from possible disruption to the mucus pattern by infection) is the motivation of the woman — you — and her partner. You can tell if you're fertile only if you read the signs, and you can avoid (or achieve) conception only if you act on this information.

For those women or couples who are aware enough of their physical and emotional needs to choose these methods, responsible use of them should be easy.

It is important to remain aware of the desire to have children, so that a continual, conscious decision is made to wait for the right time. If that is not now, then don't subconsciously forget that you are fertile. Children are precious. May all yours come when they are welcome.

The starting point

In the first few cycles, you will be learning a great deal: first, about your body and its cycles and symptoms, second, about your ability to observe them. Most attention and time is needed in the first few cycles. Luckily, this time is usually full of such interesting discoveries that your energy for the project will stay high.

As you become more familiar with the workings of your body and the implications of these changes, the whole process simplifies and you will switch to automatic pilot. Checking your mucus will become as much a part of your life as cleaning your teeth, and knowledge of mucus changes as integral to your body awareness as whether you have a cold or are well and fit.

If you are at all sensitive to your body's changes, you are probably already aware of the way you feel when your period is due. You will become equally aware of the way your body feels when ovulation is approaching. *Mucus changes are learnt experientially.*

Although you are just about to read a whole lot of information on the subject of mucus, don't expect to remember all the details immediately. The first time you read this and the following chapters on how to apply these methods, it is comprehension, not memory or obeying rules, that's important (although, of course, there are some useful rules).

Once you understand the concepts in this chapter, you are ready to start putting them into practice. Then you can return to this book at intervals (maybe once a cycle, at menstruation, for example) to reassure yourself that you are applying the principles correctly, and further your interpretation.

The understanding will come about largely through practice. Just be very careful not to make any decisions based on insufficient data or comprehension, especially in the first few months, at which time you need to be very clearly focused on the learning process. It's important to establish correct habits from the very beginning, so you don't make incorrect assumptions. Soon you will be unable to imagine a time when you didn't understand your patterns of fertility. It's a skill that, once acquired, remains with you, like riding a bicycle.

Keep returning to the source material given here until there are no more surprises for you, but everything relates directly to what you have personally experienced. Then you can be truly confident.

The cervix
The cervix (the neck of the womb) is an important organ and needs to be protected from damage. It can be adversely affected by

◆ the Pill

◆ IUD insertion and removal

◆ terminations

◆ infection

◆ dilation and curettage (D&C)

◆ laser/cauterisation/freezing

◆ cone biopsy

◆ childbirth

◆ tampons (pads are preferable for daily use).

Fortunately, the cervix is treated with a bit more respect these days since we have become more aware of how crucial its functions are to fertility. Inside the cervix there are special cells in the hundred or so gland-like crypts. These constantly produce mucus, which changes in quantity and quality throughout the menstrual cycle. They also provide a haven for the sperm that are migrating from the vagina to the uterus on their journey in search of an egg to fertilise.

When the sperm are in these crypts, they are safely sheltered and nourished, then, over a period of hours or even days, they are released up into the uterus.

Cervical Crypts

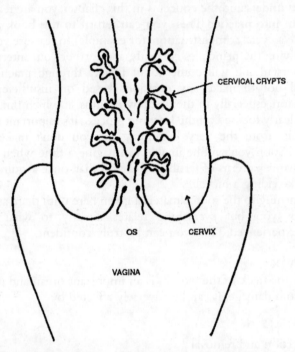

The mucus produced by the cervical crypts is controlled by the level of hormones present, with different areas in the crypts being responsible for producing different types of mucus at different stages of the cycle. Conversely, low levels of mucus may indicate low levels of oestrogen (see Chapter 12, 'Natural Remedies for Hormonal and Reproductive Health').

◆ Low oestrogen, as at the beginning and end of the cycle, results in scant amounts of sticky or tacky mucus which is opaque and contains cellular matter.

◆ As the levels of oestrogen rise and ovulation is approached, the mucus becomes more profuse, thinner, wetter and clearer.

◆ Just before ovulation, when the oestrogen levels peak, the mucus becomes jelly-like (still wet), resembles raw egg-white and can be stretched between the fingers.

Hormone Levels and Mucus Changes

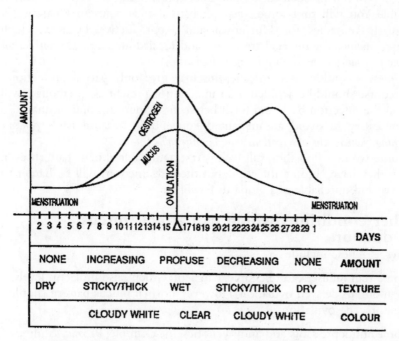

NONE	INCREASING	PROFUSE	DECREASING	NONE	AMOUNT
DRY	STICKY/THICK	WET	STICKY/THICK	DRY	TEXTURE
	CLOUDY WHITE	CLEAR	CLOUDY WHITE		COLOUR

It is these changes (part of the body's way of preparing for conception by enabling the sperm to survive and travel), that you will learn to recognise as defining the approach of fertility (or lack of it).

Every woman will experience some changes in her cervical mucus as she progresses through her hormonal cycle. These can be learnt and recognised. The presence of mucus does not mean she has an infection.

If your mucus discharge changes in quality and quantity, it is most probably your natural cervical mucus, produced in response to hormonal messages. You have probably been subliminally aware of these cyclical changes all of your adult life. Now, you can learn to recognise their significance.

Infections

If your mucus discharge is constant and does not go through changes, has an offensive smell, or causes irritation, itching or burning, then the cause is probably an infection. This may be a *yeast infection*, which is also known as *Candida albicans, monilia* or *thrush*, or one of a variety of *protozoan* or *bacterial infections.*

Since changing hormonal levels can predispose a woman to thrush, you may experience a recurring problem premenstrually. Although this may be a cyclical event, any discharge can still be easily distinguished from normal mucus changes by the symptoms experienced. Because the presence of an infected discharge disguises normal mucus changes and can make it very difficult to make decisions about fertility, mucus observations cannot be relied upon during such times. The infection should be treated as soon as possible. You will find some ideas on natural treatments in Chapter 12, 'Natural Remedies for Hormonal and Reproductive Health', which include recipes for internal treatment and local douching. *(Do not douche during pregnancy or for 10 weeks after childbirth.)*

Unless a condom is used (and this may give only partial protection), intercourse should be avoided if an infection is present as intercourse will spread the infection back and forth between partners. A condom may also be necessary to avoid an unwanted conception, because *while you are douching, your mucus observations may be unreliable.*

Some women find they still have a distinguishable mucus pattern even when they have chronic infection, but these distinctions will be harder to observe and unreliable as a guide to fertility.

Other conditions which can affect mucus production

Drugs — These include

◆ some tranquillisers, for example, Largactil, which raise prolactin levels, resulting in delayed ovulation. However, normal mucus pattern should still precede ovulation

◆ some antidepressants and antipsychotics, for example, Prozac, Valium, Thorazine, which interfere with the menstrual cycle

◆ aspirin and anti-inflammatory drugs such as Indocid

◆ some antispasmodic drugs, such as Atropine, Belladonna, Dicyclomine, Propantheline, which may dry up the mucus

◆ antibiotics, such as Ampicillin, which may increase the amount of fluidity of the mucus (these will also tend to encourage yeast infections)

◆ some drugs used for asthma or cystic fibrosis, which may also increase the amount or fluidity of the mucus

◆ cytotoxic drugs, used in cancer therapy, which prevent mucus production by suppressing ovulation and changing the whole hormonal pattern, inducing menopause

◆ some drugs such as Tagamet, which are used to treat peptic ulcers and can lead to severe hormonal imbalance

◆ antihistamines, which are also contained in some cough medicines; in some women, antihistamines may dry up the mucus

◆ some cough medicines which contain expectorants, such as Guafenesin, or potassium iodide, which may increase the quantity or fluidity of the mucus

◆ hormonal or fertility drugs, including oestrogen, which will usually cause fertile-type mucus, progesterone, which will dry up the mucus, antigonadotrophins such as Buserilin, Leuprolide or Danazol, used to treat endometriosis, but which can disrupt the whole hormonal and menstrual pattern, Tamoxifen, used to treat breast cancer, but which reduces oestrogen and fertile mucus, and Clomiphene (Clomid or Serophene), which is used to induce ovulation but — paradoxically, since these are used for infertile women — dries up the mucus. *This means that you cannot notice normal mucus patterns while on the Pill, and, in some cases, for several months after ceasing to take it.* (The IUD, however, unless causing an infection and discharge, or breakthrough bleeding, will probably not affect the mucus cycle (see Chapter 11, 'Times of Change', for more about coming off the Pill).

If a drug you need to know about is not listed here, it would be wise to check if it has any action on female hormones or the mucous membranes.

Nutritional deficiencies — You need sufficient calcium, magnesium and zinc to produce fertile mucus, and sufficient iron (not too much, not inorganic and only take if need proven) and vitamin A for mucous membrane function. Too much manganese may dry up the mucus, especially if these other nutrients are deficient.

Curettage — This procedure may damage the cervical crypts.

Underactive or overactive thyroid gland — Either of these conditions can interfere with ovulation.

Stress — This refers to stress of any kind — emotional stress, travel, illness, trauma, fatigue, excessive exercise, severe or sudden change in diet, fasting or rapid weight changes. Stress usually inhibits or delays ovulation.

Cervicitis or cervical erosion — This can cause discharge.

Cauterisation of the cervix, cone biopsy — These procedures are carried out for the treatment, respectively, of cervical erosion and cancer. Both can sometimes damage the cervical crypts which produce mucus.

Cervical cysts, polyps or warts — Any of these may damage the cervical crypts.

Polycystic, cystic or infected ovaries — Any of these conditions may cause hormonal changes.

Retained tampon — This can cause infection, with resulting discharge.

Vaginal lubricants, deodorants, douches, sprays and spermicides — Any of these chemicals may cause inflammation of the vaginal lining or an allergic reaction that could result in discharge. Their use will also disguise the mucus changes.

Under normal circumstances, douching or washing the vagina is unnecessary and undesirable. The vagina is self-cleansing and better left alone. It does not need to be sterile (unlike the womb). Douching is only useful to combat an infection, and frequent, unnecessary douching can, in fact, lead to infections by changing the pH (acidity).

Mucus and fertility

❯ *Change in the cervical mucus is the only observable symptom that precedes ovulation and, therefore, gives reliable warning of approaching fertility.*

Without this change, there is no fertility. Even if ovulation occurs, without fertile mucus the situation is infertile because the sperm cannot stay alive.

❯ *In favourable circumstances, sperm can live up to 3 days.* They have even been found alive after 6 days, but this is extremely rare, and they are generally considered to be non-viable at this advanced age. Three days is usually considered to be the maximum for viability of conception. Sperm life reduces by one-third each day, and 16–18 hours is an average lifespan. The number of sperm (sperm count) lowers each day and, even in a favourable environment, falls below a viable level after 3 days.

However, acidity immobilises sperm and vaginas are naturally acidic. Fertile mucus provides protection for the sperm from this acidity, nourishes them (it is rich in nutrients) and guides them up into the womb. Mucus present at other times in the cycle (if any) is unable to provide the sperm with this protection and is, therefore, infertile.

Different types of mucus

Four types of mucus have been identified: G-type, L-type, S-type and P-type. These are all produced in different parts of the cervical crypts.

G-type mucus is commonly called *infertile.* It is present in most women just after the period, and after ovulation in the second half of the cycle (post-ovulatory phase). It is characteristically thick and sticky, like paper paste, and forms an impenetrable barrier of protein fibres, like a natural diaphragm, across the cervix.

Since this mucus affords no protection to the sperm, the acidity in the vagina forms a natural spermicide. G-type mucus is produced while on the Pill. In fact, Mini-pills, which do not inhibit ovulation, rely on it (as well as their effect on the endometrium) to prevent pregnancy.

L-type mucus is the next type of mucus to be produced by the cervix and to appear in the vagina. It has a clumpy texture and bead-like structure, evident when stretched between the fingers. Under a microscope, this mucus shows a flower-like arrangement of perpendicularly branched crystals.

At first, this mixes with the barrier mucus and then replaces it. It neutralises the acidic vagina (it is alkaline), traps defective sperm cells and provides structural support for the S-type, or *fertile*, mucus.

S-type mucus is stretchy and lubricative, with increased water content,

G-Type Mucus as Seen Under a Microscope

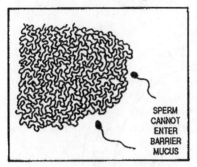

SPERM CANNOT ENTER BARRIER MUCUS

L-Type Mucus as Seen Under a Microscope

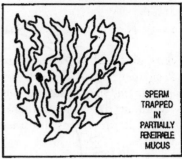

SPERM TRAPPED IN PARTIALLY PENETRABLE MUCUS

S-Type Mucus as Seen Under a Microscope

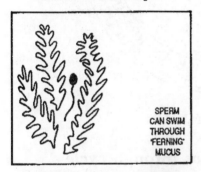

SPERM CAN SWIM THROUGH 'FERNING' MUCUS

Mucus as seen under a Microscope

resembling raw egg-white. It can be stretched to form strings, when L-type mucus can be seen as beads at intervals along it and has a ferning pattern when viewed under a microscope. This is due to the presence of channels, which guide the sperm to the safety of the cervical crypts where they go through rest and resuscitation before continuing their long swim. There, they are sealed into the crypts by a plug of mucus.

P-type mucus appears just before ovulation. It dissolves the plug, releasing the sperm into the uterus or fallopian tubes where they do not live long. After ovulation, the G-type mucus returns. P-type mucus is not evident at the mouth of the vagina.

Don't worry if you don't have a microscope. Luckily, all these changes in mucus are easily distinguishable by look and feel. Gravity does the work for us and brings the mucus down through the vagina. Mucus observations can thus be made by fingers at the mouth of the vagina.

It is not necessary (or desirable) to test the mucus at the cervix. The cervix will always have mucus on it, and the vaginal walls will always be moist, so you can get confused. Test the mucus at the entrance to the vagina: you will be able to tell if the mucus is plentiful enough to have come down through the vagina, thus providing protection for the sperm.

So, we test for changes in the *quantity* and *quality* of the mucus.

Changes in Quantity of Mucus Through Cycle

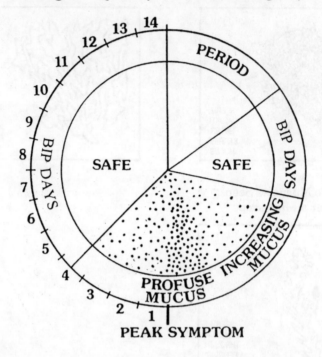

PEAK SYMPTOM

Changes in quantity of mucus through cycle

The cycle begins with a menstrual period of several days of bleeding. *Day 1 of the cycle is the first day of menstrual flow* (spotting doesn't count). During this time, even if there is some mucus present (as there can be in very short cycles), it is unlikely to be detected.

After bleeding finishes, there are usually a few 'dry' days with no apparent discharge at the vaginal entrance — which is where it is normally tested. If you have very little mucus, it may be tested at the cervix, but whichever location is chosen, the readings should always be taken at the same point; otherwise confusion will result.

You may have no 'dry' days, but always have some mucus present. Just after menstruation, this is likely to be scant and dense.

THE BASIC INFERTILE PATTERN

In average length or long cycles, there will usually be some days with either no mucus ('dry'), or continuing amounts of this very scant and sticky mucus, before oestrogen levels start to build, causing the mucus to change to fertile. *As long as the quantity (or quality) of the mucus is unchanging, it constitutes what is called the Basic Infertile Pattern (BIP).* It's what happens in the cervix when nothing is changing hormonally. For some women this is dry, for others it is small amounts of thick, tacky mucus, and for others, greater amounts of the same dense type of mucus. It's important to learn what the BIP is for you, as this is confirmation that you are infertile and your hormones have not even begun the changes that will result in ovulation. The BIP is usually evident before and after the period, when the body is at rest, before preparing to ovulate. In short cycles, it may be missing in the pre-ovulatory phase.

The cervix always secretes some mucus, but during these first days of the cycle the mucus may be so scant and sticky that it does not find its way to the vaginal entrance, resulting in the dry experience.

The walls of the vagina are always moist and give no indication of the state of the cervical mucus.

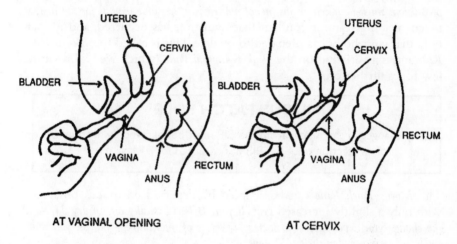

AT VAGINAL OPENING   AT CERVIX

As the cycle progresses, the mucus increases in quantity, more of it appearing at the mouth of the vagina until, around ovulation, it is usually quite profuse. After ovulation, it will lessen in quantity again, quite abruptly, and may disappear altogether, depending on the *Basic Infertile Pattern*.

Occasionally, there may be a showing of more profuse mucus just before bleeding starts, a result of the changes in hormonal levels, and this is often accompanied by a drop in the temperature readings and by an experience of the pre-menstrual syndrome (PMS), as progesterone levels dip lower than oestrogen. *This does not indicate a second ovulation.*

THE 'NOW-YOU-SEE-ME-NOW-YOU-DON'T' OVULATION

There is one other possible variation on this general pattern of increase and decrease. Occasionally, you may have gone through all the hormonal approaches to ovulation, such as build-up of mucus, and then be affected by something — such as stress or ill-health — which prevents the egg being released. The evidence shows that stress tends to delay ovulation, not precipitate it. One reason for this is that stress affects pituitary function, preventing the release of LH (which triggers the release of the egg) and raising prolactin levels (the hormone which suppresses ovulation during breastfeeding).

One of two patterns may then emerge.

◆ You simply don't ovulate that month (and, although the mucus may appear quite fertile, this anovular cycle will be evident on the temperature graph).

◆ You may have a delayed ovulation occurring a few days later. (This can result in a double peak of mucus, the first being a false peak, the second coming a few days later, when the egg is actually released. It has even been known for triple peaks to occur.)

Obviously, if a second peak of mucus builds within a few days of apparent ovulation, precautions must be taken or abstinence practised in the same way as for the first, as mucus readings cannot confirm that ovulation has occurred, and is over, only that your body has prepared to ovulate. This is called the *Mucus Patch Rule* and is a variation on the *Peak Symptom Rule* (which we will discuss a few pages further on).

MUCUS PATCH RULE

Any changes in the mucus from the BIP must be followed by abstinence or protection until the BIP has returned for 3 clear days.

The *Mucus Patch Rule* can be adapted by experienced mucus observers, with only a slightly increased risk. *If your BIP is basically one of dry days and the change you experience is to increasing levels of infertile-type mucus, you could safely reduce the 3-day wait to 2 days.*

Anovular cycles may still result in a normal-seeming period at the expected time (although the flow is sometimes reduced and this is not a true period). Cycles with delayed ovulation may be a little longer than usual, as the length of the post-ovulatory phase (the time taken from ovulation to menstruation) is usually stable, at about 2 weeks.

If you have correctly observed your mucus pattern, you will be less likely, in a long cycle, to be concerned about a possible unwanted pregnancy (or have false hopes about one that is wanted).

If these unusual patterns are suspected, temperature readings showing the day of ovulation can confirm what is really happening.

Changes in quality of mucus through cycle

Changes in the *quality* of the mucus discharge are critical, as these are what divides the fertile mucus from the *infertile*.

Fertile mucus is that which allows conception to occur. In a normal healthy woman it is present just before and during ovulation.

Infertile mucus is present at the other times of the cycle when conception *cannot* occur.

Fertile and Infertile Mucus

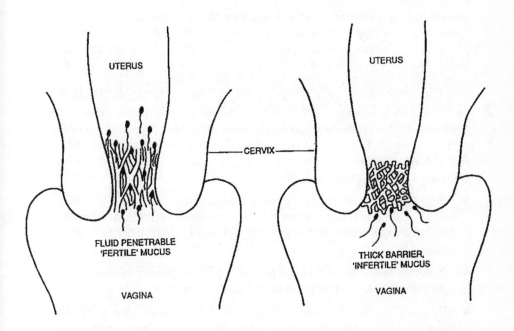

The quality of the mucus is an essential factor in the fertility or infertility of each circumstance, owing to its ability to protect and nourish — or conversely repel — sperm.

It is important to remember that each woman has a unique pattern of mucus changes as well as a characteristic type of mucus prior to ovulation. Your pattern, and the quality of your mucus, may not be exactly like 'Ms Classic-in-the-book'. This is not a problem, unless a lack of fertile mucus is compromising your ability to conceive. If you feel that your mucus changes are not as clear or as easy to interpret as you'd like, herbs and nutrients which act to balance hormones may help. See Chapter 12, 'Natural Remedies for Hormonal and Reproductive Health', or see your natural health practitioner for advice on how to achieve clearer mucus changes.

The important thing is to become familiar with *your own pattern* and learn to identify how your own body prepares for ovulation, because you are potentially fertile *as soon as the mucus is able to protect the sperm.*

Remember, sperm can live for 3 days (and very occasionally, though in reduced numbers, for up to 6) in fertile mucus, which is secreted for an average of 6 days before ovulation, during which time the follicle is ripening. After ovulation the fertile mucus ceases as a result of the production of progesterone by the corpus luteum.

Sperm can continue to stay alive in the cervical crypts even after the cervical mucus is no longer apparent in the vagina: so, you must have warning of ovulation, either for contraception or conception.

For contraception purposes — it is not enough to know that you are ovulating. If you have made love up to 3 days before, this is just bad news.

For conception purposes — it is important that the sperm are deposited *before* ovulation. The egg waits 8–24 hours in the fallopian tube to be fertilised. If this occurs, it takes about a week to travel down the tube and implant in the uterus. If it does not, it is *absorbed*, not passed out with the menstrual flow. So, you need the sperm in there, *ready and waiting*.

Whether you desire conception or not, *you need to be able to identify the fertile approach to ovulation*. This is where identifying the quality or texture of the mucus becomes important.

A TYPICAL CYCLE
A typical cycle progresses as follows.

◆ After bleeding, there may be some *dry* days, when there is no apparent mucus at all. The mucus at this time is completely infertile and forms a plug across the cervix; this may come out as a blob of sticky G-type mucus.

◆ Then, you may start to feel the presence of some *possibly infertile or slightly fertile* mucus (L-type). This is usually a damp or sticky feeling.

◆ The water content then rises and the mucus becomes wetter and more lubricative. This is the change to S-type or *fertile* mucus. It is also more profuse.

◆ Most, but not all, women then experience the *spinnbarkeit* or *spinn* mucus that resembles raw egg-white; it is wet and slimy to the touch.

◆ After ovulation there is, sometimes, quite suddenly, a return to the thick, tacky mucus, or to none at all, depending on your BIP.

◆ A typical cycle has three distinct phases which need to be identified and takes this form.

Pre-ovulatory infertile phase	Fertile phase	Post-ovulatory infertile phase
Bleeding	Increased amounts of wetter, thinner mucus	BIP (dry days or scant, thick mucus in unchanging amounts)
BIP (dry days or scant, thick mucus in unchanging amounts)	*Spinn* or egg-white type mucus	Possibly some wet days just before the period

All women do not experience all of these stages. They vary with the length of the cycle and the amount of mucus produced.

SHORT CYCLES AND THE BIP

If you have a very short cycle, the early, dry days, and even the thick, sticky mucus, may not be experienced at all. Similarly, dry days may not be experienced by those who produce greater amounts of mucus, who may have a BIP of unchanging amounts of infertile mucus.

Indeed, you may not experience the BIP at all in the first half of your cycle. In this case, you don't have what is called a *pre-ovulatory phase of infertility*, and your BIP only emerges at the *post-ovulatory phase of infertility*, when the egg is dead and gone.

A lack of early infertile days is usually a symptom of short cycles (24 days or less). In these situations, if conception is not desired, great care is needed; *the menstrual period itself can be fertile, owing to the presence of fertile mucus mixed with the blood.*

You would be unlikely to notice the presence of this mucus at menstruation, unless very experienced at mucus detection. So if there is any record of a recent short cycle or any reason to suspect that present circumstances (medication, menopause, and so forth) might cause one, the period needs to be treated, for contraceptive purposes anyway, as potentially fertile.

How to tell when you're fertile

Mucus types are best recognised through becoming familiar with

◆ amount

◆ colour

◆ texture

◆ external sensation.

We've seen how the amount changes. The colour is helpful when it comes to recognising the different stages in each woman's unique cycle but not critical for fertility. The texture is the critical and important part, and awareness through your day of external sensation at the vulva can support the direct observations.

DRY DAYS

First, we have the dry days, with no discernible mucus at the vaginal entrance and no staining or dripping in your underwear. There is no sensation of wetness, lubrication or discharge, only of *dryness*.

Mucus collected from the cervix will be very *scant, sticky* and *thick*. It is this mucus that forms the plug across the cervix. It may come out all at once or in a blob, usually when you are on the toilet, which is one good reason for testing your mucus at this time. This mucus will smell and taste *vinegary*, part of Mother Nature's plan to put your partner off at this time as *these days are infertile.*

◆ **Amount** — none evident at vaginal entrance.

◆ **Colour** — opaque.

◆ **Smell/taste** — vinegary.

◆ **Texture** — thick, dry, flaky, crumbly.

◆ **External sensation** — dry, no discernible mucus.

INFERTILE MUCUS DAYS

These days may replace the dry days, depending on your BIP, with an unchanging pattern of *thick, crumbly, opaque, flaky* mucus at the mouth of the vagina, which feels dry to the touch. It may seem very like the next type, but its *quantity does not increase*.

◆ **Amount** — unchanging

◆ **Colour** — opaque.

◆ **Smell/taste** — vinegary.

◆ **Texture** — thick, dry, flaky, crumbly.

◆ **External sensation** — dry.

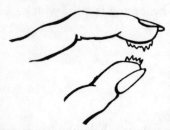

INFERTILE MUCUS

**Opaque, thick, dry,
flaky, crumbly,
holds its shape
(dense matter in it)
unchanging in quantity**

INCREASING MUCUS DAYS

The mucus at this time is increasing in response to rising levels of oestrogen and is evident externally. Although it may still feel *thick* and *dense*, the vaginal entrance may start to feel *damper* and the mucus itself is *pasty, tacky and opaque* (rather like the paste used for sticking paper). *The chances for conception are extremely low*, as the sperm find it almost impossible to penetrate this type of mucus. This mucus will form little tacky ridges when the fingers are parted (see diagram).

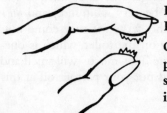

**PROBABLY
INFERTILE MUCUS**

**Opaque, thick, damp,
pasty, tacky, holds its
shape, (dense matter in it)
increasing in quantity**

The question to ask yourself is, 'Could anything swim through this?' If the sperm cannot enter the mucus, it is unprotected. However, there are a few channels open to the cervix in this mucus, and as well as filtering out deficient sperm, the mucus helps to make the vagina more alkaline (receptive to sperm). *There is, therefore, a slight chance of conception.*

This mucus is variously described as *cloudy, clotty, sticky, flaky, tacky, thick, damp, moist, curdled, dense, pasty, rubbery* and *cellular.*

It has a tendency to stiffen the underwear and is usually *opaque, white* or *yellow.*

It is important when recording the texture of the mucus that you familiarise yourself with the *appearance* of the mucus, as well as the *sensation* of touching it, which is why you should use your fingers to check it. If you have a problem with touching your genitals, you can first collect the mucus on some toilet paper, though the paper may absorb some of the moisture.

There is also the *external sensation* that you feel as you walk, sit and lie down. At this stage in the cycle, the external sensation, although probably more *damp* or *moist,* would not be described as *wet* or *slippery.* This mucus also has a characteristic *vinegary* smell (and taste).

If you *don't* want to conceive, this type of mucus should be considered, strictly speaking, as potentially fertile. The risk is small, however. In Chapter 10, 'Charting and Coordinating the Methods for Contraception', we will look at the applications for contraception and how you can make decisions about this.

If you *do* want to conceive, these days are still waiting days — the best is yet to come.

◆ *Amount* — increasing.

◆ *Colour* — opaque.

◆ *Smell/taste* — vinegary.

◆ *Texture* — damp, pasty, thick, tacky, rubbery.

◆ *External sensation* — damp, moist.

FERTILE OR WET DAYS

The change to fertile mucus heralds the approach of ovulation. The mucus *becomes more watery, fluid, wetter, thinner, clearer* and *more profuse.*

The sensation is one of increasing *wetness, fluidity and slipperiness.* The appearance is *clearer, milky-white* or *translucent,* and can even be *tinged with blood.*

Blood-spotting sometimes occurs at or near ovulation, causing mucus to appear *pink, brown* or *red.* Blood-spotting is due to the high level of oestrogen acting on the endometrium, causing seepage of blood through it. *Spotting cannot be used to define accurately the exact day of ovulation.*

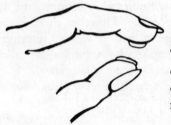

FERTILE MUCUS

**Translucent, milky-white
or pink, thin, wet, fluid,
creamy, slippery, (no dense
matter), increasing amounts**

Some women experience fertile mucus as thick, like cottage cheese, but it will still be *wet* and *slippery* — it is this characteristic which is important. Fertile mucus smells *sweeter* and, indeed, tastes sweeter, as Mother Nature conspires yet again to get you pregnant by attracting your mate. Its appearance is often accompanied by a feeling of *fullness, softness* and *swelling* in the external genitalia, almost like a fruit ripening.

The change to this kind of mucus can be very sudden. This is why it is important to check the mucus frequently, especially for the purposes of contraception (see next section). For some women, the change to wet mucus is gradual. For others, it can occur quite dramatically in a few hours. *Checks made more than a few hours previously cannot be relied upon, especially if the method is being used for contraception, in which case abstinence (or protection) is required from the first appearance of fertile-type mucus.*

This is because the sperm are protected, nourished and provided with access to the cervix and uterus (through the swimming lanes) where they may live until ovulation occurs. In other words, this mucus generally aids and abets the process of conception. This is good news if that's what you want, and a danger signal if not.

When felt on the fingers, the overriding sensation is of *wetness, slipperiness* and *lubrication*. The answer to, 'Can anything swim through this? is an unequivocal 'Yes'. The quality of this mucus will probably continue to increase, until it probably changes to the next stage, or *spinn*.

◆ *Amount* — more profuse.

◆ *Colour* — clear, milky-white, translucent (pink).

◆ *Smell/taste* — sweeter.

◆ *Texture* — wet, fluid, liquid, thin, watery, slippery, creamy.

◆ *External sensation* — wet, slippery, swollen.

SPINNBARKEIT, OR EXTREMELY FERTILE MUCUS

Spinnbarkeit (often referred to simply as '*spinn*') is German for 'ability to stretch', and is pronounced spin-bar-kite. This mucus can indeed stretch in long strands with the gelatinous consistency of raw egg-white.

Not every woman experiences this stage of mucus, and it is not essential that you do. Every woman's cycle is unique: what is important is that you come to understand the changes that take place in *your* cycle.

The sensation is still *wet* and *slippery*, but it holds together in a *jelly-like* mass, and can be spun from the thumb to forefinger, up to 10 or 15 cm (4 or 6 inches). It is not cohesive in the same sense as the sticky, infertile mucus, and remains *wet* and *slippery* to the touch.

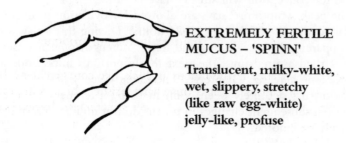

EXTREMELY FERTILE MUCUS – 'SPINN'

Translucent, milky-white, wet, slippery, stretchy (like raw egg-white) jelly-like, profuse

Usually *clear* or *milky white* in appearance, it can occur for anything up to a couple of days, although it often comes down as a single mass, as if an egg had been cracked open in the vagina. This often occurs before or during urination, which is another reason to check your mucus at this time, or it could go undetected.

◆ *Amount* — profuse.

◆ *Colour* — translucent, clear, milky-white.

◆ *Smell/taste* — sweet.

◆ *Texture* — jelly-like, raw egg-white, wet, slippery, stretchy, gelatinous, slimy, 'spinn'.

◆ *External sensation* — very wet, slippery, swollen.

PEAK SYMPTOM

Whether *spinn* is present or not, at this stage the peak symptom is experienced. 'Peak symptom' is, in a way, a misnomer, as it is not always the day of *most* mucus but, rather, the *last day of either type of fertile mucus* (wet or *spinn*).

It can coincide with ovulation, but is more likely to be followed by ovulation within 1 day (85 per cent of women) or 2 (a further 10 per cent, making 95 per cent of women). The most fertile — and healthy — state is when the peak symptom occurs just before ovulation, as this ensures that fresh, healthy sperm are ready to meet a fresh, healthy egg if conception is attempted. Whether you wish to conceive or not, this optimum condition can often be restored, if not evident, through the use of natural remedies to balance the hormonal state.

Since the sperm can live for 3 days in the cervical crypts, they can wait for the 1 or 2 days between the peak symptom and ovulation as well as for the 24 hours of the life of the unfertilised egg.

The peak symptom, the last day of fertile mucus, is only recognisable retrospectively, after the mucus has dried up or become sticky again as a result of the increase in progesterone, reverting to the BIP.

This delay in recognition is no problem as *it is necessary to leave 3 days after the peak symptom before infertility is assured for contraception* purposes, and intercourse for conception will already have begun.

After the peak symptom, 2 days are allowed for ovulation to occur and 1 more day for the life of the egg (8–24 hours). During this 3-day wait, it becomes apparent that the last of the fertile mucus has been observed. Infertility is then assured until the next fertile period (unless your lunar fertile days come here, see Chapter 7, 'The Lunar Cycle').

If ovulation has definitely been confirmed (by a temperature rise, for example), then subsequent changes in mucus do not indicate a fertile time and can safely be ignored.

PEAK SYMPTOM RULE

The post-ovulatory infertile phase begins after 3 consecutive days of non-wet mucus or dry days following the peak day.

Mucus checking

The easiest routine is to check the mucus on each visit to the toilet. This ensures that you are checking frequently, so you are aware of any sudden changes. It is also easier to remember as a routine than trying to keep to a set time each day, or timetable, which can be upset by changes in daily habits. (Ten o'clock may be fine one day, but the next it may coincide with an inappropriate situation.)

It's also convenient. You have a couple of minutes to spare, and you have privacy and access to the vaginal opening.

Collect some mucus on your fingertips when you sit down; the check for quality and quantity can take the place of reading the cartoon books.

It's preferable to use your fingers, not toilet paper, as the latter will absorb moisture and may give a distorted reading. It's also important to check *at the mouth of the vagina*, not the walls (which are always moist).

If you find it difficult to tell the difference between mucus and vaginal secretions, you can do the solubility test. Dip a sample of mucus (or secretion) into some water. If it is cervical mucus it will form a blob and sink, whereas vaginal secretion will dissolve.

Although you can check mucus at the cervix, where there will always be some, it's important to always check at the same site. Cervical checks are usually reserved for times when you can't get the information you require at the vaginal opening because there is too little of it present. Remember that one of the functions of mucus is to protect the sperm from vaginal acidity, and to do that it needs to be present in the vagina.

After a while, the routine becomes automatic and requires little thought, as does the differentiation of the separate types of mucus. This, initially, may be confusing. *Don't panic! If you keep a record of the amount and texture of the mucus (these are the most important characteristics as far as fertility is concerned), you will be amazed at how quickly a recognisable pattern emerges on the charts.* As with anything new, it's really a matter of familiarisation.

During the process of learning to recognise your unique pattern, you will also learn which words are appropriate for you to use to describe it. Words you use at first may be discarded later as you settle into your own vocabulary that accurately describes the different stages you tend to go through (see Chapter 10, 'Charting and Coordinating the Methods for Contraception', for more on charting).

With some women, the changes are dramatic and obvious. With others, they are more subtle, taking a little longer to learn.

Patience is quickly rewarded: most women in a normal, healthy situation feel pretty confident after about three cycles.

Mucus checking and intercourse

Frequent checking ensures that sudden changes are observed. It also means that when sexual excitement initiates lubrication, thus confusing mucus detection, a recent reading will still give reliable information. However, *morning intercourse can be dangerous if you do not want to conceive.* This is because the change to fertile mucus could have occurred during the night. Once you are already aroused and lubricating, this check cannot be made. Certainly, it is unlikely to be reliable while you are still prone, as the mucus will not descend to the mouth of the vagina, though it will do so in less than half an hour once you are standing up again.

Pelvic-floor exercise (also called *Kegel* exercise) can help here if you don't want to get up. The repeated tightening and relaxing of the muscles surrounding the vagina (such as is done when trying to prevent the flow of urine, or when preparing for childbirth) will help to push any mucus down to the vaginal opening. This little trick can be useful at any time to make mucus more available. It will also help to expel other fluids, such as semen.

Residual seminal fluid from a previous act of intercourse, with or without the addition of spermicide, can also be confusing. This can often be a problem with morning mucus checks, as most sexual activity occurs at night (or first thing in the morning). Seminal fluid will only drain out of the vagina once you get up from your bed. Since different vaginas tilt at different angles, they also drain at different rates.

The difference between seminal fluid, spermicide, lubrication and mucus should become evident with experience. Some women claim that they can differentiate mucus types even in the presence of other fluids. But if you are in doubt, *24 hours should pass after intercourse before checking mucus.*

For some women, it becomes evident that they drain faster than this: experience will tell. Other women feel dry all day, even directly after intercourse. If this is so for you, you could rely on the next evening being infertile.

Washing or douching the vagina is not recommended, except in emergency situations or to treat infections, as it alters the natural environment of the vagina and can give rise to yeast proliferation (thrush). Also, you might wash away all the mucus and make an inaccurate assessment of fertility. Anyway, vaginas are self-cleansing and better left alone.

The *Kegel* exercise can also be used to help eliminate residual fluids after intercourse, but if you feel that you need to wait 24 hours to make a safe mucus check, then you should use the *Early Days Rule*.

This rule allows intercourse only every other night (and not in the morning) in the first half of the cycle, to allow for confident mucus checking. This is particularly important for contraception.

EARLY DAYS RULE

Dry day, safe night, skip a day.

The only exception to this rule is if you have a completely dry day straight after intercourse.

Keeping records

Recording observations is very important: it speeds up the learning process enormously, enabling the comparison of one cycle with the next. In the first few learning months, you will discover how to distinguish the different *types* of mucus, the *pattern* of these types and an appropriate *description* for each distinct variation that you experience. It's easier, at first, to simply describe what you see and feel, rather than try to make decisions about whether it is fertile or not.

You don't need to write a novel, just jot down a word, symbol or code for the *amount* and *texture* (important), *colour* and *external sensation* (less important), at the end of each day. If you've noticed more than one kind of mucus that day, *describe the most fertile*; that way you always make the safest decision. As your unique pattern emerges, you will soon find that the differences become clear.

Don't despair if, for the first few months, the mucus observations seem obscure. Keep checking every time you go to the toilet, and write down the observations. After you've been doing this for a few months, you should be able to use a consistent description for each type of mucus that you normally experience (see Chapter 10, 'Charting and Coordinating').

As is the case with anything with which you are unfamiliar, subtle differences only become apparent upon familiarisation. Just as an elderly person may say, 'But all these pop groups sound the same to me, dear!', so too will you take a little while to differentiate the mucus types. They will soon become familiar, and it will be second nature to know where you are in your cycle.

You will come to know whether to normally expect any *spinn*, and when, and how many days of wet mucus to anticipate. You will learn if your BIP is one of no mucus (dry days) or if you always have some mucus present.

Everyone's cycle is unique, and you will become familiar with yours once you see it repeat in a similar pattern, cycle after cycle and month after month. Individual patterns may change, of course; it cannot be expected that any situation will remain entirely consistent.

Abstinence during the first few months (at least in the first half, or pre-ovulatory phase, of the cycle) is helpful in enabling you to learn mucus patterns more quickly (as well as making you more confident of avoiding unwanted pregnancies). However, a rigid rule to abstain for at least 1 month may not be realistic.

Always be aware of any previous sexual activity which may have compromised the mucus readings. If in doubt, leave the reading (and the sexual activity) for at least 24 hours.

The more you abstain, the faster you learn (and then the less you need to abstain). Take it at your own pace and write down all possible conditions affecting your body, along with your mucus record (see Chapters 10 and 13 on how to chart for contraception and conception).

Extra helpful hints

◆ Wear loose underclothes so you can more easily feel sensations of dryness and wetness.

◆ Beware of mid–cycle spotting. Don't confuse it with a period.

◆ Charting is usually necessary for at least 12 months. After that, you make your own decision on your need for written records.

◆ Flexibility comes with experience, but *may* involve greater risk for those not wishing to conceive. Make your decisions wisely.

◆ Recovery from taking the contraceptive pill can cause abnormal mucus patterns, which may take several months to settle down (see Chapter 11, 'Times of Change').

◆ Patience is rewarded. Take the first few months of mucus checking at your own pace. All will become clear.

◆ Sudden irregularity can cause confusion as your patterns change. However, a new pattern will emerge. A little extra attention at these times will see you through.

Simplicity itself

As you can see, the mucus method is really very simple. Fertility is defined as starting as soon as the mucus changes and lasting until 3 days after the last day of any type of fertile mucus (wet or *spinn*). These are the days to be avoided for contraception. As we shall see in Chapter 13, 'Conscious Conception', some refinement of this is helpful in optimising chances of conception.

It has been confirmed in laboratory tests that, 'The woman's own awareness of her cervical mucus could indicate ovulation even more accurately than oestrogen measurements.'

The efficiency of the mucus method (correctly applied) is around 98.5 per cent, and with good teaching and motivation, even higher.

CHAPTER 5

Basal Body Temperature Changes

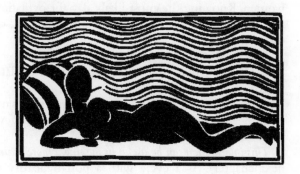

The temperature method relies on the measurement of body-at-rest temperature, sometimes called *basal temperature*.

Temperature readings, although they do not *warn* of the approach of ovulation the way the mucus observations do, can still be extremely useful. This is particularly true during the learning period, and the method is an ideal back-up if there are times of confusion in mucus checking.

You can confirm through checking your temperature graph whether or not ovulation has occurred, and if you have entered into the post-ovulatory infertile phase.

Mucus observations and their usefulness in identifying fertility may be compromised in a number of situations, as we saw in the previous chapter. Even though the mucus changes are still evident, you may become less confident if any of the following occurs:

◆ your menstrual pattern changes

◆ your cycle becomes irregular (see Chapter 11, 'Times of Change')

◆ you are suffering from an infected vaginal discharge

◆ your level of sexual activity suddenly increases

◆ you are taking any of the drugs or are experiencing any of the conditions described in the previous chapter as affecting mucus production.

The first few months of learning, especially if recovering from taking the Pill, is also a time of relative uncertainty.

At this time, if conception is not desired, it may be necessary to avoid unprotected sex during the pre-ovulatory phase (first half) of the cycle, and rely on temperature changes alone to confirm post-ovulatory infertility.

Temperature changes also help to confirm that ovulation did, indeed, take place. They also represent one of the most accurate ways of telling when ovulation occurred, this information usually being more specific than that obtained from mucus checking and accurate for about 80 per cent of women. Knowing the most likely day for ovulation gives a more accurate figure for the length of the luteal phase, or post-ovulatory second half of the cycle.

Fifty per cent of women have a luteal phase of 13 or 14 days most of the time. The other 50 per cent experience a post-ovulatory phase of 10–12 or 15–16 days.

Each individual tends to keep to the same interval, although, occasionally, there is a difference in alternating cycles as the ovaries take turns (usually) to release an egg.

This information can be useful in making a more accurate rhythm calculation (see next chapter). As a cycle with a post-ovulatory phase under 10 days is regarded as infertile (not enough progesterone is produced to prepare the endometrium for the fertilised egg), knowing the length of the post-ovulatory phase can also be helpful in diagnosing fertility problems. Of course, if you know when you ovulate, you will also know the length of the pre-ovulatory (follicular) phase and, as you will find out in Chapter 13, this can be important information to avoid miscarriage and defective ova.

As part of the process of learning about your cycle, temperature readings can be invaluable. Knowing fairly accurately when ovulation took place can help you see where this occurred in your mucus pattern.

This speeds up the recognition of mucus patterns and confidence will come much sooner. You may then, if you wish, discard temperature readings as a regular part of your fertility identification, preferring to rely on the mucus readings.

For those trying to conceive, knowledge of where ovulation comes in the mucus pattern can be crucial to success (see Chapter 13, 'Conscious Conception').

You may prefer to keep taking the temperature readings as back-up for the mucus observations. For some women, the temperature graph will show very clearly when ovulation is over, and this can certainly increase confidence, especially for those using the method for contraception. It may also cut down on waiting time if the change back to the *Basic Infertile Pattern* is not very clear.

Do not play one method off against another, especially if you don't want to conceive.

To understand more about using the different methods together for contraception or conception, see Chapters 10 and 13.

Why does the temperature rise?

As ovulation occurs, the increased production of progesterone generates greater heat in the body and the body-at-rest temperature rises. This is what is measured to ascertain whether or not ovulation is over and when it occurred. A strong, immediate and sustained rise indicates healthy progesterone levels.

In a classic graph, the temperature jogs along with small changes in the first half, or pre-ovulatory phase, of the cycle. It drops slightly just before ovulation, and then rises by up to 0.5° Celsius (1° Fahrenheit) and stays up until just before or during the menstrual period, when it falls again. If this doesn't occur, the first thing to do is check your thermometer and your technique.

If ovulation doesn't occur, then the temperature won't go up, and if menstruation doesn't occur, then the temperature won't come down.

If your body-at-rest temperature has been elevated for more than 20 days and is continuing to rise, you can consider yourself pregnant. Let's hope this is *good* news.

Hormone and Basal Body Temperature Levels

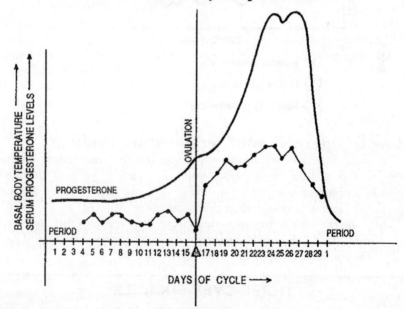

When does ovulation occur?

Ovulation is generally considered to have occurred *at the beginning of the temperature rise*, which is sometimes called the 'thermal shift'.

This is *usually* also the lowest reading, as the temperature does in fact drop (by 0.12–0.3° Celsius (0.25–0.6° Fahrenheit) just before ovulation takes place. However, this drop can take place during a shorter interval than the 24-hour gap between one reading and the next (for example, overnight), and may not show on your graph. Therefore, the *most likely* day for ovulation is at the beginning of the rise, which is not always the lowest temperature recorded in the cycle.

Although this is the *most likely* time for ovulation, up to 3 days prior to the rise is reasonably common, and it is possible for the egg to have been released up to 5 days before the rise, during the rise, or up to 2 days after. In the healthiest and most fertile situation, the rise will follow directly after ovulation. If there is a discrepancy between the temperature readings and other indicators, such as mucus, you may want to use natural remedies to improve hormone balance. See Chapter 12 for more information on how to achieve this. Here is a diagram showing the possibilities.

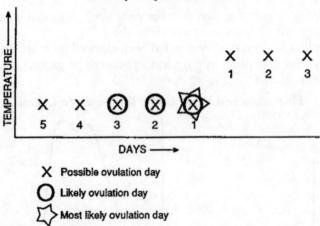

How to interpret your temperature readings

As with the mucus observations, when you use the temperature method there is also a 3-day wait before you can consider yourself definitely infertile, and before you can be confident that you have ovulated and that you know fairly accurately when this occurred.

This time the wait is for three consecutive daily readings that are at least 0.1° Celsius (0.2° Fahrenheit) higher than the six previous readings. This is called *Thermal Shift Rule*, or the *Three-Over-Six Rule*.

THREE-OVER-SIX RULE

You can be confident that you have finished ovulating and that you are infertile when there have been three consecutive temperature readings that are at least 0.1° Celsius (0.2° Fahrenheit) higher than the previous six readings.

◆ The first four readings in a cycle do not count as they may still be falling from the previous cycle.

◆ The rise will generally be from between 0.1–0.5° Celsius (0.2–1° Fahrenheit). However, this can vary a great deal from woman to woman, and may depend on the level of hormone production.

◆ Because there are several factors which may send the temperature up, as well as hormonal changes, it is necessary to ensure that the rise experienced is not a *freak high*, caused by

  • infection (however slight), medication or drugs (including prescription)

  • moving quickly across time-zones (as in air travel)

  • severe overheating in bed (from an electric blanket, for example)

  • activity before taking temperature (such as a visit to the toilet)

  • disturbed sleep, hangover, stress or late rising time.

This is why you must be sure you have a *sustained* rise of at least three consecutive higher readings before you can consider unprotected intercourse safe, if you don't want to conceive.

If one of these freak highs occurs in the 6 days prior to the sustained rise, you include 1 more day in the count of six, as you will see.

There is a simple way to apply the rule.

No mathematics required

When you have recorded what you feel is a shift in temperature and want to make sure that it complies with the *Thermal Shift Rule* (*Three-Over-Six Rule*), draw a line one space above the highest of the last six readings. This is called a *cover-line*; you need *three consecutive readings above the cover-line*.

So let's redefine the *Three-Over-Six Rule*.

SIMPLIFIED THREE-OVER-SIX RULE

You can be sure you have entered the infertile post-ovulatory phase of your cycle when you have recorded three consecutive temperatures that are above the cover-line.

Especially after a little experience, the graphs will usually be easy to interpret at a glance. You may well find that you only need to use the *Three-Over-Six Rule* in the less obvious cases. However, if you do need to use the rule, *remember*:

◆ Your 6 days are always counted *backwards* from today, so that, day-by-day, they are recounted to see if a rise has occurred.

◆ The first 4 days of a cycle don't count.

◆ Ignore any freak highs.

◆ If you are trying to conceive, it's the approach to ovulation that is important. This means temperature readings will be most useful for identifying the most likely day of ovulation retrospectively, and seeing where this falls in your mucus pattern.

Now let's see how this all looks on the graphs. Don't panic. It all becomes easy with very little experience.

Example temperature graphs

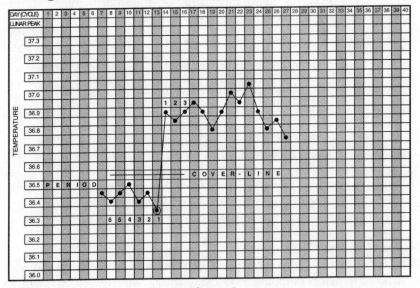

Chart 1

In Chart 1, the rise after ovulation is immediate and clear. It's what I call a 'Whoosh' chart, because the temperature shoots right up in 1 day. The three higher readings, therefore, come at once on the first, second and third days after the probable day of ovulation, which is the circled day at the beginning of the rise.

This type of graph is very clear and useful for contraception purposes in that it gives immediate information on the start of the post-ovulatory infertile phase. It also indicates good levels of progesterone.

If you consistently have this type of graph and are trying not to conceive, you will need to decide

◆ that temperature readings are helping you to learn that the fertile time is over in a clearer way than that afforded by your mucus observations and that you will continue to use the temperature method on a permanent basis, *or*

◆ that although it is giving you this information more clearly, it's too much hassle and you would rather rely on the mucus method — even though this may involve you in more abstinence days (or use of barrier methods), *or*

◆ that although the graph gives you clear information, your mucus readings are just as efficient and, therefore, sufficient, *or*

◆ that the graphs you are drawing up cycle by cycle are sufficiently consistent to be able to reduce the number of days on which you take your temperature.

If you consistently ovulate at the same time in your cycle, you could learn to anticipate this by enough days to use your *Three-Over-Six Rule* (which may be at the onset of your fertile-type mucus) and cease taking your temperature after the third higher reading. Or, if you could interpret your graphs by look alone, you could start taking your temperature as the mucus indicates that you are approaching ovulation, confirm that you have, in fact, passed it and then stop again.

This last option will only be possible if you have a regular cycle, but you may prefer to take a daily reading anyway, a daily habit being easier to maintain than one that is sporadic.

If you consistently have this type of graph and your aim is to conceive, your need to continue taking your temperature would be based on the regularity of information that you were receiving.

Of course just because you have decided to use the temperature method in one of these ways doesn't mean that you can't change your mind if the circumstances alter. *Adaptability equals success.*

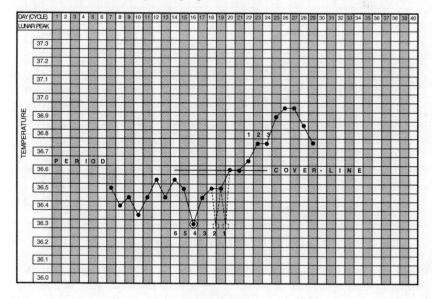

Chart 2

Chart 2 has two possible interpretations: which one you choose may depend on other symptoms, such as mucus and cervical changes.

It may be what I call a 'Step' graph, with the rise taking place over a number of days. Ovulation (circled) is at the beginning of the rise, but the three higher readings do not occur until almost a week later, on Days 22, 23 and 24, which are 6, 7 and 8 days after ovulation.

This gives a very short elevated phase, deficient progesterone and a limited use for this method for contraception (unlike Chart 1), as mucus observations will indicate post-ovulatory infertility more accurately. However, you'll still learn the day of ovulation, which will help you to refine rhythm or mucus timing for conception or contraception. Once you know this, you may choose to discontinue taking your temperature, unless patterns change.

If this is a correct interpretation, mucus should peak *before* Day 16. If it peaks *afterwards*, ovulation may happen later, just before the graph goes over the cover-line, with the dip occurring *between two readings* (for example, overnight between Days 18 and 19, or 19 and 20). This would substantially alter the visual appearance of the graph. In this case the post-ovulatory phase is very short and indicates insufficient progesterone production.

If the cover-line goes through a point, then that day does not count as one of your three higher or six lower readings. It is not necessary to know the exact day of ovulation for contraception purposes.

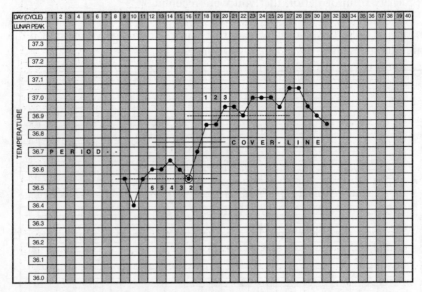

Chart 3

When you first look at this chart it may be difficult to distinguish the two distinct phases, as the rise appears to commence from the very beginning. As a result, you might feel confused as to which day is the most likely day for ovulation.

If a chart is not easy to interpret visually, a pencil or some other straight object may be lined up horizontally along the readings. This will nearly always clarify the chart into two distinct plateaux, or what is called a biphasic pattern, with the rise between them starting at the most likely day of ovulation. On this chart, the ovulation day is circled as in Charts 1 and 2, and I have marked in the two average temperatures for the first and second half with dotted lines. The solid line is the cover-line.

The first day after ovulation (Day 17), the reading is not higher than the cover-line, and would not have been if you had counted back 6 days from the circled day, in which case the cover-line would have run straight through this reading. So, the cover-line has to be redrawn to include Day 17 in your count of six.

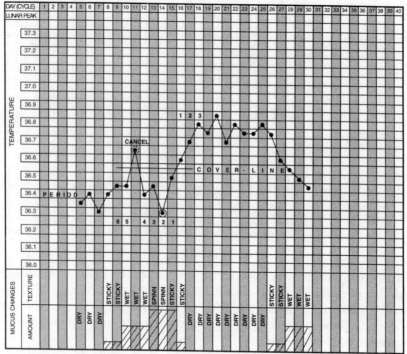

Chart 4

In this chart there is a freak high reading in the pre-ovulatory phase. For some reason, the temperature has risen for 1 day and then dropped again. The cause of this may or may not be obvious at the time of recording the temperature, but, if it is, it should be noted.

This freak high *is not* included when you make your count of six, it being obviously abnormal. If the freak high readings were included, the three higher readings might never arrive.

As it is in this graph, by ignoring the reading on Day 11, the readings start to count on Day 16. If the freak high had been included, you would have needed to wait until Day 18. On a slightly different graph, you might never get any readings 0.1° Celsius (0.2° Fahrenheit) higher than that on Day 11.

In this chart, the temperature drops sharply before menstruation and this is accompanied by wet mucus, as discussed in Chapter 4.

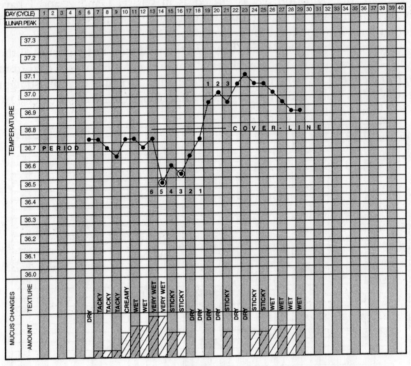

Chart 5

In Chart 5 it is difficult to tell whether the rise starts on Day 14 or 16. The peak mucus symptom coincides with Day 14, but may occur up to 2 days before ovulation. Previous (or future) charts may clarify the issue, though, for contraception purposes, you don't really need to know. If it's Day 14, progesterone is slow to rise.

Chart 6 shows a long cycle with the post-ovulatory second half remaining at approximately 14 days (here it is 13), and the pre-ovulatory phase being extended at 27 days. It would be unwise to attempt conception on this cycle (see Chapter 13, 'Conscious Conception').

Chart 7 shows an anovular cycle (one with no ovulation), resulting in a monophasic graph (a graph without a rise and with only one plateau). This can occur even though you experience a build-up of mucus — ovulation being arrested at the last minute — and may well result in a bleed, although this is not a period and may be lighter than usual. This cycle may also be an unusual length.

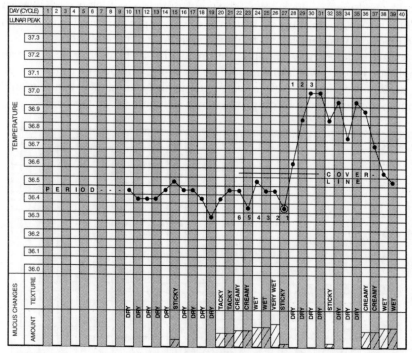

Chart 6

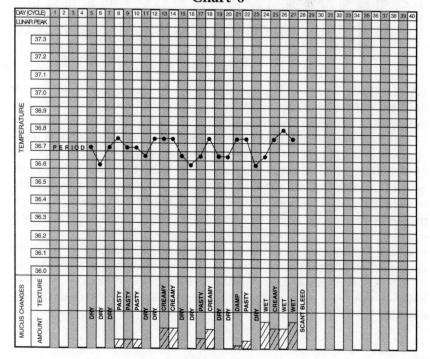

Chart 7

The only reasonably sure test of ovulation is a temperature rise (or a blood test). An occasional cycle such as this need not concern you, although frequent or persistent failure to ovulate would require attention.

Chart 8 shows how unstable the pre-ovulatory phase can be. All freak highs are ignored when making the count of six. The post-ovulatory phase is nearly always more stable, as very little is likely to happen which would cause the temperature to drop, other than deficient progesterone.

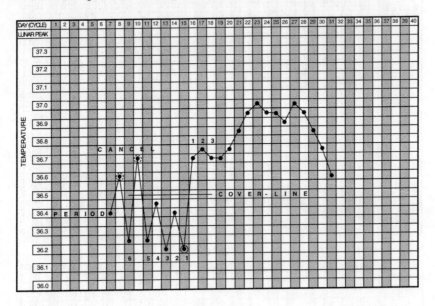

Chart 8

Chart 9 shows a very short cycle, still with a 15-day post-ovulatory phase but with the pre-ovulatory phase ending at ovulation on Day 9. This may indicate low oestrogen levels, though mucus is adequate and fertile as soon as bleeding ceases, and possibly also during the period. In this cycle abstinence would need to be practised during menstruation.

The six previous readings can only be assumed to be low, as only four have been recorded, the other 2 days being during menstruation. Many women don't take their temperature while they are bleeding, although only the first 4 days of the cycle are actually unreliable (as the temperature may still be falling from the previous cycle).

Chart 10 shows another long cycle with ovulation too late for a healthy conception (see Chapter 13). This may be due to oestrogen imbalance or to the hypothyroid condition indicated by the low temperatures. Note, however, that the most likely day of ovulation is *not* the lowest temperature recorded.

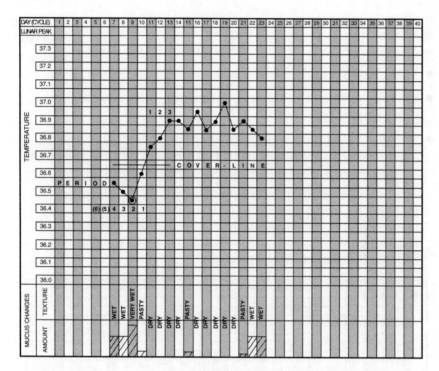

Chart 9

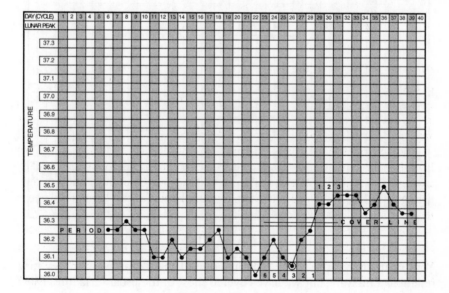

Chart 10

In Chart 11, a mistake has been made. It would have been possible for this woman to think that she had ovulated on Day 15, with the next two readings being higher. There are three reasons why she shouldn't.

◆ There are only two higher readings.

◆ She had the 'flu during the temperature rise, which could also have delayed ovulation.

◆ She still had wet mucus. There could be ten higher readings, but if you still had wet mucus that had not ceased since the rise, you should not consider yourself infertile (see Chapter 10 for more information).

The correct count for the cover-line has been shown; the high readings on Days 16 and 17 can be ignored because of the 'flu. However, the woman may have been misled (or been trying to conceive) as the extended and increasing (triphasic) temperature rise indicates that she is probably pregnant.

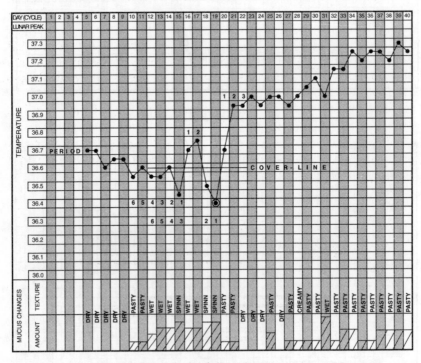

Chart 11

Your charts may or may not look like one of these examples, or they may resemble a mixture, but we have covered most of the usual variations. *Don't be concerned if your charts are unique. You can still easily learn to interpret them.*

How to take your temperature

Mercury thermometers are cheaper and more reliable than most of the digital variety. There are two different types of thermometer: normal fever thermometers which read to very high temperatures, and basal or fertility thermometers which only read basal or body-at-rest temperatures.

The difference between the two types is that the fertility thermometer usually has no markings above 38° Celsius (100° Fahrenheit), leaving more room on the stem for the degrees to be marked in small gradations. This makes it easier to distinguish small changes. If your thermometer is marked in gradations of 0.05°C (0.1°F), each gradation will represent one box on the chart illustrated in Chapter 10 (and which is supplied with all Natural Fertility Management kits). Some fertility thermometers also show a scale of 0–60 (starting at the lowest mark). Although this may seem easier than counting the degrees, it can get confusing as not all thermometers are similarly marked.

Fertility thermometers tend to be rather more expensive and can be more difficult to find, so you may prefer to buy a standard fever thermometer. In this case, you should make sure that it is marked in at least 0.1° Celsius (0.2° Fahrenheit) gradations as you will need to read to 0.05° Celsius (0.1° Fahrenheit). Although it is possible to distinguish if the mercury is halfway between markings, any greater distinction would be too difficult to discern.

If you have no experience in reading thermometers, here are some clues. The temperature is indicated by how far up the stem the mercury rises. The mercury in the bulb heats up when placed under the tongue (or wherever you are taking the temperature), and expands up a tiny capillary tube which can only be seen clearly through magnifying glass.

Thermometers

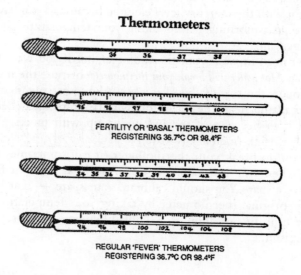

FERTILITY OR 'BASAL' THERMOMETERS
REGISTERING 36.7°C OR 98.4°F

REGULAR 'FEVER' THERMOMETERS
REGISTERING 36.7°C OR 98.4°F

There is magnifying glass down one side of the thermometer and this is why you need to hold it at a special angle when reading it. It should be held horizontally and turned until a silver line appears. The top of the line can then be read off against the temperature it has reached.

There's a break in the mercury near the bulb, which is a constriction in the tube that prevents the mercury falling back down until you shake the thermometer with a flicking motion. *This ensures that the mercury will stay up until read.*

To take the temperature, place the bulb under your tongue in good contact with the flesh, close your mouth and leave the thermometer in place for about 3 minutes. Individual thermometers take different times to register. Whenever you buy a new one experiment with it by testing the reading after 1, 2, 3, 4 and 5-minute intervals.

Some women prefer to take their temperature vaginally or rectally. This is supposed to be more accurate. Nearly everyone finds the oral reading adequate and easier. *It is important always to take the temperature the same way.* This is because vaginal and rectal temperatures are, on average, 0.5° Celsius (1° Fahrenheit) higher than oral temperatures.

You need to take your temperature first thing in the morning (it is the body-at-rest temperature you are recording). So keep the thermometer by your bed, put it in your mouth as soon as you awake and spend the next 2–5 minutes waking up as the thermometer registers.

Falling back to sleep can present a hazard as your mouth may open, letting the thermometer fall out and possibly break (and the reading will be false if your mouth is not closed).

After you take the thermometer out of your mouth, you can put it down and wait until later (when your eyesight may be clearer) to read it. The mercury stays up until it is shaken down — for at least an hour and, in some thermometers, all day. After you have read it, shake it down and put it away. Don't leave it with the mercury level elevated because, if you have to shake it down the next morning before taking your temperature, *you may send your temperature up.*

You don't need to wash your thermometer, but if you want to, use the cold-water tap. *Hot water will break your thermometer* because the mercury will expand through the top of the glass stem. Also, don't put it on a sunny ledge, under a lamp, near a heater or follow the example of a client of mine who tested it in her cup of tea and ended up with pieces of mercury floating in her drink (mercury is toxic).

In case you do break your thermometer (it can sometimes fall out of your hand when you are shaking it down, so hold on to it firmly), it's good to have a spare. You should calibrate your spare — that is, check it against your original thermometer by taking your temperature on both at the same time in case there is a slight difference in the temperatures that they register.

Conditions for taking your temperature

◆ You should take your temperature before undertaking any activity, preferably before getting out of bed or having conversations and definitely before having a hot drink or hot food. If something needs to be done before you get a chance to take your temperature, for example going to the toilet, move slowly and gently and take the temperature as soon as possible after returning to bed.

◆ When marking the temperature on the graph, note any special circumstances. Individuals respond in different ways.

◆ At least 4 hours sleep is required for your body to have reached the at-rest state, so if your night was short or disturbed, note it down.

◆ Read your temperature at the same time of day (approximately). The basal temperature is much higher later in the day and lower earlier, regardless of how much sleep you've had. There is a useful rule to adjust early and late readings. First, you need to decide on a set, usual, rising time, based on your most frequent experience.

TEMPERATURE ADJUSTMENT RULE

If you rise *earlier* than usual, adjust the temperature *up* by 0.05° Celsius (0.1° Fahrenheit) for each half hour before recording it. If you rise *later* than usual, adjust the temperature *down* by 0.05° Celsius (0.1° Fahrenheit) for each half hour before recording it.

Some women have a greater or lesser variation than that given in this formula, which is based on an average woman's expectation. Experience will tell. If you use the graph in Chapter 10 (which comes with all Natural Fertility Management kits), you will find that 0.05°C (0.1°F) is equivalent to one box on the graph. So the adjustment is one box, up or down, for each half hour.

If changes in rising times are frequent and the difference is great, you may want to find out how much your temperature tends to rise each hour. Take your temperature at your earlier rising time and go back to sleep. Then take it at the later time and see how much difference there has been per hour.

It is necessary to use an adjustment to avoid the freak highs associated with late rising. Otherwise you may end up with 'weekend syndrome' (strange bumps). For shift workers who rise in the afternoon or evening, note that by 5.00 pm, the temperature will have peaked, and then it will start to drop again. Mark both the measured and adjusted temperatures on your graph using different marks, say, a dot and a cross, and note the rising time.

Always take your temperature under all circumstances. Just make sure you note on your graph what any unusual circumstances were.

Here is a list of other conditions you may need to note.

◆ Ill health.

◆ Extreme temperature changes (such as leaving your electric blanket on all night and waking up in a sweat).

◆ Stress.

◆ Hangovers.

◆ Medication or drugs.

◆ Air travel across time zones.

The temperature method is really very simple to use and can be a great help to give you some idea of what is going on while you learn to distinguish mucus changes or if these are unclear. It will also give you clear information about the timing of ovulation and if this is, in fact, occurring. You cannot use it to warn of the approach of ovulation which means it has limited application on its own.

The effective rate of the temperature method correctly applied with abstinence in pre-ovulatory phase has been assessed as 99 per cent.

CHAPTER 6

Rhythm Calculations

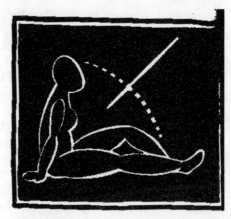

The purpose of another method

The rhythm method, notorious though it has been, can have a useful part
to play. We have all heard the jokes about the rhythm of the pitter patter of
little children's feet and, certainly, as a contraception method used on its
own, rhythm leaves a lot to be desired (frequent love-making, for one
thing). You may find, however, that *rhythm has a role to play as a warning, back-
up and fail-safe method, especially for contraceptive use.*

The more you come to understand the workings of your body, the more
you will be able to make the rhythm calculations appropriate to your cycle.
This will render them more accurate and effective, and less prohibitive of
unprotected intercourse.

If you are trying to conceive, rhythm calculations can be useful as a
warning that ovulation is approaching, and that it is time to put into effect
the preparatory measures discussed in Chapter 13, 'Conscious Conception'.
You can then use the mucus readings to identify more accurately the best
time for conception attempts.

However, the *rhythm method is not enough on its own for confident
contraception or conception.* This is because in the rhythm method, your
calculations are based on your experience and the recent history of your
cycle — when you *think* you are likely to ovulate. When you use the
sympto-thermal approach, you find out what is happening in reality, not by

supposition. This reduces the role of the rhythm method to warning, fail-safe and back-up.

WARNING

Having calculations written up in advance means that you are less likely to pass into or through your fertile time without being aware of it. It will also remind you to be thorough in your body observations at these likely-to-be-fertile times and, if your cycle is short, indicate if your menstrual period is potentially fertile (see Chapter 4).

FAIL-SAFE

If you find yourself in the (hopefully rare) situation where there are problems with both your temperature and mucus observations, it's good to have another method, apart from wishful thinking, to resort to. Be careful to ensure that the condition affecting your mucus or temperature will not also affect the timing of ovulation and compromise your calculation.

BACK-UP

Rhythm calculations provide helpful back-up while mucus patterns are first being learnt, but only in situations where there are sufficient records of a natural cycle.

Although temperature readings can be useful at this time for giving the all-clear (for contraceptive purposes) that you are into your post-ovulatory infertile phase, the temperature method gives you no warning of the approach of ovulation. Until you are familiar with your mucus pattern, rhythm calculations are the only way you can tell when you start to become fertile.

DISADVANTAGES

There are two main problems with relying on rhythm method for contraception.

◆ *The rhythm method does not account for unpredictable changes in the cycle.*

◆ *The rhythm method's effectiveness relies on fairly large safety margins and will always involve more abstinence (or days when protection is required) than the sympto-thermal approach.*

This is because, with the rhythm method, you are basically making an informed guess as to what is likely to happen, whereas when you use the sympto-thermal approach, you are observing what is actually happening.

If you are trying to conceive, there are other disadvantages in relying solely on rhythm.

◆ *You are less likely to time your conception attempt accurately, and may miss it altogether, or conceive with old eggs or sperm, which is less healthy.*

◆ *Even if you do have intercourse on the right day for conception, you are likely to be spreading your attempts over too long a period of time (see Chapter 13). This may result in a lowered sperm count and reduced fertility.*

However, for a fairly regular woman, rhythm method can be reasonably reliable for contraception (which is the application most under consideration here) especially if

♦ you have become aware of the likely effects on your cycle of different circumstances and allow for these

♦ you have come to a fairly good understanding of the unique rhythms of your own cycle

♦ you combine the use of the rhythm method with observance of the lunar cycle (see Chapter 7, 'The Lunar Cycle', in which we will see how the original research into this cycle was conducted in combination with rhythm calculations, and raised considerably the effectiveness of the method).

Rhythm formulae

There are two possible ways of making your rhythm calculations. The first is the traditional, very cautious approach that is applicable to all women. This takes into account all fertile days associated with any possible repetition of the longest and shortest cycles experienced in the last year (or at least the last 6 months — anything less will be unreliable).

This formula works by subtracting 18 days from the shortest recorded cycle to give the earliest possible beginning of fertility; and 10 days from the longest recorded cycle to give the end of the fertile period. It is generally recommended that cycles need to have been recorded for between 6 months to 1 year before the calculations can be made.

TRADITIONAL RHYTHM FORMULA

S-18 TO L-10

S-18 gives you a calculation for the *first possibly fertile day* by allowing for the earliest possible ovulation (16 days before the earliest recorded menstruation, therefore 15 before the last day of the shortest recorded cycle) and subtracting 3 more days for the lifespan of the sperm. This gives the first possibly fertile day as 18 days before the end of the shortest recorded cycle.

L-10 gives you a calculation for the last possibly fertile day by allowing for the latest possible ovulation (12 days before the latest recorded menstruation, therefore 11 before the last day of the longest recorded cycle) and adding one day for the lifespan of the egg. This gives the last possibly fertile day as 10 days before the end of the longest recorded cycle.

First Possibly Fertile Day — 'S-18'

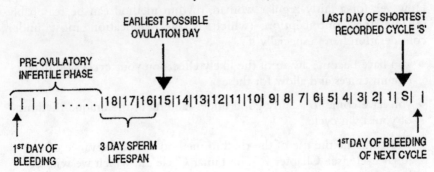

Last Possibly Fertile Day — 'L-10'

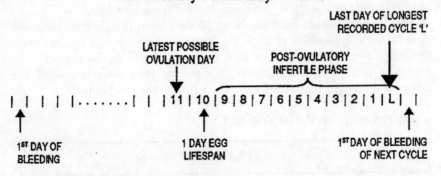

For example, a shortest recorded cycle of 24 days gives Day 6 as the first possibly fertile day, and a longest recorded cycle of 32 days gives Day 22 as the last possibly fertile day.

First and Last Possibly Fertile Days using
Formula S-18 to L-10

Number of days in shortest cycle 'S'	First possibly fertile day 'S-18'	Number of days in longest cycle 'L'	Last possibly fertile day 'L-10'
22	4	22	12
23	5	23	13
24	6	24	14
25	7	25	15
26	8	26	16
27	9	27	17
28	10	28	18
29	11	29	19
30	12	30	20
31	13	31	21
32	14	32	22
33	15	33	23
34	16	34	24
35	17	35	25
36	18	36	26

Two considerations may cause the ultra-cautious among you to make an even more conservative calculation.

◆ On very rare occasions, sperm have been known to survive for up to 6 days. There is great doubt as to whether such geriatric sperm could survive the trip to the egg in viable health, however, if you wish to be extremely careful in avoiding conception, you would need to revise the first half of the formula to S-21 to account for this.

◆ Post-ovulatory (luteal), phases have also been known with reasonable frequency, to be less than 12 days long and as short as 10 (if they are less than 10 they will be infertile). So once again, to be even more sure, you could need to revise the second half of the formula to L-8. *Your ultracautious formula is then:*

S-21 TO L-8

First and Last Possibly Fertile Days using Formula 'S–21 to L–8'

Number of days in shortest cycle 'S'	First possibly fertile day 'S–21'	Number of days in longest cycle 'L'	Last possibly fertile day 'L–8'
22	1	22	14
23	2	23	15
24	3	24	16
25	4	25	17
26	5	26	18
27	6	27	19
28	7	28	20
29	8	29	21
30	9	30	22
31	10	31	23
32	11	32	24
33	12	33	25
34	13	34	26
35	14	35	27
36	15	36	28

This traditional formula relies on two assumptions.

◆ The first is that the post-ovulatory phase is always between 10–16 days and usually between 12–16. The latter figure is true of the vast majority of women. Fifty per cent have a post-ovulatory phase 13 or 14 days long; nearly all the remainder have a phase of 10–12 days or 15–16 days. There are a very few women for whom this is not true. A second half that is shorter than 10 days will, in any case, be infertile. For most women, the length of this half of the cycle will not vary by more than a day or two. Through personal experience of monitoring a cycle (with temperature observations) it becomes possible to be a lot more specific about what each individual can reasonably expect.

◆ The second is that the cycle will continue to behave as it has done in the recent past. Once you have some information about how your cycle behaves under different conditions, you will be able to make a much more accurate assessment of the chances of it changing its pattern.
The longest cycle in the last year's records may well have coincided with a particular set of circumstances which you know tends to lengthen your cycle, but which no longer prevails. Or, your whole pattern may have changed dramatically which means that records as far back as a year ago may have become irrelevant.

So, the second way to make your rhythm calculation involves a more personally relevant approach.

PERSONAL RHYTHM FORMULA

◆ Take the shortest cycle length experienced in the last year, *excluding* freak cycles from known causes, as long as these no longer prevail.

◆ Add 1 day to take you to the first day of bleeding of your next cycle.

◆ Subtract the longest duration of the post-ovulatory phase of your cycle that you have experienced during the last year.

◆ Subtract 3 more days for the lifespan of the sperm. *This is the first possibly fertile day.*

◆ Then take your longest cycle length experienced in the last year, *excluding* freak cycles from known causes, as long as these no longer prevail.

◆ Add 1 day to take you to the first day of bleeding of your next cycle.

◆ Subtract the shortest duration of the post-ovulatory phase of your cycle that you have experienced during the last year.

◆ Add 1 day to account for the lifespan of the egg. *This is the last possibly fertile day.*

You can increase these safety margins if there is any reason to suppose that present conditions may lengthen the cycle, or if there seems to be a trend for your cycle to be lengthening or shortening. No external conditions, except breastfeeding, are likely to shorten your cycle, although any health condition which upsets the balance of your hormonal system may do so.

Rhythm calculations must not be relied upon in unstable conditions. Experience will tell what these are for each individual. Watch out for

◆ stress

◆ any major physical change

◆ diet or weight changes

◆ travel

◆ trauma

◆ drugs (prescription or otherwise)

◆ shock

◆ excessive exercise

◆ ill health

◆ any major psychological or emotional change

◆ perimenopause.

Long and short cycles

In cycles that are longer or shorter than the average of 29–30 days, the pre-ovulatory (follicular) phase will be where the expansion or contraction takes place. This is assuming that the post-ovulatory phase remains fairly stable (and this is nearly always the case, although sometimes you may experience alternating lengths as the ovaries take approximate turns). Thus

Average 29-Day Cycle

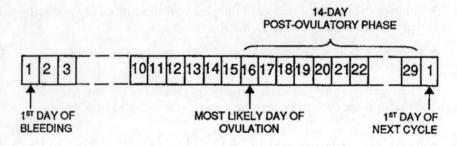

Long 36-Day Cycle

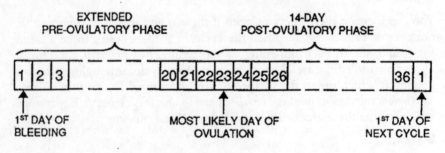

Short 24-Day Cycle

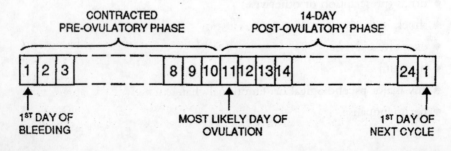

◆ a long cycle is nearly always the result of a delayed ovulation, not a delayed period, giving a long first half

◆ a short cycle is the result of an early ovulation, if there is an ovulation at all, resulting in a short first half.

Sometimes an abnormally long (greater than 16 days) or short (less than 10 days) post-ovulatory phase is caused by a hormonal imbalance, or dysfunction of the ovaries, and these can usually be corrected with natural therapies (see Chapter 12, 'Natural Remedies for Hormonal and Reproductive Health').

Until you have verification from your temperature readings of the length of the second half of your cycle, you should assume that it lies somewhere between 10 and 16 days, and use the traditional formula.

In a very short cycle, if the length of the post-ovulatory phase lies within the normal range, ovulation can come very soon after menstruation.

This may mean that the fertile mucus which precedes ovulation, and enables the sperm to survive, may well be present during bleeding.

The flow of blood is not sufficient to expel either the mucus or the sperm. Therefore, *in a very short cycle, menstruation is potentially fertile.* (The only other possibility for this to occur is when it coincides with the lunar cycle. See Chapter 7, 'The Lunar Cycle').

This is perhaps another reason why it may be a good idea to use rhythm calculations as back-up and warning, so you are aware of this possibility. Mucus detection is difficult, if not impossible, while you are bleeding, but rhythm calculations can bring the likelihood of this situation to your notice.

IS MENSTRUATION A DANGER TIME?

Because mucus readings are unreliable during menstruation, most teachers of mucus method will answer 'Yes'.

If you normally have regular and long cycles and use rhythm calculations to warn you of the possibility of a short cycle, there is a very small risk involved. You must decide for yourself if you are prepared to take this risk.

If you have occasional or frequent short cycles, your rhythm calculations will make it clear that menstruation is risky.

If you are in an unstable situation, you should consider that you are at risk of having a shorter cycle than usual and, as a result, of being potentially fertile during menstruation.

Using rhythm for conception

The rhythm method is not the best way to time conception attempts as it is not accurate enough to ensure that fresh sperm meet a fresh egg (see Chapter 13, 'Conscious Conception', for how to use mucus and temperature observations). However, in case calculation is the only option open to you, here is a table showing you the probable days of ovulation. It is based on the rhythm calculation and on the assumption that the luteal phase is between 10 and 16 days long. *Conception attempts should start the day before ovulation is due.*

Most Likely Ovulation Day

Length of cycle	Possible ovulation days	Most likely ovulation day	Possible ovulation days
22	7– 8	9	10–13
23	8– 9	10	11–14
24	9–10	11	12–15
25	10–11	12	13–16
26	11–12	13	14–17
27	12–13	14	15–18
28	13–14	15	16–19
29	14–15	16	17–20
30	15–16	17	18–21
31	16–17	18	19–22
32	17–18	19	20–23
33	18–19	20	21–24
34	19–20	21	22–25
35	20–21	22	23–26
36	21–22	23	24–27

Rhythm's (limited) use for contraception will be explored in Chapter 10, 'Charting and Coordinating the Methods for Contraception'. Rhythm method calculations, although useful as warning, fail-safe and back-up, are not sufficient on their own, and should never be followed if they contradict body symptoms. *Body symptoms always take precedence over calculations, as they tell you what is really going on.*

CHAPTER 7

The Lunar Cycle

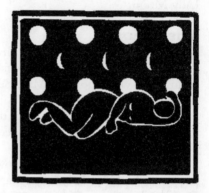

So far in this book, we have explored the advantages of being in tune with your personal rhythms. You will have become aware — if indeed you weren't already — that women are cyclical creatures.

We all, men too, change and grow all the time, but with women the greater life changes are grafted onto this underlying and very obvious monthly cycle, which affects us in endless ways. Change and pattern are integral to a woman's existence.

In this chapter, these ideas of personal cycles are extended into the cosmos to include the cycles of the phases of the moon.

Most women seem to have very little difficulty with the idea that the moon influences their fertility. It's as if this were obvious and required little proof. You may already delight in being able to connect your personal cycle to those of the planet, in being aware of your interconnectedness with other living things.

The information in this chapter brings you the chance to establish your personal relationship to the moon while extending your awareness of, and attunement to, your own physical changes. It will also add to the sum of knowledge that you have to help you feel in control of your own fertility.

In my experience, the use of the lunar cycle has increased the effectiveness of the other methods described in this book, giving an extra edge to their success for those trying to avoid or achieve pregnancy.

Astrology?

Objections to the use of the lunar cycle have often arisen from the use of the term 'Astrological Birth Control'. In fact, the lunar cycle is not really astrological in that it deals merely with a monthly repeating cycle, and the relationship is between two heavenly bodies, the sun and the moon.

To some extent, the title 'astrological' is a misnomer which may alienate those who otherwise might be prepared to consider the moon's role in influencing fertility.

The lunar cycle itself is not based on traditional astrological philosophy, but on proven fact. Some of you may enjoy astrology, others may deplore it, but whatever your position, it is difficult for anyone to ignore the effect of Lady Moon.

The moon

Throughout the ages, the moon has symbolised two things. First, woman — her femininity, and her special characteristics, distinctive from and contrasting with those of Man. Second, fertility — reproduction in the animal world and growth in the kingdom of plants.

The roots of these beliefs about the moon run deep in many cultures and religions, and are invariably connected with an appreciation of the special powers of women.

They occur in many races all over the world including the Indigenous people of Australia, Polynesia, Asia, Africa, the Americas and the people of Greenland.

The folk tales and legends of European peasantry also have a large lunar content. It is a tradition which extends world-wide. Religions in India, China and Mongolia, Ancient Greece and Rome, South America, Arabia and Syria and in the old religions of Judaism and the Celts in Northern and Western Europe have all centred on the moon.

It's understandable that such a large and obvious heavenly body should play such an important part in myth and religion; we find again and again, in widely dispersed and different cultures, that *the moon is inseparably linked to woman and fertility*. These beliefs have a basis in the experiences and observations of people all over the world from time immemorial.

Most primitive people have considered the moon's influence as necessary for growth. This applies to a woman's capacity to bear children in relation to both conception and birth, the reproductive ability of animals, and the germination and growth of seeds and plants.

These beliefs may well have been based on the observation that the moon's cycles affected fertility and growth, but they were often taken even further by some who saw the moon as the fertilising power, actually giving life to a previously inert substance.

The kingdom of plants

The special relationship between women, the moon and growing things was often manifested in peasant cultures by women being given charge of the cultivation of the crops — which were, of course, sown and harvested at certain phases of the moon.

The germination and growth of plants was seen to have a relationship with these phases, as was the woman's menstrual cycle. This could even result in menstrual blood itself being thought to have properties of fertility; in some cultures it was used as a fertiliser for plants.

Beliefs such as these, although primitive and in some respects foreign to scientifically sophisticated levels of understanding, perhaps can be perceived as tuning in to more subtle levels of energetic influence than modern science has yet recognised, and certainly as arising from observable truth.

Indeed, modern research bears out the idea that different phases of the moon have varied influences on plant growth and germination. The waxing moon is commonly held to coincide with the period of growth for all things, and the waning moon as being the time to gather, prune or harvest and prepare the ground for the next planting. *See here the parallel with the common experience of ovulating at the full moon and bleeding at the new.*

In many less developed societies these beliefs are still part of agricultural practice today and are also being used increasingly by those who feel the need to tune into Nature's cycles rather than basing their confidence on their ability to overcome them.

You may conclude, as I do, that the absence of such practice in modern Western agriculture has more to do with this misplaced confidence in modern technology to override Nature than in any greater understanding of the presence or absence of natural fertility cycles.

Hopefully, our new green consciousness will swing the pendulum — not 'back' the other way, but into some higher level of awareness which can integrate the good and constructive approaches of both the new knowledge and the old.

The animal world

The effect of the moon on breeding cycles is also clearly demonstrated in animal life. Many different forms of marine life, worms, fish, some types of seaweed and even coral, breed with specific phases of the moon. The previously held belief that it was the tides that gave rise to these patterns has now been disproved. *It is now obvious that animals, as well as plants, respond directly to the moon's phases.* The metabolic and sexual activity of oysters, salamanders, worms, rats, mice, monkeys, cows, bats, hamsters (and even vegetables such as potatoes and carrots) has been found to vary with the moon.

Dr Eugen Jonas, a Czech psychiatrist whose work in the 1950s gave rise to our understanding of the lunar cycle's effect on human reproductive capacity, said,

> Up to the present, science has recognised the influence of the moon on lower-order animals. This influence affects their capacity for existence and reproduction ... This possibility has not yet been investigated with respect to Man. *However, should the possibility that the moon affects the reproductive function of Man be completely excluded? ...* The unicellular ovum of the mother's womb in no way differs from the most minute living creatures which are so strongly affected by the moon. On this basis alone, it no longer appeared impossible to establish a correlation between the influences of the moon and the reproductive ability of Man.

Then, Jonas claims, 'After several years of research it was possible to demonstrate this connection.'

It is Dr Jonas' research that will enable you to extend your understanding of your personal lunar cycle.

Humans, too

Women, lovers, bleeders and lunatics have the acknowledged power of the moon in common. With lovers, there is a proven increase in sexual activity, with bleeders, there is an increased flow of blood, and the moon is seen to affect sanity and levels of excitement of lunatics. With women, it's the menstrual cycle. For some of you who suffer from PMS this may well also relate to your sanity!

The word *menstruation* is derived from Latin and Greek words for *month* and *moon*. In many languages, the word for menstruation is even more direct in its reference to the moon, and many myths abound of the moon touching (or even having intercourse) with women to trigger their monthly bleeding.

From Ancient Greece to modern times, beliefs and evidence have connected the hormonal cycle with the lunar month and its phases of waxing and waning. It seems that the moon affects natural phenomena in four main ways.

Ways in which the moon may affect fertility
GRAVITY

The moon affects us through its gravitational pull on fluids, most obviously observed in tidal flows. Its effect on fluid content in animal and plant life has also been demonstrated. There is no reason why humans should suppose that they are immune, or that the essentially fluid release of menstruation and the liquid in which the ovum is suspended are less likely to be affected than animals and plants.

LIGHT

Depending on whether the moon is full or new, we have more or less light on the earth. Of course this difference is less directly experienced by urban dwellers than their country cousins, but it has been shown that the light of the full moon increases levels of the follicle stimulating hormone (FSH) via the hypothalamus and the pituitary glands (see Chapter 3, 'Your Bodies').

We also know that light is absorbed via the optic nerve and used as a nutrient for the endocrine system, and that the pineal gland (the 'third eye') is also light-sensitive. Indeed, blind women menstruate earlier, on average, and their cycle is shorter. City dwellers, exposed to long periods of artificial light (such as street lighting), mature sexually earlier than rural people.

Further evidence showing the relationship between light and the reproductive system includes

♦ an increase in gynaecological abnormalities in women who live in Polar regions, particularly during the long Arctic winter of darkness

♦ the complete cessation of ovulation in female rats which are exposed to light for the 24 hours before ovulation is due

♦ the ability in women to influence the timing of ovulation by leaving the light on all night to simulate full moon (lunaception).

IONISATION

Although less well known, it appears that the moon influences atmospheric ionisation, the electrical charging of atoms. Positive ions, which build up prior to a storm, are notorious for their deleterious effect on mental and physical health, causing headaches and a stuffy, faint feeling of listlessness and unease.

Negative ions (as generated by ionisers), which are prevalent *after* a storm or near the sea, cause a feeling of physical and psychological well-being.

Full moon brings an increase in positive ions, while the negative ions proliferate as the moon wanes.

Brain serotonin levels and adrenal functions (both part of the complex hormonal interaction in the body) are affected by air ionisation.

ELECTROMAGNETISM

The earth's magnetic field changes slightly with the positions of the sun and the moon, and the electrical potential of living organisms increases at new and full moons.

It has also been established that reduced geomagnetic activity (that of the Earth) is more likely to coincide with the onset of menstruation and, conversely, increased activity less so. The duration of the menstrual period is also affected.

Once a month, coincident with ovulation and subject to daily fluctuations, the body's electrical field shows a huge increase in voltage for 24 hours. This voltage surge comes also at times of extreme agitation in mental patients, notably at new and full moons, and demonstrably affects the nervous system.

See how the picture builds for the symbiotic relationship between the moon, the hormones and the emotions?

We are all lunatics

Is it the moon? Is it our hormones? Is it our nervous system? It is not known (as yet) whether the controlling factor of the moon over the menstrual cycle is gravity, light, ionisation, electromagnetic fields or, more probably, a combination of all of these (and perhaps other) effects. But as the Ancients and primitive peoples in touch with Nature have all known — and as science is finding out — this connection is obvious and undeniable.

The moon has been worshipped by many as the Great Mother, and women's connection to it has seen them rise and fall in status. Women's power has often been seen as being derived from the moon, a power welcomed in some societies, a reason for persecution in others.

That women's power waxed and waned not only with the moon but also with their own menstrual cycles, has been a cause for celebration as well as taboo, depending on who's in charge of a society at any given time.

Let us, as women — cyclical 'lunatics' that we are — use this connection with the moon to understand our bodies and ourselves better. Let us use it to create a situation where we can express ourselves sexually without detriment to our physical and psychological health, and in tune with natural cycles, both personal and planetary.

You will find it immensely rewarding to understand your reproductive cycles, tune in to them for fertility awareness, and acknowledge their physical, psychological and psychic patterns.

By understanding your hormonal cycle, you can feel in control of your fertility and in touch with your physical self through observation of your body changes.

By understanding the moon's influence on your fertility, you not only increase your chances of avoiding or achieving pregnancy, but you extend yourself to acknowledge your contact with, and part in, the corner of the universe in which you dwell. You can bring meaning and joy to your relationships with yourself, your partner and your world.

The lunar cycle

As well as the lunar orbit, which takes 28 days and is the time taken for the moon to travel around the earth, and the lunar month, which is the time from one full (or new) moon to another, there is also your personal lunar cycle or lunar phase cycle.

The repetition of the phase of the moon at which you were born has a strong influence on your fertility. This is a biorhythmic cycle. (This does not signify biorhythms, a specific term relating to a certain system popular in the 1960s and 70s, but signifies a recurring rhythmic cycle which affects your body.) This cycle commences at birth, becomes effective at puberty, and will continue to influence your fertility throughout your fertile life.

The Lunar Cycle

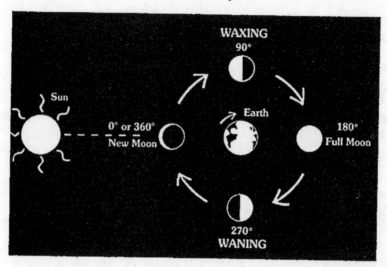

How and when the lunar cycle was discovered

The lunar cycle (or lunar phase cycle) was discovered (or re-discovered) by Dr Eugen Jonas, who had an understanding of astrology (or as he preferred to call it, astrobiology). This was a fairly unusual combination of skills for a doctor practising in Czechoslovakia in the 1950s. However, it was precisely this mix of interests that led to his discovery.

Although he was unable to work with this information for more than a short period of time, it has been inspirational to many others all over the world.

Jonas was working with Catholic women who were using the rhythm method — with characteristically little success. He became concerned about the harmful effects of termination, which had recently been legalised in nearby Hungary, and seemed likely to jump the border.

Being a Roman Catholic himself, Jonas did not agree with termination on religious and ethical grounds. Indeed, as a doctor, he recommended surgery only when absolutely necessary. As a psychiatrist, he was also concerned with the possible harmful psychological effects.

Jonas became interested in discovering why the rhythm method had such a low success rate. He felt that if there were any truth in the ancient ideas of astrologers that Man and Universe were part of the same harmonic unity, then as important an event as conception must surely be subject to these same cosmic laws.

In 1956, Jonas discovered a statement that started him on a new journey. From the writings of the ancient astrologers of Babylon and Assyria, he unearthed the following: *Woman is fertile during a certain phase of the moon.*

But which phase? He started studying, calculating and researching to find the patterns that connected the conception dates of his many patients, which frequently fell well outside their expected mid-cycle ovulation times.

Jonas eventually formulated three fundamental rules on conception, the determination of sex and the life capability of the foetus.

RULE 1
The time of a woman's fertility depends on the recurrence of the angle between the sun and the moon that occurred at the woman's birth.

In other words, a woman is fertile at the same phase of the moon that was present at her birth.

RULE 2
The sex of the child conceived depends on the position of the moon at the moment of conception.

This echoes the traditional belief that a child conceived when the moon is in a male (positive) sign of the zodiac, will be male, and vice versa. (This rule is examined further in my previous book, *The Lunar Cycle*, which is available by mail order; see Appendix 1).

RULE 3
Certain configurations of the nearer celestial bodies, and the resulting unfavourable distribution of gravitational forces, at the time of conception, can affect the viability of pregnancy and foetus. (See Chapter 13, 'Conscious Conception', for more on this.)

So, according to Jonas, you are fertile when the sun and moon are at the same relative angle as they were at the exact time of your birth, *whether or not this coincides with your mid-cycle ovulation.*

Jonas' Rule 1 is the basis of the lunar cycle (the lunar phase cycle) and its use for contraception and conception. This is the aspect of his work which has received most attention worldwide and been tested most thoroughly.

His other ideas, as set out in Rules 2 and 3, although investigated fairly thoroughly by Jonas, have not been so extensively used.

Jonas was amazed by the patterns he had uncovered. He could not ignore what appeared to be indisputable facts, so he set out to verify his findings. For 2 years he collected data to investigate this cycle. He met with much support as well as plenty of opposition; the unconventional nature of his ideas touched a few raw nerves.

In 1958, Dr Kurt Rechnitz, a professor of gynaecology in Budapest, tested the combination of abstinence at the lunar-phase return with the rhythm method and verified Jonas' findings.

The normal success rate of the rhythm method (between 30 and 85 per cent) jumped to approximately 98 per cent.

As Jonas' career swung up and down with the extent to which his ideas fascinated or alienated his superiors, popular interest grew. The data supporting his theories continued to pile up. Eventually, in 1968, the Astra

Clinic, a centre for planned parenthood, was established in Nitra, Czechoslovakia, with Jonas as director. It offered the following services.

◆ *To calculate the sterile days on which no conception could take place.*

◆ *To calculate the days on which the conception of a boy or girl might be expected.*

◆ *To calculate the days of increased susceptibility to conception in cases of unexplained infertility.*

◆ *To calculate the days on which a healthy child might be expected to be conceived.*

Lunar cycle effectiveness

In the first few months of the Astra Clinic opening, almost 10 000 applications flooded in, 2300 of which were for birth control. The scientific board at Astra evaluated data received from 16 000 women who used the method for 4 months. *The success rate was 98.5 per cent.*

Although the use of the method for birth control was what Astra tested most thoroughly, the service most widely requested concerned infertility, while sex selection and conception of viable children were least requested. All categories achieved excellent results.

Rechnitz continued to obtain similar results in his Budapest practice.

In 1970, the board at Astra evaluated 1252 cases of women using its method for contraception for a full year. These women abstained at both their lunar days and at mid cycle as calculated by themselves using the rhythm method. Only 28 cases proved negative, which gave *a success rate of 97.7 per cent.*

Nowadays, by combining observance of the lunar phase cycle with the more scientific and precise sympto-thermal method instead of rhythm, we can expect an even greater degree of reliability.

These statistics (and others of similar degree obtained since) certainly support Jonas' assertion that he had discovered something important about female fertility. Several other findings are also of interest.

◆ Many, if not most, of the pregnancies reported in the tests on the use of the method for contraception were in women whose menstrual cycles were irregular, and who were relying on the rhythm method to calculate when ovulation occurred.
   Since rhythm method relies on regularity to work, it is very likely that these conceptions happened at the mid-cycle ovulation.

◆ In instances where women are either trying to conceive, or are well in touch with their bodies (for example, through using other natural birth control methods involving body awareness), and are fairly unstressed and healthy, *there is a marked trend towards the hormonal cycle ovulation occurring at the lunar phase fertile time.*

◆ The rhythm method, which was used in these tests, has a success rate on its own which has been evaluated as low as 30 per cent. (These findings are based on a 1969 study of 2300 American and Canadian women.) *This is a long way from 90 per cent.*

◆ Women who were trying to conceive were also asked by Astra for information regarding the times when intercourse occurred. Many who were successful in conceiving (often after years of failure) had intercourse only on the lunar cycle days, showing that *some ovulation must have occurred at that time.*

◆ Monthly cycle charts kept by the women attending our Natural Fertility Management clinic also show that a significant number of conceptions appear to be due to intercourse at the lunar peak. These charts will also often show *symptoms of ovarian activity* (such as changes in mucus and temperature, and ovulation pains) t*hat normally accompany mid-cycle ovulation, recurring at the woman's lunar return.*

◆ With some women there seems to be a *relationship between their lunar peak and the onset of labour* (or false labour). This seems to be particularly likely if conception occurred at the lunar peak, since pregnancy is, of course, 9 lunar months long, from conception to birth.

◆ In *The Natural Birth Control Book*, the Aquarian Research Foundation of Pennsylvania, USA, claims that when a woman is using the Pill in the 'proper' manner, then conceptions (or failures) *are almost always the result of intercourse taking place at the lunar fertile time.*

How does the lunar cycle work?

There are still a lot of unanswered questions about how and why conception can take place at the peak time on a woman's personal lunar cycle. That the lunar cycle is connected to, and has an effect on, fertility is well established, but how does it have that effect? And what is its connection to the hormonal cycle?

There are many clues and theories. My book, *The Lunar Cycle*, explores these more thoroughly.

Jonas had no answers to the many criticisms that arose from the improbability of his discovery, and spent little time in examining the underlying connections between the hormonal and lunar cycles. He was more concerned with the effects. Indeed, his work on infertility, sex selection, chronic miscarriage and congenital abnormalities was even more astrological, requiring the calculation of full horoscopes (or cosmograms, as he preferred to call them).

On the other hand, Dr Rechnitz, being a gynaecologist, was more disposed to connect the lunar cycle with a real physiological event involving ovulation. After studying the question of conceptions that occurred outside the expected ovulation time, even during menstruation, he wondered if 'increased levels of agitation' (including physical sexual activity) could have brought on an irregular ovulation.

Spontaneous ovulation

Spontaneous ovulation has always been the rogue in the pack when we are trying to identify our fertile times, especially for purposes of contraception.

Certain of the smaller mammals such as the cat, the rabbit and the hare, do not have a fertility cycle as such. Mature follicles, ready to burst, are always present in the ovaries of these animals. This happens during copulation, resulting in conception virtually whenever intercourse takes place. If this happened in humans, the only form of effective natural birth control would be celibacy.

In humans, the egg is usually released mid-cycle. However, there is a capacity for this to occur at other times. Modern research shows that intercourse (particularly at times of high stress) is most often the trigger for this event.

When conducting their research into human sexual responses in the 1970s, William Masters and Virginia Johnson discovered through laboratory observations that 'the very occasional woman ovulates out of cycle after orgasm'. What is needed now is for some research to be done to see whether these occasions occur at the return of the natal lunar phase of the woman involved. Dr Harold Saxton Burr, working at Yale University in the late 1930s, showed that 70 per cent of the women tested sometimes ovulated outside the expected ovulation time. The results of the work on the electronic detection of ovulation carried out by Saxton Burr and his student Leonard Ravitz suggest that these 'extra' ovulations are often the result of intercourse.

Dr Rechnitz speculated that perhaps the effects of the moon predisposed women to this reaction:

> Biologically there is a possibility that tension, due to the effect of certain moon phases, builds up in the woman's nervous and hormonal systems, which in the event of sexual intercourse, leads to the rupture of the follicle and thus conception. It is no accident that this connection was recognised by a psychiatrist [Jonas] and not by an obstetrician.

Indeed, Jonas first became interested in the subject because of the appearance of symptoms similar to PMT outside their expected time.

If Rechnitz is correct, *sexual intercourse at the lunar return can trigger a spontaneous ovulation and lead to conception.*

The evidence is all there, as we saw earlier, revealing how the moon can effect our nervous and hormonal systems in order to set up such a situation. The assumption that we make, on the overwhelming evidence of the effectiveness of the method, is that *spontaneous ovulation does not seem to be triggered at other times during the lunar month.*

Mystery conceptions

Over and over again in clinical use of the lunar phase cycle, instances have occurred where it seems to explain otherwise puzzling phenomena. Conceptions have been frequently known to occur when, according to orthodox medical models of fertility, this is considered totally or virtually impossible. They have occurred during menstruation, during pregnancy, and while on the contraceptive pill, among other instances.

◆ Many women feel sure that they know when they have conceived, only to be told by doctors that they are mistaken.

◆ Ultrasound tests often give results that show the pregnancy to be 1 or 2 weeks at variance with the expectations of the doctor.

◆ Many women feel sure that they know when they ovulate, have regular cycles, and yet have conceived against their wishes, even though they felt quite sure that they were safe. Doctors are often all too ready to assume that the woman has made a mistake, and although some doubtless do, it's also possible that the lunar cycle may be responsible. Indeed, in my experience, retrospective calculations often show this to be the case.

◆ Conception often occurs during menstruation where there has been no history of short cycles and no reason to expect one.

◆ Menstruation, often avoided by those trying to conceive as unlikely, unaesthetic or taboo (for religious reasons), has been used with great success by those aware that it coincides with their lunar return (see Chapter 14, 'Case Histories').

◆ There is the suggestion that 'failures', or conceptions on the contraceptive pill are nearly always due to lunar fertility.

◆ Further conceptions have been known to occur during an existing pregnancy, when hormonal states should preclude an ovulation.

Is spontaneous ovulation detectable?

Certainly — if you have instruments to record surges in electrical potential. Otherwise, there is no warning in the body, as there is with a mid-cycle ovulation, of mucus changes and so forth; the body is taken by surprise. However, *many women, experienced at detecting mid-cycle ovulation, having had intercourse at a lunar time (either protected or for purposes of conception) report symptoms of ovulation pains, a sudden, temporary dip or rise in temperature and increased mucus following the sex act.*

It is possible, of course, to mistake semen for mucus, though most experienced observers would not make that mistake. Further studies are needed to verify the clinical data.

If spontaneous ovulation does change the hormonal situation, it would explain how sperm survive in an apparently hostile situation and eggs implant in an apparently unsuitably prepared endometrium. While the egg travels down the tube before it implants, there is a period of at least 6 days for changes to occur in the endometrium.

More research is needed — but if you desire to be as effective as possible in your attempts to understand and control your fertility, it's perhaps foolhardy not to take seriously the impressive proven evidence.

Is one cycle more fertile than the other?

This seems to vary, and certainly more research is needed to answer this question. Jonas claimed that a great majority of conceptions occurred at the lunar time, but this may have had a lot to do with the Catholic religion of his patients, who were in all probability using rhythm method and avoiding the mid-cycle ovulation. The question is, for all practical purposes, spurious.

If you don't want to conceive, avoid both your mid-cycle ovulation (as assessed by yourself) and your lunar cycle fertile time (as calculated in advance), unless they coincide. If you do want to conceive, fertility seems to be enhanced if the mid-cycle ovulation coincides with the lunar peak.

Synchronising cycles

All users of the lunar cycle, from Jonas onwards, agree that if mid-cycle coincides with the natal lunar phase recurrence, this provides optimum conditions for conception.

Fertility is greatest if you experience your mid-cycle ovulation at your lunar fertile time. The combination of menstruation and the lunar phase comes a close second.

Although one would expect that a time when both cycles indicate fertility would be most highly fertile, it's not so easy to see how a seemingly unsuitable time such as menstruation should also provide such a fertile combination with the natal lunar phase.

From Jonas onwards, however, practitioners and clients alike have found it to be so. *Menstruation, far from being an infertile time, is a likely time for conception to occur* — if it coincides with the natal lunar phase. This is important news for those trying to avoid or achieve pregnancy.

Mid-cycle ovulation is not only the most fertile combination with the lunar return, but also the most common. The menstruation/lunar combination comes second (in both cases).

It seems that the recurring moon-phase cycle works like a biological clock — a biorhythm beginning at a woman's birth, becoming effective at puberty and influencing fertility through its effect on the hypothalamus, pituitary, glandular hormones and nervous state. Perhaps, as well as the link to the ability to spontaneously ovulate, there is another — with the ongoing hormonal cycle.

There is a marked tendency for the two cycles to synchronise. A much higher than probable rate of synchronisation occurs in certain types of cases.

◆ In women who are trying to conceive, especially when efforts have been ongoing for at least 6 months. Conception is often successful when the synchronisation finally occurs.

◆ In women who are in tune with their bodies, especially those practising natural fertility awareness methods, who are unstressed, in good health and have rhythmic, hassle-free lifestyles. (There are still some people like this!)

The lunar cycle may well be a blueprint for the hormonal cycle. If this is so, it would mean that in a truly natural state we would only have one fertility cycle.

It seems that when the rhythms of life are disturbed and the hormonal cycle subjected to the stresses and strains of modern lifestyles, or we are in ill-health, or suffering from poor nutrition, the dislocation of frequent travel, excessive exercise or drug abuse, the cycles are less likely to come together. The next chapter will discuss techniques for achieving synchronisation.

How to use the lunar cycle for contraception

Using the lunar cycle for contraception is very simple. You avoid unprotected intercourse when the moon is at the same phase as it was at your birth. For example, if you were born 3 days before a full moon, then you will be potentially fertile 3 days before each full moon.

When you have your natal lunar phase calculated, safety margins will be added for sperm and egg life, giving a total of 4 days each lunar month. These can be calculated in advance and marked on a calendar chart. Then all you have to remember is to *avoid unprotected intercourse on your lunar fertile days whether or not they coincide with your mid-cycle ovulation* (see Chapter 10 on how to combine this with your sympto-thermal observations).

How to use the lunar cycle for conception

This is also very simple. If your lunar time does *not* coincide with your mid-cycle ovulation, you have two chances in a month. If it does, you have one *superchance*.

You would prepare for each of these occasions in the ways described in Chapter 13, 'Conscious Conception'.

One more factor emerges here as an extra aid in overcoming infertility.

Men have a lunar cycle, too

Ongoing fertility has often been used to explain why some men might be less discriminating in their sexuality than women, who are only fertile at certain times in the month, during which they definitely seem to experience heightened sexuality.

Male sexuality does not appear to peak in this way. Men's fertility is not thought of as cyclical, either, although it's acknowledged that it changes — sperm count goes up and down according to many factors. It does appear, however, that there is a cyclical aspect to male fertility and that it is connected to the moon.

With a woman, of course, she is either fertile or she isn't, and much of the time, she isn't. With a man, it seems that there are degrees of fertility. Evidence (patchy so far, it's true) shows that *sperm count can be up to ten times as high during the man's lunar return.*

Now, when the aim is contraception, this is not really of concern. But when the issue is infertility due to low numbers of sperm, it may be (see Chapter 13).

There is an ancient Chinese traditional belief that the lunar birthday is, for both sexes, a time of heightened *chi* (life force or energy). It may be this which causes the release of increased numbers of sperm rather than a specific effect on the generation of sperm, which takes place in the previous 3–4 months, during which time their health and quality is also determined.

It takes two to tango, and two to perform the dance of creativity. Babies have fathers, too! And those paternal instincts (if they have motivated any men to read this book) may well be feeling a little neglected by now. Here is where we rectify that.

The reason men have such a small slice of this book is simple. Male fertility behaves differently to female fertility. Most men who have a healthy and viable sperm count and good sperm motility and morphology (see Chapter 13, 'Conscious Conception') are fertile *all the time.* Therefore, there is very little need to study the patterns of their fertility. It's usually enough to know whether or not the woman is at a fertile time.

But, if a low count is part of an infertility problem, then it may be that the man's lunar phase return provides the best time for conception to occur.

Of course, in order for this to be achieved the woman must be fertile then, too. So, in the next chapter we will look at ways of synchronising ovulation with *either* the woman's lunar cycle *or* that of her male partner.

Calculations

You may be able to make the calculations for the lunar cycle for yourself. You will probably find it easier (and safer and more accurate) to have them done for you by a consultant. Either way, it's good to know how they are done.

Let's suppose that you were born when the angle between the sun and the moon was 60°. This occurs about 5 days after the new moon, when the moon is a traditional crescent shape in the sky. You will then be fertile, according to Dr Jonas' findings, 5 days after each new moon, and for a period either side of this peak time.

To calculate the natal angle (in this case 60°), the time, date and place of birth need to be reasonably accurately known.

As the sun–moon angle only increases by approximately 1° every 2 hours, you don't need to know your birth time as accurately as you would for, say, your horoscope. Birth time is valid even if the birth was induced or performed by caesarean section. If the birth took place in a hospital, the records are often still available. Many mothers (and fathers) can remember at least an approximate time, for example 'early morning', which is better than no information.

In the absence of any information, a noon time is taken and safety margins added to allow for error. Astronomical tables are then consulted to find the *natal angle* and when this will recur (once a lunar month).

This diagram shows how the angle between the sun and the moon increases during the lunar month, and how the moon appears in the sky, at each stage.

A Lunar Month

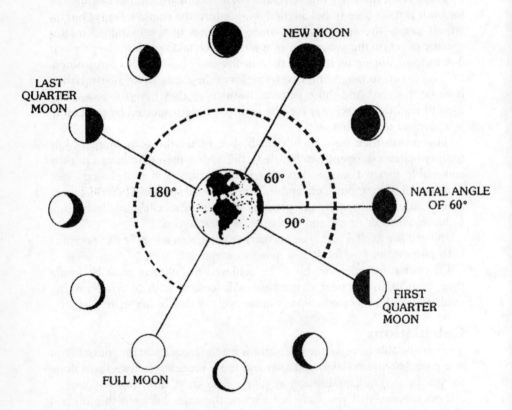

At new moon — the angle is 0°. The moon is in a direct line between the earth and the sun, and there is no light falling on the reflective face of the moon.

Five days later — the angle is 60°. The moon is a fatter crescent.

At the first quarter — the angle is 90°. The moon is at right angles to the sun (as seen from the earth) and the light falls on *half* the reflective face.

At full moon — the angle is 180°. The moon is opposite the sun, and the whole of the reflective face is illuminated.

At the last quarter — the angle is 270°, and the other half of the moon's face appears.

Then, at 360° (which is the same as 0°), an average of 29.5 days after the first new moon, there is another.

The lunar month

The lunar month is approximately 29.5 days long. This differs from the length of the moon's orbit around the earth, which takes about 28 days. This is because in the 28 days the moon takes to complete its orbit, the earth has moved around the sun a little, so the relative angle between the sun and the moon is different from that at the beginning of the moon's orbit. Thus, to complete the same angle with the sun that it had at the beginning of its orbit around the earth, the moon has to travel a little further.

This means that the length of time between one new moon and the next, one full moon and the next, or (for example) one 60° angle and the next, is about 29.5 days. It varies a bit because the earth's orbit around the sun is elliptical, not circular. Interestingly, an average menstrual cycle is also 29.5 days, not 28 as is commonly believed.

If you are confused, perhaps this diagram of how the example natal angle of 60° repeats 1 lunar month later will make it clearer.

Change in Sun and Moon Positions during a Lunar Month

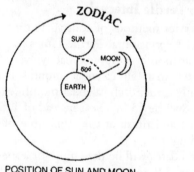
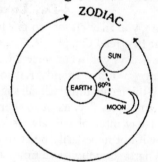

POSITION OF SUN AND MOON
5 DAYS AFTER A NEW MOON
(60 DEGREES APART)

POSITION OF SUN AND MOON
ONE LUNAR MONTH LATER,
5 DAYS AFTER THE NEXT NEW MOON

One result of this is that the moon is in a different part of the sky after an interval of 1 lunar month. This is why a full (or new) moon is in a different sign of the zodiac each lunar month. It is whether this sign is male (positive) or female (negative) when 'your' moon recurs that gives us Jonas' technique for sex selection. This can also be calculated from astronomical tables.

This may all seem very complicated. But, *all you need to know is your natal angle (for example, 60°), when it occurs in the lunar month (for example, 5 days after a new moon) and on which dates this recurs each calendar month.*

Once this has been calculated, safety margins are added for sperm and egg life (and possible error).

After some initial experimentation, a general formula has been found to be safe and workable.

The 24 hours before the exact recurrence of the natal angle is the most fertile time.

This is the time best used for conception purposes.

Three days is added before the peak time to allow for sperm life, and 1 day afterwards to allow for egg life. This makes a 4-day interval in total. Since sperm can live for up to 3 days in the female genital tract under favourable conditions, and since a spontaneous ovulation could possibly be triggered by an event other than intercourse, *unprotected intercourse should be avoided for the whole 4 days for contraception purposes.*

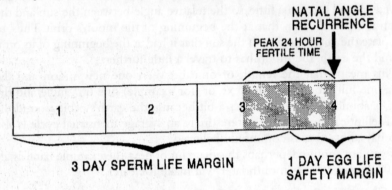

4-Day Lunar Fertile Interval

Of course, you may choose to use barrier methods of contraception at this time, but first read Chapter 9, 'Sexual Expression at Fertile Times'.

These 4 days will recur once a lunar month, or approximately every 29.5 days. Since a lunar month is shorter than all calendar months except February, the fertile time will fall slightly earlier each calendar month (except March), and every 3 years or so there will be 13 in a year instead of 12.

The 4-day interval will always start and finish at the same time of day, which will not necessarily be at midnight.

Any charts showing these times and dates will be drawn up for a specific time zone, and must be adjusted for different time zones and daylight saving. For example, if your natal angle were 60°, this might recur at 10.00 pm Eastern Standard Time in Australia, which would be the equivalent of midday Greenwich Mean Time in England, and 6.00 pm the day before in California. Differences in time zones can always be ascertained from international telephone exchanges.

These charts can be drawn up by any Natural Fertility Management counsellor who uses the lunar cycle. They can also be drawn up by astrologers, although they may not have the information on the fertility applications and may just give the exact time of the natal angle returns. This leaves it up to you to add the safety margins and apply the information in this book.

In Appendix 1, 'Available Services', you can find out how to go about seeing a counsellor or ordering a Natural Fertility Management kit, which includes a computer-calculated personal lunar chart.

For further reading about the lunar cycle and astrological birth control, also see Appendices 1 and 3.

CHAPTER 8

Synchronising Cycles

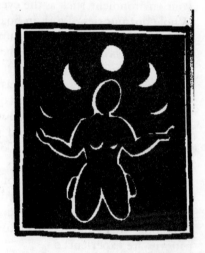

Why synchronise?

Although it seems that it may be natural to have your hormonal cycle synchronised with your personal lunar rhythms, it is in no way necessary. Many aspects of our lives are not rhythmic or seasonal any more. For urban dwellers in particular, the earth's natural cycles can seem very remote.

We pay a price for all of this, of course, but we also learn to adapt. Although the perfect scenario may be to have regular cycles averaging 29.5 days, with ovulation coinciding with the lunar fertile peak, it is not essential to your health.

Synchronisation is a little like eating organically grown vegies which are raised in a pollution-free back garden — an ideal which is really a dream. So, although synchronisation is desirable — and often achievable (unlike a pollution-free city garden) — don't worry if it doesn't always happen.

If you are using these methods for contraception, it will certainly be more convenient for you if you only have to concern yourself with one fertile time each month.

If you are using these methods to try to achieve conception, then the need to synchronise your cycles has another purpose. Although there are many ways that you can raise your levels of fertility (see Chapter 13, 'Conscious Conception') and achieve conception at either the lunar time or mid-cycle ovulation, very often the breakthrough seems to come when the two fertile times eventually coincide.

Which cycle shifts?

Your lunar cycle is, of course, fixed. Unless the moon is blown off course, it won't change. (And then you will have other concerns!)

Your hormonal cycle is constantly affected by all manner of influences. Stress, trauma, travel, ill-health, sudden changes in weight or diet, drug taking and excessive exercise are some of the things that can change the timing of ovulation (and, therefore, your cycle).

You may also find that you have a tendency to tune in to other cycles in your environment, such as the cycles of the women you work or live with. Whole dormitories of girls in boarding schools have been known to bleed (and therefore ovulate) at the same time as each other. This is due to the presence of *pheromones* — which cause you to smell attractive to your mate when you are fertile (ovulating). As you can see, Mother Nature is at it again, trying to get us pregnant as often as possible.

Some women even tune in to other women whom they are emotionally (but not physically) close to, although they may be some distance apart.

You may be very aware of and affected by new and full moons, and tend to ovulate or menstruate at one or the other time. In the Zambeze valley, populated for thousands of years by people with a stable culture, women expect to ovulate at the full moon and menstruate when the moon is new. Their houses are so constructed that there is an opening in the roof through which the full moon can shine. In other societies, where new or full moons are significant for cultural or religious reasons, similar communal patterns are experienced.

Lunaception — a technique for controlling the timing of ovulation — uses this effect of light on the endocrine system to induce ovulation. This technique involves simulating the full moon by leaving the light on all night.

If you tend to ovulate at full moon, you could use this technique to synchronise your cycles. By moving a simulated full moon (your bedroom light) closer and closer to your personal peak time in the lunar month, the timing of your hormonal cycle could be changed.

Another possibility is that as you become more aware of your body by using these methods, your cycles will automatically start to fall in line with each other. As you will remember, this is often the case with women who are not even aware that they have a lunar cycle. In other cases, awareness of the lunar rhythms can itself be the stimulus required.

The menstrual cycle is affected by both conscious and subconscious processes. To be most effective, you should focus on raising your awareness of your lunar peak time consciously, and use suggestions to affect your subconscious. Conscious activities which seem to affect the process of synchronisation are:

◆ working to get your hormones balanced and your cycles regular (see Chapter 12, 'Natural Remedies for Hormonal and Reproductive Health')

◆ becoming aware of the hormonal rhythms of your body (for example, when charting or trying to conceive)

◆ avoiding or preventing situations which disturb your cycle (such as stress, travel, or ill-health)

◆ charting your lunar peak dates in your monthly cycle chart to see how they fit together

◆ watching the moon as it waxes and wanes, and looking out for 'your' moon

◆ putting a lunar calendar on your wall (there are many well-illustrated versions available, and one comes with every Natural Fertility Management kit).

Subconscious processes are at least as important as conscious processes, and these are what are involved when you tune in to other women, new and full moons or other cycles in your environment. You can effectively program this level of awareness through autosuggestion.

Autosuggestion techniques

Autosuggestion techniques are a way of reprogramming your body through your mind. By the use of visual and verbal affirmations and suggestions, physical responses can be changed.

Just as the hormonal cycle is so obviously sensitive to all the random and negative effects of various kinds of stress, so it can be programmed positively and helpfully.

This is made easy for us in two ways.

◆ The menstrual cycle is not static; it is always in a state of change.

◆ The menstrual cycle is governed by the pituitary and the hypothalamus, which are deeply influenced by, and attached to, the higher centres of the brain, which are involved in thought, senses, memory and creativity. (This, of course, is also why thoughts, feelings, memory and so forth, are affected by the menstrual cycle, and why the menstrual cycle is affected by stress.)

A program of visualisation and affirmation can be done in a deeply relaxed or alpha state. Hypnosis, induced either by a therapist with the use of a recording, or self-induced, has the same effect, although stronger. These states can be induced by whatever method you find acceptable and enjoyable, though if the suggestions are to be effective, you should listen to them (or create them) on a regular basis (say, four or five times a week). See Appendix 1 for further details of a Natural Fertility Management kit — including relaxation and suggestion tapes.

Here is a text that you can follow to conjure the images in your mind's eye. Or you can record it on tape. If you order a Natural Fertility Management kit for contraception, this visualisation will be on the tape you receive. If you already have a favourite relaxation or meditation technique, you may prefer to use that rather than the imagery presented here.

RELAXING AND AFFIRMING

First find a comfortable place to sit or lie, where your body is well supported, including your head, where there is no light shining in your eyes, you are warm enough, and unlikely to be disturbed for the next 10 minutes or so.

Don't wear any tight clothing, belts or shoes, and ensure that your arms and legs are uncrossed. Then, just lean back, close your eyes, relax and *focus on your breathing*.

Follow the breath down into your body and out again. Become aware of your lungs expanding and contracting as they pull the air in and push it out. Fill your lungs thoroughly, and completely expel the air.

Tune in to the rhythm of your breathing — deep but gentle — and that other rhythm of your body, your heartbeat.

Let your mental energy come down with each breath and merge with your physical energy, right down at the base of your lungs, around your stomach and your diaphragm, where emotional tensions can gather. *Let them go.* You don't need them any more. Relaxation is something that you allow, not do. Just let go and it happens all by itself.

Imagine that with each breath you are *inhaling new, positive and healthy energy*, and exhaling old, negative and stale energy, letting go of old patterns, old beliefs, stresses and the past, and embracing new possibilities, clarity, flexibility and the future, moving forward with each breath, moment by moment, in present time, always changing, always growing.

With each breath, each moment, you relax more and more deeply, coming down into that central place where you are calm, at peace, self-contained, safe and uniquely yourself.

Imagine yourself floating on a cloud. The cloud is very soft; it puts no pressure on your body whatsoever. It supports you completely. *It's just like being weightless.*

You are floating, weightless, on your cloud, in the clear blue sky, with no particular place to go, and no particular time to get there in. The sun is shining down on you from above. *The warmth and light of the sun are spreading up your body like a glow, bringing relaxation and strong, vital energy.*

Feel the warmth and see the light in and around your feet, spreading up towards your heels and ankles, relaxing the arches and insteps.

Feel the tensions drain out of your toes, into the cloud and gone. Feel the new, healthy energy flooding in to take its place.

Let the glow spread up to your lower legs, around your knees and through your thighs. Feel tensions being absorbed by the cloud as if by a giant sponge, leaving your legs feeling *very relaxed, quite weightless, warm and light.*

Now the warmth and light are spreading through and around your lower body, relaxing your buttocks, hips and tummy. *Feel the warmth, see the light. Leave the tension behind as you float on through the sky towards total relaxation.*

Imagine now your reproductive system. See clearly your ovaries, tubes, womb, cervix and vagina. See the health-giving warmth and light enter through your vagina and spread up through your cervix, womb, and tubes, and around your ovaries, bringing *health, relaxed activity and positive energy*.

Imagine now any reproductive organ that is diseased or dysfunctional, clearing and becoming healthy, relaxed and vital.

Feel the muscles on either side of your spine warm and relax. Let the glow spread all the way up your back to your shoulder-blades.

The warmth and light are filling your whole body, relaxing the areas around your stomach, your diaphragm, your chest and shoulders.

Your body is filled with warmth and light, and is more and more relaxed with each breath you take.

Now the glow is relaxing your upper arms, your lower arms, the backs of your hands, the palms of your hands, your thumbs, index fingers, middle fingers, ring fingers and little fingers. Tension is draining out of the ends of your fingertips. You leave it behind as you float on.

Now let the glow surround and fill your throat and your neck, relaxing your jaw, your chin, tongue, lips and mouth.

Feel it spread over your face, releasing tensions in your nose, cheeks and ears, and coming up to your eyes. *You can see the warm pink glow through your eyelids and you welcome the warmth and light right down into your head* where they release the tensions in your eyelids, eyeballs and the muscles around your eyeballs. Feel the glow fill your head with clarity and light, releasing the tensions, fears and anxieties in your mind and bringing peace and quiet.

Let your glow spread up and over your eyebrows, forehead, and all over your scalp, releasing all the little tensions and closing over the top of your head like a cocoon.

Wrapped in your cocoon of warmth and light, you are safe, secure, calm, peaceful, relaxed and full of joy.

In this relaxed state, you are *recharging* with new, positive energy, like a battery.

Release the tensions. *Relax* your mind and body. *Recharge* your energies. *Renew* yourself.

Now you feel your cloud very gently come floating down towards the earth, drifting softly like a feather. As it does so, the sun begins to set, and you, warm and safe in your cocoon, float down through the colours of the sunset. As you drift down towards the earth, the yellow light spreads up, around and through you.

As the yellow light floods through you, you feel it bring clarity to your mind, releasing old patterns of thought.

You float on down through the yellow light and into the orange, clear and bright. *The orange light surrounds and fills you, bringing vitality, joy and courage to your heart.*

Drift further down now, into the red light, warm, clear and bright. *You can feel it and you can see it.* The red light is all around you and through you, *activating your physical energy.*

The red light gives way now to the soft, soft pink, so comfortable and warm, and coming further and further down through the pink light, you float deeper into purple.

Coming down through the purple light to this place, *here and now*, your cloud dissolving underneath you, you are left lying absolutely relaxed, warm and safe.

Imagine that you are looking out through the window of the room. The colours of the sunset are dying away and the night sky emerges.

The sky is deep, deep blue.

The stars are bright and clear.

The moon is very bright and the same shape as it was at your birth. (If, for example, you were born at 60° or 5 days after new moon, it will be a fat, crescent-shaped moon.)

You can see a calendar on the wall of the room you are in. You have marked the days off up to the present.

You can see the new (or full) moon printed on the calendar, 5 (or however many) days before (or after) the last day that you have crossed off. This confirms that this situation you are visualising is indeed the same phase of the lunar month at which you were born — *when your fertility peaks.*

Now, see clearly again your whole reproductive system — *ovaries, fallopian tubes, womb, cervix and vagina.* The organs and tubes are still full of warmth and light, relaxed and healthy. See the vagina and cervix full of *wet, fertile mucus,* and know your body is preparing for its mid-cycle ovulation.

See one of your ovaries release an egg, which is captured by the tiny filaments at the end of the fallopian tube and passed down into the tube.

(Here, the visualisation continues differently depending on whether you wish to conceive or not. The following version can be used for contraception; you can find the text for conception in Chapter 13, 'Conscious Conception'.)

The egg is not fertilised, it lives for a little while and is absorbed. You see the lining of the womb thicken, detach and pass out through the vagina with the menstrual blood.

Return to your breathing, in and out.

Follow the rhythm of your breath. Sink right down into your centre, *deeper and deeper,* further down with *each breath, each moment and each word.*

Come at last to your most central, private and unique place, where you are *your essence.*

In this place, you know exactly who you are, what your real goals are, and that you can, and will, accomplish them.

Say to yourself, in your mind, in this central place, substituting your own phase of the moon.

My reproductive system is becoming healthier and healthier every day. I will ovulate mid-cycle [n] days before (after) the new (full) moon. I will continue to do so cycle after cycle. I will not conceive unless (until) I consciously decide to do so. I am quite clear about my intention not to conceive in the near future, and am confident in my ability to observe and record my fertile times.

Return to your breathing, in and out.

Feel the energy return to your mind and body with each breath.

Feel your normal body muscle tone return.

Feel your circulation speed up.

Feel your heart-beat and breathing speed up.

Feel your mind coming back up to normal wakefulness and consciousness, alert and full of energy.

Open your eyes! Wide awake! Take a *big* yawn and a *huge* stretch.

WHEN SHOULD I DO MY VISUALISATION?

This kind of technique has other benefits besides synchronising your lunar and hormonal cycles. Full body and mind relaxation is very therapeutic in all sorts of ways. One of the obvious results is that your cycle, if it isn't already, will become more regular. (This, of course, will also depend on your reproductive health; see Chapter 12, 'Natural Remedies for Hormonal and Reproductive Health'.)

To get maximum benefit from the suggestions of these visualisations and affirmations, they should be done, if possible, once a day. They can be done at any time *except in the car, while operating machinery, using sharp knives or being involved in any other activity which could be dangerous if you get drowsy.* This is particularly important if you are using a relaxation recording, which may take you down to a deep level of consciousness and may also *affect anyone else within earshot,* even if they are not aware of hearing it. *So don't listen to a recording in a car, even if you're the passenger.*

You will find the whole exercise takes only about 10 minutes and can be easily fitted into your day.

If you do it in bed at the end of the day, you will also benefit from a relaxed, dream-filled sleep. It may be easier, at the end of the day especially, to listen to a recording that you have made of the exercise rather than creating the pictures and words in your head. Otherwise you could tend to fall asleep before completing it.

Lying in bed is a comfortable and convenient place to listen to your recording, with no deadlines to cause anxiety. If you are tired, you may still fall asleep while listening to the recording. However, if there is a suggestion at the end to wake up as the tape finishes (as in the script in this chapter), and if you respond to this suggestion, you can be confident that you have at least received the messages subconsciously. You will then drift back into a deep, relaxed sleep.

SYNCHRONISING WITH YOUR PARTNER'S LUNAR RETURN

This is achieved in exactly the same way. If low sperm count seems to be the primary fertility problem, then you can attempt to synchronise with your partner's peak time in the lunar month as sperm count may be higher at these times. This is calculated in exactly the same way — from his birth data.

Using the extended version of this text that you can find in Chapter 13, 'Conscious Conception', you then visualise your hormonal ovulation happening at that point in the lunar month when his lunar peak time comes.

The lunar peak times always stay the same: it's only your hormonal cycle which can be influenced and changed.

Unless your lunar peaks are at the same time of the lunar month as your partner's (unlikely, but possible), your hormonal cycle will need to be moved to achieve synchronisation. Sperm count seems to rise over a few days, towards the peak, and then decline again slowly, so it's not as critical to synchronise with the exact peak time as it is when attempting this with the woman's lunar peak

Since lining up with your partner's peak time takes you out of your natural rhythm, it is best to avoid this strategy unless your fertility is robust, with regular cycles and no reproductive problems. The quality of the sperm seems to be unaffected by the lunar peak, as their generation has been taking place during the previous 3–4 months, and the conditions that prevail during this time will determine how healthy they are. The numbers generated will also be determined during these months, but the quantity released into the semen can be affected by the conditions that prevail at the time of ejaculation. If a man is very stressed he may not release many, if any, sperm, but at times of high energy, such as the lunar peak, the count can be up to ten times higher than usual. This is not true for all men, so to avoid unnecessarily disturbing the natural patterns of your menstrual cycle, a sperm count can be performed at the male lunar peak and again 2 weeks later, at a trough. If the difference is not significant, then you may prefer to stay with your own rhythms, which is known to enhance the chances of conception.

HOW LONG DOES IT TAKE TO WORK?

Some women find that this way of achieving synchronisation brings instant results and their cycle, if ovulation is not already synchronised with their lunar peak, has a great hiccough, then, in one extra long or short cycle, it catches up.

More often, your cycles will tend to get a little longer or a little shorter for a while, until they are in tune with your lunar rhythm (or your partner's).

Some women have cycles that are marching to a different drum; they are so affected by other conditions that the response to your attempts to influence their timing may be negligible or absent. If the influence is physical, say, a hormonal imbalance, natural remedies may well do the trick (see Chapter 12). If your cycle is tuning in to a different rhythm in your environment, such as another woman's menstrual cycle, it's worth trying hypnotherapy, because the suggestions go in at a deeper level. The approach is exactly the same, but the therapist would be able to guide you to a deeper level of relaxation, so that the suggestions act on the subconscious, rather than the conscious, mind.

Never feel afraid that in hypnotherapy you will lose control. You remain aware at all times of what is happening. The therapist is quite unable to place thoughts or commands in your mind that you do not welcome. Indeed, you can open your eyes and talk normally should you so desire.

If you use any of these approaches, they are likely to work, so don't be surprised if your cycle length changes, either dramatically or bit by bit over several months.

Of course, it's not essential that your cycles synchronise, although for conception it gives you a better chance, and for contraception it's really a matter of convenience to have to worry about only one fertile time in a month.

You may feel that you have quite enough to do familiarising yourself with your body changes and the other ideas in this book. It may happen all by itself.

But what a wonderful way to create change, just by relaxing and dreaming!

CHAPTER 9

Sexual Expression in Fertile Times

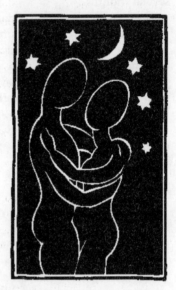

'What, me? Natural birth control? Doesn't that mean holding an aspirin between your knees?'

You can practise natural birth control and still have fun — and sex.

Many people consider natural birth control methods inappropriate for them because they are under the impression that it will be necessary to abstain for long periods of time. There are two misconceptions (an unfortunate choice of word, but the correct one!) here. First, that there is no choice but abstinence, and second, that the fertile period is necessarily long.

Abstinence is not the only choice available

It may be quite unrealistic for most couples to even consider that they can voluntarily abstain at all fertile times, however, many teachers of natural birth control methods insist that the method only works if abstinence is maintained throughout all fertile times.

Often, centres that teach natural birth control methods are funded by the Roman Catholic church, and exist principally to give advice to couples who cannot, for religious reasons, use any other method of contraception. Obviously, these centres do not give advice on the use of barrier methods at fertile times, so if and when couples do use them — as many will — they may be confused. This may well be why statistics can show that the use of barrier methods decrease the effective rates of the method. Indeed, these very statistics don't include 'user problems', which are the highest cause of unwanted pregnancies.

The term *user problems* means incorrect use of the methods, and includes couples who, because they have no other contraception available, make unprotected love at fertile times.

Unless you have a total commitment to abstinence at fertile times (for religious reasons, for example), it is recommended that you have access to some form of mechanical contraception which can be used when required and discarded when not. It is preferable to have a diaphragm or a packet of condoms sitting waiting in the bathroom cupboard than a baby coming unwanted into the world. Many women and couples overestimate their capacity to abstain. It's better to underestimate it, and then be surprised!

All statistics on effective rates of natural birth control methods are taken from couples who abstain at all fertile times.

More and more counsellors are finding that a combination of fertility indicator techniques and barrier methods can be a highly effective method of birth control, *as long as the barrier methods are used correctly and with awareness of possible interference to mucus checking.* However, there will always be a risk, albeit slight, compared to abstinence, which has no risk attached to it all. This combination of techniques is often called 'natural fertility awareness' rather than natural birth control.

The effective rates of the barrier methods used in this way (only at fertile times) should be the same as those outlined in Appendix 4, that is, in situations where they have been assessed by couples using them continuously through the cycle. The theoretical rate will apply as long as the barrier method is used correctly.

The reason there is such a big gap between the theoretical success rate and the actual (or user) success rate with the use of barrier methods is because they are often incorrectly employed. Many people simply do not know how to use them. These are referred to as 'teaching-related failures'. If you do opt for barrier methods, it is very important that you receive proper instruction.

The higher failure-rate among users also results from laziness setting in about the correct use of barrier methods when people have to use them all the time.

If you only need these methods for a short period each month, then the lack of spontaneity and embarrassment that you may feel their use involves is much less likely to tempt you into occasional risk-taking.

These failures are usually called 'informed choice failures'. The couple is conscious of taking a risk, even though their stated aim is to avoid pregnancy. This category may also include failures resulting from unresolved desires for children, when mistakes are made at the subconscious level. Couples are less likely to fall into this category if they have barrier methods available.

Advantages of flexibility

The advantages of this approach of combining natural fertility awareness with barrier methods is that it becomes a viable method for those who

◆ feel that continual use of the barrier methods is inhibiting their sexual expression

◆ feel that they want to discontinue use of the Pill or the IUD but do not feel happy with full-time barrier methods or feel unable to commit to abstinence at fertile times

◆ are attracted to natural birth control methods but are concerned about the effect of abstinence on their relationships or are unsure of their partner's willingness to cooperate

◆ feel able to commit to abstinence for much of their fertile time but feel the need for an alternative under certain conditions.

Even if you consider that abstinence is the way for you, there may be occasions when full sexual expression of your relationship is important. If alternative contraception is available, then the choice is yours.

In this way, these methods can be adapted to suit different needs at different times. Fertility awareness methods offer choices and options. *The more flexible you are within safe guidelines, the more likely it is that these methods will prove successful for you.*

It is important that you understand the limitations different methods impose on your fertility indicator techniques. However, with a mix-and-match approach, a combination of a barrier method and a suitable way of observing fertility can be found in most, if not all, situations.

How often will I need to use abstinence or contraception?

Well, the good news is — certainly not all the time! Traditionally, men and women have felt that contraception was a full-time requirement, but now you are equipped to tell when you are fertile and when you are not. All full-time methods of birth control are overkill. *Remember, you are only fertile for a few days each month.*

Of course, you will need to use abstinence or protection for a few extra days. There may be times when you are not absolutely sure and choose not to take a risk. And there are those days approaching ovulation when the sperm can stay alive and the days after ovulation when you are waiting for the all-clear.

The number of fertile days in a cycle can vary from woman to woman and cycle to cycle.

As far as your mid-cycle fertility is concerned, ascertaining this may depend on which method you use. Calculations will create many more possibly fertile days than mucus observations, while the temperature method may help you to determine more quickly when ovulation is over.

◆ If you are using mucus observations on their own to determine mid-cycle fertility, it will depend on how many days of fertile-type mucus you tend to get in the pre-ovulatory phase.

◆ If you are using the temperature method, it will depend on how quickly your temperature rises to satisfy the *Three-Over-Six Rule*.

◆ If you are using rhythm calculations, it will depend on the regularity of your cycles.

◆ It will also depend on whether or not your lunar and hormonal cycles coincide, overlap or come at different times in the month.

If you have very clear and immediate signs of mid-cycle fertility and these coincide with your lunar cycle fertile phase, the number of days that you need to abstain or use protection could be as little as 1 week in a month.

If you have less clear indications or lots of fertile mucus in the pre-ovulatory phase, a long, slow climb of temperature readings, and your lunar and hormonal cycles don't coincide, you might have to consider yourself potentially fertile for up to 2 weeks in a month.

The good news is — you get better at determining your unique pattern. The number of possibly fertile days will reduce considerably as you become more confident at observing your body symptoms, and if you manage to synchronise your lunar and hormonal cycles. So, we need to look at our contraception needs for

◆ when you are starting out, and

◆ when you have it all under control.

Starting out

There are two mottoes you should remember for the first few months of learning natural fertility awareness methods: *Be Patient*, and *Don't Panic!*

Although all may seem very obscure at first and you may need to use quite a bit of contraception and/or abstinence, it rarely takes more than three cycles to feel reasonably confident that you can recognise the fertile state and significantly reduce the number of possibly fertile days.

Your experiences in the first few cycles will vary depending on what method of contraception you previously used.

Coming off the Pill — It is imperative that you stop taking the contraceptive pill before starting these methods, as body symptoms are masked by the action of the chemicals. You will have no record of your cycles and will need to be very careful (see Chapter 11, 'Times of Change').

Having your IUD removed — You don't have to have your IUD removed before you start observing temperature and mucus changes. Some people find that the patterns change slightly after the IUD is taken out, but much can certainly be learnt while you are still 'safe', helping you to feel more confident about the changeover. The only problems might be that the extensive bleeding which sometimes occurs with the IUD in place may mask the initial build-up of mucus. The fact that you are 'safe', may encourage greater sexual activity and make it more difficult to learn your mucus changes.

Using your diaphragm or condoms less frequently — This is bound to be a good experience, because even in the very first cycle you will have a few days when you can be sure that you are infertile (after your temperature has risen).

Using something when you were using nothing — This is an excellent idea — things can only improve.

There are two significant things to remember — *the more you abstain the faster you learn; the faster you learn the less you abstain!*

Since abstinence interferes least with mucus checking, it is the preferred option for the learning cycles. A condom is the next best choice as it interferes only slightly (see next section). A diaphragm is the last choice.

Even in the very first cycle, you may feel well able to interpret your temperature graph and be confident of infertility in the post-ovulatory phase (if, of course your lunar peak does not occur at this time). This may involve abstinence in the pre-ovulatory phase to help you feel confident about both your safety and your mucus interpretation.

Remember, the first cycle may not have a typical mucus pattern if you have just finished taking the Pill. In this case, a resolve to abstain for all or part of the first cycle in order to learn your mucus pattern may be a waste of time. You may simply prefer to use barrier methods until your cycle has settled down (see Chapter 11, 'Times of Change').

After your first period (not the withdrawal bleed that comes within a few days of stopping the Pill), you can consider the first 6 days of your next cycle 'safe', *if*

◆ your temperature readings in the previous cycle shifted enough for you to be confident that you ovulated and that the subsequent bleeding was a true menstruation (one that follows an ovulation)

◆ you have no signs of fertile mucus

◆ your cycles do not tend to be short (24 days or fewer) and you have a consistent record of their length

◆ you are not experiencing your lunar fertile time.

In order to be sure that you have no signs of fertile mucus, you may need to practise the *Early Days Rule*, that is, you only have sexual activity on *alternate evenings*.

By the evening, you will know whether or not any mucus has dropped down during the day. If you have intercourse that evening, the next day is suspect because of residual fluids in the vagina which mask any mucus. Remember, *dry day, safe night, skip a day.*

The *Early Days Rule* may become modified with experience. Different vaginas tilt at different angles which means they drain at different rates. This process can be sped up by urinating straight after intercourse and by employing the *Kegel* (pelvic floor) exercises (see Chapter 4, 'Cervical Mucus Changes').

If you have felt dry all day after sexual activity the night before, you can feel 'safe' that night.

Make your decisions only after a few cycles when you have gleaned more experience.

Once you discover mucus, you must consider yourself fertile, and *until you are experienced, you must consider any mucus to be fertile.* Later on, you may be able to tell the difference between your *Basic Infertile Pattern* (BIP) and the start of fertile mucus.

Until you have some experience, however, it's best to consider any change from a positive feeling of dryness as a possible approach to ovulation.

Your choice of back-up contraception may change as you become more experienced in what suits you and in detecting mucus. Don't feel stuck with your first choice. You can change your mind or have more than one option available.

Back-up contraception choices

The choice you make for back-up contraception may have a great deal to do with personal preferences and tolerances. Many couples provide themselves with all the alternatives and make the choice they deem suitable on each separate occasion.

Just as flexibility leads to success when deciding what method to use to identify your fertile times, the same applies to back-up contraception. For example, since some methods interfere with mucus detection more than others, they might be chosen only when necessary. Since different methods favour the pleasure of the male or female partner, there may be a need for a balance in this respect.

There are five methods available to you. In order of effectiveness they are abstinence, diaphragm, condom, spermicide, withdrawal.

Not all of these are recommended.

WITHDRAWAL

When a couple comes to consult me, and in response to my question, 'What are you presently using for contraception?' responds, 'Nothing' — they usually mean withdrawal! Sometimes they mean that they assess roughly when their fertile time is and only use withdrawal when they think they are at risk.

Some couples do, in fact, have success with this kind of approach, but it's always possible that their fertility is very low. The success rate of withdrawal in avoiding pregnancy is assessed at 83–85 per cent.

Withdrawal is not enough. All one can say is that maybe it's better than nothing at all (when nothing really means nothing), but you have to bear in mind that some fluid, called pre-ejaculate, is often lost from the penis before ejaculation. So sperm may already be in the vagina before the penis is withdrawn. Also, sperm deposited on the outside of the vagina often find their way in. Even after or during withdrawal, it's possible for some sperm to be left in a danger spot.

The other problem with withdrawal, especially if used frequently, is a psychological one. In this respect, it is perhaps the least satisfactory sexual experience for many (men in particular).

There is an interesting alternative to withdrawal. Called the *Diamond* method, it is an approach that was recently rediscovered by Harvey Diamond in California. The *Diamond* method is an ancient technique found in certain Eastern countries and also practised by the Saxons in England, hence its scientific name, *coitus Saxonicus*.

In this method, as ejaculation is approached, the man places his index finger under the penis and presses on the urethra (the tube through which the sperm travel). This is easy to find, as it is very close to the surface. Pressure is applied at the base of the penis, just in front of the testicles.

In this way, the man can experience orgasm normally, but ejaculation will not occur. *The penis is withdrawn before pressure is released.* If intercourse is to be resumed, the man should urinate to clear remaining semen.

The method is comfortable and allows sexual climax to be experienced fully, as orgasm is felt as the semen passes through the testicles. However, no statistics are available on the reliability of the technique. It is included here for your interest only; there is no recommendation to use it. If you do decide to use it, perhaps some practice could occur during masturbation to find out how much pressure is required and how to allow the fingers to move in rhythm with the penis (see Appendix 3 for further reading).

SPERMICIDES

The first problem with spermicides is that, on their own, *the effective rate is not reliable enough.* The foam-based spermicides are most effective, as they hold the active ingredients against the cervix. The creams and jellies, on the other hand, will fall into a pool at the back of the vagina if you are lying on your back, and to the bottom (and out) of the vagina if you are upright. Standing on your head might be the only safe position!

The second problem is that you may be using natural methods to get away from chemicals. Spermicides have been known to have side-effects (see Chapter 2, 'The Unnatural Approach').

The third problem is that spermicides reduce spontaneity (they usually need to be inserted just before sex takes place) and sensation (some are greasy). This can be a plus if lubrication is a problem.

The fourth problem is that you may have, or develop, an allergic reaction to them. Sometimes the allergy is limited to a certain brand. Allergies may manifest as itching, discharge or rashes.

The fifth problem is that spermicides interfere with mucus detection, as they can actually change the consistency of the mucus for some time after application.

If you use spermicides during your pre-ovulatory phase, you may need to

◆ practise the *Early Days Rule* in order to keep track of mucus changes, *or*

◆ you may prefer to forget about mucus and use calculations, or use contraception from the very beginning of the fertile phase until your temperature has given you the all-clear on the *Three-Over-Six Rule, or*

◆ as an emergency only, wash the vagina out with warm water (remember, too much douching can lead to yeast infections). If you douche you may also wash away any mucus. Six to eight hours should have passed before you attempt to monitor the state of your mucus, during which time you should not be prone (or gravity can't help bring it down through the vagina) but you may use the *Kegel* (pelvic floor) exercises to speed up this process.

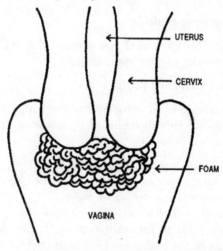

UTERUS

CERVIX

FOAM

VAGINA

Spermicidal Foam acting as a Barrier as well as Killing Sperm

Your willingness to use a chemical spermicide may well be dependent on how often you need to use any kind of back-up contraception. Spermicides, of course, are also used in conjunction with barrier methods, especially the diaphragm, and some condoms are actually impregnated with them.

There is a natural alternative spermicide. Some promising research has been done into the use of vitamin C. Since vitamin C is highly acidic, it is hostile to sperm but natural to the body. The only research done so far was carried out in the Ukraine, with 300 women over a 2-year period. This is a fairly large sample, and the success rate was impressive — 96 per cent. This was using a 200 mg tablet of vitamin C inserted into the vagina 10 minutes before intercourse. Success rates might be considerably higher if used with a diaphragm.

Although it seems highly probable that vitamin C is preferable to chemical spermicides with regard to possible detrimental local effect, no research has been done so far on its effect on vaginal membranes.

If this method appeals to you, it might be best to use it in conjunction with a diaphragm, otherwise the vitamin C may not be close enough to the cervix to be effective. However, since vitamin C is acidic, it may corrode the diaphragm, so you will need to check frequently for holes in the rubber.

You may be able to find a brand of vitamin C tablet which dissolves in the vagina, in which case it must be inserted in good time for this to occur (at least 10 minutes before intercourse). The sperm will then be immobilised, but the vitamin C may only remain effective for half an hour, so timing is obviously critical.

A tablet would need to be loosely enough packed to dissolve in the vaginal fluids and must be free of colouring. The vitamin C must be acidic (some vitamin C comes in a non-acidic form). If this is difficult to find, try the following.

Recipe for alternative spermicide

◆ Take 1000 mg (1 g) vitamin C powder (ascorbic acid) and enough *Slippery Elm* powder for five applications.

◆ Mix with water to form a paste.

◆ Keep the spermicide in an airtight jar in the fridge and use it as you would a spermicide jelly or cream — by smearing on both sides of the diaphragm.

The *Slippery Elm* powder makes a good base for the paste and protects your vaginal membranes. *Do not keep the spermicide for longer than 1 week or the vitamin C will deteriorate, and store in the fridge.*

Neem is a herb, the oil of which acts as a powerful spermicide. It is used in the Indian subcontinent for contraception. Traditionally, cotton soaked in *Neem* oil is kept in the vagina for 15 minutes before intercourse. Recent studies have shown that both in vivo and in vitro, an intravaginal dose of 1mL of *Neem* oil killed sperm within 30 seconds. Histopathology failed to show any side-effects.

Acid fruits have been used traditionally as spermicides. An ancient Egyptian medical text advises the use of fresh dates and figs (equal parts) to two parts of *Myrrh* powder, inserted 12 hours before intercourse. Apparently this is effective for 3–7 days, as it breaks down to produce lactic acid (it probably tastes good, too!). The Essenes used rosehips (an excellent source of vitamin C) for contraception for over 400 years. Rosehips are supposed to increase the acidity of the vagina to pH2; a wash with pure soap (pH8) and water the next day would restore the natural environment (pH5).

I include these stories here for interest only: although the theories seem sound, there are no reliable statistics on effectiveness.

Commercial spermicide jellies, creams and foams are available from pharmacies. Test on the inside of your elbow for allergic reaction before use.

CONDOMS

The theoretical success rate of condoms is very high (95–99 per cent). This means condom will be effective if used correctly.

Guidelines for effective use

◆ Use by the use-by date; 2 years is the limit. But even 2 years could be too long if the condoms are kept in warm or damp conditions, such as a glovebox in a car. They will only be reliable if the cover is intact (it can get worn or torn if the condom is kept in a wallet, for example). Open the packet carefully.

◆ Buy a brand that conforms to a required testing standard. Most well-known brands are very thoroughly tested. In Australia, the packet will say if it's approved by the Australian Standards Association (ASA). This means that less than 0.1 per cent of them have burst during very rigorous testing.

◆ Be careful of rings, sharp fingernails and such like as you handle condoms. They are made of very thin rubber and can easily tear.

◆ As it's rolled on, squeeze the tip of the condom to expel air. Then it is less likely to burst. Room must be left at the tip of the condom for the semen. Most condoms have extra space at the end for this purpose.

◆ Put the condom on before any genital contact (not just before ejaculation), but after the penis is fully erect.

◆ Don't use oils or oil-based lubricants with the condom. Water-based lubricants are readily available.

◆ After orgasm, the penis needs to be withdrawn *before the erection subsides*, and the condom should be held firmly onto the penis as withdrawal takes place. Otherwise, semen can leak out or the condom may even be left behind. (Although this means conception could occur, don't worry that the condom will be lost — you can find it with a finger.)

◆ Roll the condom off *away* from the vulval area, and wipe the penis with a tissue.

One of the main reasons why condoms aren't used properly is that people get fed up with them if they need to use them all the time. With fertility awareness this is becomes unnecessary. Also, if you have been sufficiently motivated to consider natural methods (and have read this far), there is a high probability that you will take the care to be sure that you follow correct guidelines.

Advantages of condoms

◆ They protect against disease. This was one of their first uses in the seventeenth century, when they were made of animal skin or gut. This protective aspect has become even more important now that we have the threat of AIDS among us.
Although natural methods of birth control are perfectly easy for a single woman to use, she may prefer to insist upon a condom until it is established that she and her partner are free of disease.

◆ They are easily available. Pharmacies, mail order and vending machines are the most common sources. Since the concern over AIDS has grown, condoms have become much easier to obtain, their use is encouraged, and they don't any longer carry the stigma that used to be associated with their use.

◆ They can be used without spermicides (make sure they aren't impregnated if you want to avoid them). This helps allergy problems and mucus checking. For an even higher rate of effectiveness, they can be used with spermicides.

◆ Semen is contained, so mucus checking is facilitated even more, and can be relied upon much more quickly after intercourse than with a diaphragm. If you use a diaphragm, you will have to wait for residual fluids to drain away (see next section). When you are keeping track of mucus changes, sex with a condom is actually less of a problem than unprotected sex.
This makes condoms the method of choice during the first few months when you are learning the changes that take place in your cycle.

◆ Condoms allow the male to contribute to contraception.

Disadvantages of condoms

◆ The woman has to rely on the man to use them (correctly) and, in some cases, to acquire them.

◆ There may be some embarrassment at their purchase. This is becoming less of a problem since the campaigns to promote them have resulted in them being on open display. You don't have to ask for them, just go to the shelf and select them yourself.

◆ They can cause embarrassment, lack of spontaneity and loss of tactile experience (especially for the male). The embarrassment is usually swiftly overcome. The loss of sensation may mean that you take turns with abstinence or a diaphragm.

◆ They often have a chemical lubricant that can cause an allergic reaction. Try another brand, perhaps one that's not lubricated.

There are many different kinds of condom available — ones with ridges, funny colours, even some that taste and smell delicious. There are almost as many variations as there are names — sheath, French letter, rubber, franger, prophylactic, protective — so it goes on.

After you have used it, do not dispose of your condom down a toilet, as they contribute to pollution problems. Wrap it in toilet paper or a tissue and put it in the rubbish.

DIAPHRAGMS

As with condoms, *diaphragms have a very high success rate — if* correctly used. Again, if you are motivated (of course you are!) and don't have to use them too often, this should be easy.

The theoretical success rate of diaphragms is not quite as high as for condoms (92–98 per cent) but the user rate is higher (see Appendix 4). This may be due to the fact that the woman, who is responsible for its use, is often more highly motivated.

Guidelines for effective use

♦ Your diaphragm should be regularly checked for deterioration in the rubber by holding it up to the light to check it for holes. Replace your diaphragm every 2 years.

♦ Your diaphragm should be refitted (checked to see if it is still the right size for you) every 2 years, or after considerable weight change (more than 3 kilos or 8 pounds), or a after pregnancy (or termination).

♦ Your diaphragm should be fitted by a doctor or at a clinic to make sure it is the correct size. If it's properly fitted, there should be just enough space to insert one finger between the inside of the pubic bone and the anterior rim of the diaphragm.

Correct Insertion of a Diaphragm

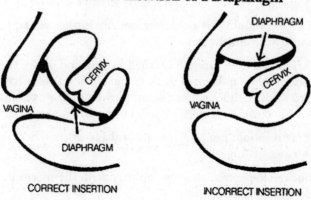

CORRECT INSERTION   INCORRECT INSERTION

◆ It is crucial that your diaphragm is inserted correctly (over your cervix) as it can easily slip in the wrong way, leaving you with no protection. *When you are fitted for your diaphragm, make sure that you are shown how to insert it correctly.* Many doctors are too rushed — it's best to go to a family planning clinic or a women's health centre.

◆ *After insertion you must check with your finger to see if you can feel your cervix through the rubber.* If you can feel the bump of your cervix directly, it is not in correctly — you might as well wear it as a hat!

◆ If possible, ask for a practice diaphragm to try out for a week (use further protection such as a condom during this time) and return for a repeat fitting. You may be more relaxed at the second visit; you may also need a larger size.

◆ Your diaphragm should be left in place for a considerable time after intercourse. The amount of time depends on whether you used a spermicide or not, but don't leave it in indefinitely. Usual recommendations are

   • 6–8 hours with a spermicide

   • 6–12 hours without a spermicide.

◆ Many authorities now claim that it is not necessary to use a spermicide (one study carried out with 100 women by the Family Planning Association in Sydney showed no difference whether a spermicide was used or not). However, most studies on effectiveness have been carried out including their use, and the manufacturers still recommend it.

◆ If you don't use a spermicide you will be relying on the acidity of your vagina to kill the sperm. Some authorities claim that this takes longer, so your diaphragm needs to be kept in place for a longer time. Others have found this to be unnecessary (the Sydney study mentioned above).

◆ More spermicide should be inserted before any further sexual acts — do not remove your diaphragm.

◆ Your diaphragm must be carefully washed in soap and water, rinsed and dried thoroughly, and stored in its container in a cool place. It can be powdered with cornflour (not talcum powder as this can harm your vagina).

◆ Your diaphragm should not be bent out of shape or stretched, or snagged on rings or fingernails.

◆ Do not douche after intercourse or you may wash the sperm in under the rim and the spermicide out.

How to Insert your Diaphragm

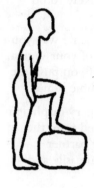 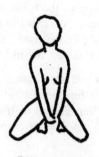

FIND A COMFORTABLE POSITION

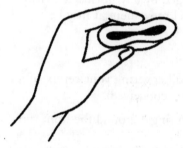

SQUEEZE THE DIAPHRAGM

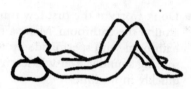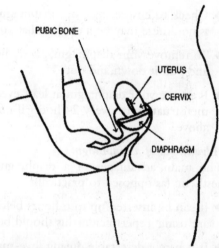

PUBIC BONE

UTERUS

CERVIX

DIAPHRAGM

SLIDE THE DIAPHRAGM SO IT FITS OVER THE CERVIX AND BEHIND THE PUBIC BONE

How to insert your diaphragm

◆ First urinate and wash your hands.

◆ You can lie (with legs raised), squat or stand (with one leg raised, say, on the edge of the bath or the toilet seat) to insert your diaphragm. Whatever is most comfortable for you.

◆ Squeeze your diaphragm into a long, oval shape, smear about a teaspoonful of the spermicide (if you are using one) over the inside of the dome so that it is covering the cervix. Spermicide placed around the rim will make it slippery, harder to hold and more likely to be dislodged during intercourse.

◆ Insert your prepared diaphragm into your vagina in the same way you would a tampon. If you slant it down towards the floor of your vagina, it will slide easily over your cervix (see diagram), then, if you push the front edge up with your finger, it will rest behind the pubic bone.

◆ Don't worry if the first few times you are chasing a slippery diaphragm around the bathroom. Many a first-time user has emerged from the bathroom with spermicide up to her elbows to find her partner snoring soundly! You will learn to insert your diaphragm easily and quickly in no time.

◆ Once it's inserted, your diaphragm should not hurt or be particularly noticeable to either partner if it is the correct size. If it is noticeable, have the size checked. It cannot be dislodged by any normal activity, but if there is severe straining with a bowel movement, it may be advisable to hold it in place with a finger.

How to remove your diaphragm

◆ Check to ensure that your diaphragm is still covering your cervix (if it is not, there may be a chance that you have conceived).

◆ To remove your diaphragm, gently hook a finger around the front rim and pull it down and out.

◆ Remove your diaphragm at least every 12 hours if you are menstruating or every 24 hours if not. Clean and store as directed above.

Advantages of a diaphragm

The main advantages of a diaphragm (as opposed to a condom) are aesthetic (as opposed to practical).

◆ It can be inserted up to 6 hours before intercourse, in privacy (if you are using a spermicide, this should be reapplied before intercourse).

◆ It is barely detectable during love-making:

◆ It is controlled by the woman.

◆ You can use it during a period to reduce the seepage of blood during intercourse.

◆ Diaphragm use has been linked to a decreased incidence of cervical dysplasia because it prevents the sperm coming into contact with the cervix.

Disadvantages of a diaphragm

◆ Some women can't use diaphragms because their vagina is too long (they can't reach their cervix), their cervix is too short (it won't stay in place), their cervix has been damaged, or their vaginal muscles aren't strong enough (as a result of childbirth or prolapse).

◆ You may have an allergy to the spermicide (try another brand, try vitamin C, try without).

◆ You may be allergic to rubber (try a plastic diaphragm).

◆ You may find you develop a tendency to cystitis if you use it too often.

◆ It can interfere with mucus checking. This is because there is much residual fluid in your vagina (semen, lubrication and, possibly spermicide), and also because of the effect of the spermicide on your mucus.

You may feel that to be sure of maximum effectiveness you would prefer to use a spermicide (or vitamin C), which may mask cervical mucus changes *even after you have removed the diaphragm.*

To eliminate semen and spermicide, you can try the pelvic floor exercise, even douching (remember, you will then have to wait for the mucus to collect), *but only after you have removed the diaphragm.*

Even if you don't use a spermicide (no statistics are available for this type of approach) you can't check the mucus while the cervix remains covered by the diaphragm, since this is where the mucus comes from. You may also need to keep it in place for longer than if you do use a spermicide.

There are several different types of diaphragm (or Dutch cap, as they are sometimes called), including the flat spring and coil spring; there are also cervical caps, which fit directly over the cervix. If the first type you try is not suitable, see your local family planning clinic or women's centre to find out what else is available.

Types of diaphragm are known to have originated in many parts of the world. Disks of oiled silk paper were used in China and Japan, moulded wax wafers in Europe, and moulded opium cups in other parts of Asia. In some societies, a fruit such as a lemon was halved and hollowed out for use. These days they are made of vulcanised rubber and have been widely used in this form since the 1880s.

Remember, frequent use of the diaphragm is incompatible with mucus checking, and if it is used often you may need to rely on rhythm and temperature methods, or the alternate dry day rule. Some women find that by checking the cervix directly, they avoid the greater effects of the spermicides.

A Cap fitting directly over the Cervix

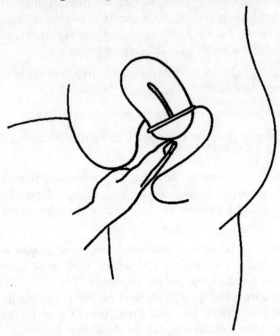

ABSTINENCE

Totally effective! Not necessarily difficult, either. Most couples find abstinence for a few days each month not nearly such a problem as they had anticipated.

There is much physical sexual expression that does not rely on genital contact; there is also a place in every relationship for expressing affection in a non-sexual way. To be cuddled and held is often quite satisfying.

Abstinence means no genital contact (internal or external) because of the ability of the sperm to find their way through any fertile mucus, even from the external genitalia. So use this time to be creative (rather than procreative). You'll find you enjoy the full sexual act even more when it's resumed after a few days. (Some religions prohibit all contact during certain times of the cycle, often the *in*fertile times, as sex is only allowed for reproductive purposes.)

You may feel that in order to tune into your natural cycles you need to abstain from full sexual intercourse at all fertile times, as an affirmation of your intent not to conceive. This may require that you make a fundamental re-evaluation of how you express your sexuality and love for your partner. *Experiment.*

Reminders

Remember, all methods of contraception are open to risk and failure, and can be used improperly. They won't work if you don't use them properly, whether you are using natural methods or are on the Pill.

Always be clear about your intentions. People who harbour secret or repressed desires for children will (subconsciously) make mistakes. Those who intend to have a baby 'some time soon' (spacers), do not traditionally have such good contraception results as those who definitely don't want a baby yet.

It's also possible to have a desire to 'become pregnant' as opposed to 'have a child'. Women who feel this seem to need a confirmation of their fertility, either as part of their sexuality or to ensure that they can have children in the future.

If you feel either of these two conditions apply to you, try doing a clearing meditation at each period, affirming your intentions *for the next cycle only*. This way you can feel free to change your mind in the near future and it will be easier to commit to a firm decision for the present. There is a flower essence, *Fig*, which helps to clear conscious and subconscious confusion about conception desires, which you may find helpful.

Always be aware that semen and spermicides and even lubrication, though a lesser extent, look very like fertile mucus. While these are present, no competent assessment can be made of the state of the mucus.

One of the reasons that barrier methods fail is that they are neglected because the user (you) becomes intolerant of them. If you are only using them occasionally, this becomes less of a deterrent to their effective use.

Always remember that *all contraception methods have a higher risk than abstinence, and all statistics given for use of natural methods are taken from cases where abstinence was practised at all fertile times.*

Whatever protection you choose, making mutual, responsible and caring decisions that are appropriate for your circumstances will enhance most relationships, bring couples closer together and help to make them more physically and sexually aware.

CHAPTER 10

Charting and Coordinating Contraception Methods

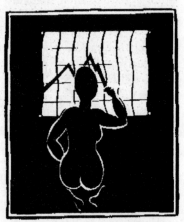

If it all seems a little confusing by this stage — don't panic! Just jump in at the deep end and you'll find you can swim. These methods are really learned experientially, not by reading this book.

You will find that until you actually start *looking* and *feeling*, mucus changes and other variations will be obscure. Once you start charting, you will be amazed at how quickly it all starts to make sense.

Then you can return to this book and read it again to exclamations of 'Oh, I see now!', 'That's what she meant!' and 'Well, I never noticed it before, but that really did happen in my last cycle.' Then, the day will arrive when you will know it all so well that you can write a book, too.

Mix and match

Natural Birth Control, Natural Fertility Awareness, Natural Family Planning — there are lots of names applied to these approaches. Some of them apply to one method only (for example, *Ovulation Method* means mucus observations), while others apply to various combinations (for example, *Sympto-thermal* means body symptoms and temperature).

There are teachers who think that a mix-and-match approach is confusing and that it is better to stick to one method. There are others who feel that a certain combination works best. I find it most successful to dispense with as many rules as possible, give you the information and let you find out what works for you.

Individual methods give slightly different information which means they can complement each other; they may not, and need not, all be used continuously. One method may be ruled out by a particular circumstance, and then it is useful to have other ways of determining fertility.

Different methods may be appropriate in different situations. If we can avoid making too many rules (some are necessary) and offer as many options as possible, your approach can remain flexible and appropriate in conditions which might otherwise be difficult. *Just remember that greater flexibility may come with experience, but it may also require greater caution.*

INFORMATION IS MUCH MORE USEFUL THAN RULES

With sufficient information at your disposal, you won't be left without guidelines when your circumstances vary from the norm. For example, let's say you generally rely on mucus observations to tell when you are fertile and you suddenly find yourself suffering from an acute yeast infection with a large amount of discharge. You can, if familiar with either rhythm or temperature methods, use these until you have treated the condition.

Similarly, a sudden bout of frequent love-making could compromise mucus observations, or your pattern might change dramatically from your normal experience, making you feel insecure about your interpretation.

If you have a fever, the temperature readings can be quite useless, and irregular cycles invalidate rhythm. Luckily, all methods are not usually affected simultaneously.

DIFFERENT OBSERVATIONS GIVE YOU DIFFERENT INFORMATION

Mucus observations will tell you that you are preparing to ovulate, but only your temperature graph (or a blood test) can confirm that this has taken place, and roughly when it did so.

Temperature readings will also give you an accurate idea of the length of your post-ovulatory phase and enable you to make a more accurate rhythm calculation.

To all of these ways of determining fertility on your hormonal cycle, you will be adding your awareness of the lunar cycle.

Motivation

The only limiting factor for the use of these methods is your motivation (and, to some extent, that of your partner).

You can only tell if you are fertile if you read the signs, and you can only successfully avoid (or achieve) conception if you act on this information.

The most common reasons for failure in using these methods correctly (if we ignore delusions of invulnerability) are a subconscious desire to conceive or a lack of clarity on this issue. *Be very clear about your desire not to conceive* and under what conditions you will change your mind; reappraise and reaffirm this as necessary.

Most women (and most men, too, despite the 'happy bachelor' syndrome) have a strong drive to reproduce. Mother Nature ensures it. Maternal (and paternal) instincts are very deep; conscious decisions to delay (or omit) childbearing in our lives may not be effective on subconscious levels.

Many women or couples may be very split on this issue, or may have a strong desire for children, even though their present circumstances preclude the possibility of having them.

I have known women who fall into this category to perform the most amazing juggling feats with their dates and observations, without consciously acknowledging it. This, not surprisingly, usually results in an (un)wanted pregnancy.

Of course, this same woman, if on the Pill, could 'forget' to take her Pill, or to use her diaphragm or other method of contraception. If you choose to use natural methods, your personal responsibility for doing it right is obviously more complex and critical than that of your sisters on the Pill, and more easily abused.

So, make clear decisions, revise them as and when required, and you can then use these methods for natural family planning. These methods can be used to help you avoid or achieve conception. Make sure you know which you want.

If you have decided that children can wait, then you need to be able to define very clearly your *pre-ovulatory and post-ovulatory infertility*. To revise: there are three main methods for doing this.

Mucus method — revision

◆ You can consider the first 6 days infertile, unless

- your cycle has a history of being less than 25 days long

- you have fertile mucus, or your mucus pattern is unreliable

- you are at your lunar fertile time.

◆ You can define the first 6 days of your cycle as beginning on the first day of bleeding of a *true* period (one preceded by an ovulation). Spotting does not count.

TRUE MENSES RULE

A true period is one which follows a cycle in which your temperature shifted by at least 0.2° Celsius (0.4° Fahrenheit) from the last lower temperature before the rise.

◆ You may then need to apply the *Early Days Rule*, to continue to check your mucus.

EARLY DAYS RULE

Dry day, safe night, skip a day,

or you may find, through experience, that your vagina drains more quickly and that the day after intercourse is mostly dry. This can be helped by urinating after intercourse, and *Kegel* (pelvic floor) exercises. You can then change the rule to the

SIMPLIFIED EARLY DAYS RULE

Dry day, safe night.

Once you are confident that you know what your *Basic Infertile Pattern* (BIP) consists of (for example, small, unchanging amounts of infertile-type mucus), you may (as long as your cycle is stable) further adapt this rule to the

EARLY DAYS RULE FOR THE EXPERIENCED

BIP day, safe night.

◆ Assessment of the beginning of the fertile phase can be made in a number of ways, depending on how experienced you are and how safe you want to be.

- To be *really* safe, you should cease unprotected love-making as soon as you stop having a *positive* sense of *dryness*.

- If you are experienced in recognising your BIP of continuing small amounts of sticky mucus, you may, with care, wait until this changes to *increasing* amounts of mucus.

- If you feel able to take a *slightly* greater risk — and have experience of your mucus pattern and how it generally behaves as you approach ovulation — you may wait for the *texture* of the mucus to change to a *wet* feeling and a *wet* sensation on the outside of the vagina. This approach relies on the conception being unable to take place in the absence of fertile mucus, and *in your ability to detect this.*

◆ From this time on, as soon as you have determined that you are fertile, you must abstain or use protection until you have determined that you are not.

◆ While you are fertile, your mucus will be wet, or slippery and stretchy, culminating within 2 days of ovulation at the peak symptom.

◆ You can determine the peak symptom *retrospectively* as the last day of any type of fertile mucus.

◆ You can resume unprotected sex on the morning of the fourth day after the peak symptom or, with a marginally greater risk, on the evening of the third.

PEAK SYMPTOM RULE

The post-ovulatory infertile phase begins after 3 consecutive days of non-wet mucus and/or dry days following the peak day.

If non–BIP mucus recurs after the *Peak Symptom Rule* has been satisfied, it will need to be considered fertile and abstinence or protection resumed for a further 3 days (*Mucus Patch Rule*). Mucus cannot confirm ovulation; it only tells you that your body has been preparing for it. If, however, the temperature has risen for 3 days, ovulation is confirmed and days of wet mucus need not be considered potentially fertile.

MUCUS PATCH RULE

Any change in the mucus from the BIP must be followed by abstinence or protection until the BIP has returned for 3 clear days.

◆ *The Mucus Patch Rule can be adapted by experienced mucus observers. If your BIP is basically one of dry days and the change you experience is to increasing levels of infertile-type mucus, you could safely reduce the 3-day margin to 2 days.*

HOW TO CHECK

◆ Ask yourself, 'How does the outside of my vagina feel?' Is it wet, dry?

◆ Collect some mucus and look at it. Is it clear, opaque, milky, white, yellow?

◆ Feel it. Is it pasty, flaky, crumbly, thick, dense, sticky, fluid, wet, watery, slippery, slimy, stretchy, gelatinous? Is there a lot of it, a medium amount or very little?

◆ Use your own words. It is as important to find the right words to describe the unique changes that you go through, as it is to learn to recognise them.

REMEMBER

◆ Get into the habit of checking each time you go to the toilet so that you keep pace with changes.

◆ Morning intercourse can be dangerous, as changes can occur during the night and mucus may not have dropped down (try the pelvic floor exercise).

◆ Now-you-see-me-now-you-don't ovulation can give false peak symptoms. Always wait for the full 3 days after any wet mucus symptoms have ceased.

◆ You will quickly become familiar with your mucus changes and the words needed to describe them, so have patience.

◆ Mucus checking can be compromised by douching, arousal and infections, among other things.

◆ Lunar fertile days may come at any point in your hormonal cycle.

See Chapter 4, 'Cervical Mucus Changes', for detailed information.

Temperature method — revision

◆ You can ignore the first four temperatures.

◆ You can ignore freak high readings (those that occur for less than 3 days) in the pre-ovulatory phase.

◆ You cannot tell when ovulation is approaching, only when it is over. If relying on temperature method alone, you must abstain or use protection until you have entered the post-ovulatory phase of infertility.

◆ You can resume unprotected sex on the morning of the fourth day after the thermal shift, as determined by the *Three-Over-Six Rule* or, with a marginally greater risk, on the evening of the third.

THREE-OVER-SIX RULE

You can determine that ovulation is definitely over and that you are infertile when there have been three consecutive temperature readings that are at least 0.1° Celsius (0.2° Fahrenheit) higher than the previous six readings (not including freak highs).

◆ Your temperature may start to come down before you bleed or during menstruation.

HOW TO CHECK
When checking the temperature, take the reading at these times.

◆ First thing in the morning before activity.

◆ After at least 4 hours sleep.

◆ At approximately the same time each day (adjust if necessary).

◆ Leave the thermometer in the mouth for 2–5 minutes.

REMEMBER

◆ Your probable ovulation day is the day at the *beginning of the rise*.

◆ Fevers will not only distort your temperature readings but may delay ovulation, which could occur during the fever, disguising the thermal shift.

◆ Temperature can be thrown out by time of day, illness, hangover, severe overheating in bed and crossing time zones at speed.

◆ Lunar fertile days may come at any point in your hormonal cycle.

See Chapter 5, 'Basal Body Temperature Changes', for detailed information.

Rhythm method — revision

◆ You need records of your cycles for at least 6 months to 1 year.

◆ Depending on how much information you have regarding these cycles, you can either

• use the extremely cautious formula S-21 for the first possibly fertile day (allowing for 6 days sperm life), and L-8 for the last possibly fertile day (allowing for a post-ovulatory phase of 10 days), or

• use the conservative formula S-18 (allowing for 3 days sperm life), and L-10 (allowing for post-ovulatory phase of 12 days), or

• with more information at hand, personalise the calculations by excluding freak cycles in your assessment of shortest and longest cycles, and assessing the shortest and longest post-ovulatory phases experienced in the last year.

REMEMBER

◆ The first day of full menstrual flow counts as Day 1 of your cycle.

◆ Ovulation can occur any time from 10–16 days before menstruation (and in exceptional cases may even be outside this range).

◆ Rhythm calculations alone are not enough for a full-time method. Use them only as *fail-safe, back-up* and *warning*.

◆ The post-ovulatory calculation is even less reliable than the pre-ovulatory formula as ovulation is more likely to be delayed than precipitated.

◆ There is more need for you to use rhythm as back-up for your determination of pre-ovulatory infertility because temperature cannot be used for this purpose.

◆ Rhythm method should not be used if your cycle is irregular and unpredictable, or if you are travelling, ill, under stress, taking drugs (prescription or otherwise), fasting, experiencing great changes in weight or diet, or going through similarly unsettling experiences.

◆ You must add your lunar fertile days to your rhythm-calculated days.

See Chapter 6, 'Rhythm Calculations', for detailed information.

Lunar cycle — revision

◆ You need to avoid unprotected intercourse for the whole 4 days that are calculated in advance as being potentially fertile. This will include safety margins for sperm and egg life.

◆ You can have these calculations made for you by a Natural Fertility Management counsellor who works with the lunar cycle or by an astrologer, in which case you may need to add the safety margins yourself (see Appendix 1 for details on obtaining a Natural Fertility Management kit).

REMEMBER

The recurrence of your natal lunar phase each month is potentially fertile, wherever it falls in your hormonal cycle, including during menstruation.

See Chapter 7, 'The Lunar Cycle', for detailed information.

Which method do I use?

If you start off by using all the methods in the learning months, you will soon find a combination that works for you.

It's important to learn first-hand how to use each method, and how useful each method is for you — what information you can glean in which way.

PRE-OVULATORY PHASE

There are two ways of determining the beginning of your fertile phase — by *calculation* and/or by *mucus detection*.

Making the calculation will give you warning of when you are likely to become fertile. *Your body symptoms are much more reliable.* If the state of your mucus changes before the calculations indicate that this is likely to occur, you'd better believe it!

If the state of your mucus changes later than the calculations indicate that this is likely to occur, you'd better be sure!

Once you are confident about interpreting your mucus changes, these will be the primary way for you to assess the beginning of your fertile phase. Use calculations only as warning, back-up and fail-safe if your mucus readings are compromised.

Right at the beginning, before you feel confident about assessing mucus changes, you may feel it is necessary to abstain or use protection for the whole of the pre-ovulatory phase.

Using the different methods to determine the phases of your hormonal cycle

Pre-ovulatory infertile phase		Fertile phase		Post-ovulatory infertile phase	
Bleeding	BIP (dry days OR thick, scanty mucus in unchanging amounts)	Increased amounts of wetter, thinner mucus	Spinn or egg-white type mucus	BIP (dry days or thick, scanty mucus in unchanging amounts)	Possibly some wet days just before menstruation
Temperature may still be falling during first few days of cycle	Low temperature readings (with possible freak highs)	Temperature begins to rise somewhere in this phase (close to ovulation)		Temperature remains high	Temperature may begin to fall just before menstruation
S–18, or S–21 if extra cautious, or amended formula from personal records				L–10, or L–8 if extra cautious, or amended formula from personal records	

POST-OVULATORY PHASE

There are three ways of determining the end of your fertile phase — by *calculation, mucus detection* and/or *temperature graph*.

Making a rhythm calculation will again give you *warning, fail-safe* and *back-up*, but as it is less reliable at this time than it was for assessing the beginning of your fertile time, *use it only as a last resort.*

Usually you will determine the end of your fertile phase by applying

◆ the *Three-Over-Six Rule* to determine the thermal shift, or

◆ the *Peak Symptom Rule* to determine the return to the BIP or the dry days.

For the first few cycles, while you are still learning to interpret the mucus changes, you will probably rely on the temperature readings for this assessment. You may in this instance need to abstain until you have this confirmation. The French call this *la methode dure* (the hard way).

Later, as you gain confidence, you may find that you prefer to use one method or the other, or that you make choices according to the situation.

If you continue to use both mucus and temperature methods as back-up for each other, you may find that sometimes they give you slightly different information. *Never play one system off against another.*

If your temperature readings give you the all-clear first, then you need to corroborate your three higher readings by at least 2 days of no wet mucus.

If your mucus observations indicate that you are infertile, then your 3 days of return to BIP or dry days should be confirmed by at least three readings in a rising pattern, with the last reading being above the cover-line.

Unprotected intercourse can then be resumed on the evening of the day indicated.

Never assume that you are infertile if any system definitely indicates fertility.

REMEMBER

◆ One system will nearly always work for you.

◆ If in doubt, abstain or use protection.

◆ If your period is late, check when you ovulated. You need only be concerned about pregnancy once the temperature has stayed high for 20 days or more.

◆ Don't play one method off against another.

◆ As your confidence in mucus checking increases, you may choose to limit your temperature taking, starting as you experience fertile mucus and continuing until you experience the thermal shift, then ceasing until the next cycle.

◆ As you gain in experience and confidence you may find that you can be more flexible. (This could possibly involve you in slightly greater risk.)

◆ You may find that the necessity to record all of these observations diminishes in time as you become more intuitive in your approach.

◆ It all becomes very easy with experience!

Secondary symptoms

There are several secondary symptoms which you will become aware of as you pay more attention to your cycle. Some of these you may choose to record as you experience them so you learn their patterns and significance.

CERVICAL CHANGES

Changes that occur in the cervix are sometimes thought of as primary symptoms rather than secondary, and they can certainly give you quite clear indications of the approach and finish of your fertile phase, though these are not as clear-cut or reliable as mucous or temperature observations. The signs that you receive from these changes can act as a double check for you, if you feel you need this. However, it is perfectly possible to use natural methods to control your fertility without observing or recording the changes in your cervix.

◆ If you do decide to record these changes, you will be surprised at how clear they are.

◆ You may be reluctant to touch inside your vagina. You can be quite confident that you will not damage yourself, although it may be better not to have your nails too long or your hands too dirty. Your vagina does not need to be sterile, neither do your hands when examining your cervix. After all, you don't sterilise your partner's penis before intercourse!

◆ You may have been to self-help groups where a speculum is used in conjunction with a mirror to see the cervix. This is not necessary. You can get all the information you need from touch alone.

◆ You may have already found your cervix when you checked your diaphragm or felt for the string of your IUD. If you have no idea where your cervix is, it may be best to locate it first during your infertile phase, as it is lower then. If you try to find it around ovulation, you may get the impression that it has disappeared!

Your cervix goes through the following changes.

Cervix Changes

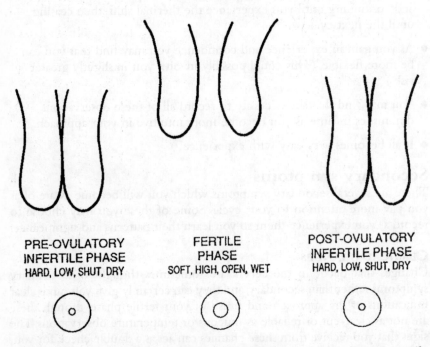

PRE-OVULATORY INFERTILE PHASE	FERTILE PHASE	POST-OVULATORY INFERTILE PHASE
HARD, LOW, SHUT, DRY	SOFT, HIGH, OPEN, WET	HARD, LOW, SHUT, DRY

Soft/Hard — The changes in the firmness of the cervix can be quite easily felt and can be likened to a ripening process. As you approach ovulation, increased oestrogen production softens the cervix, whereas during the infertile phases it feels smooth and firm like the tip of your nose. This is the most obvious change that takes place.

High/Low — In the early infertile phase, the cervix is low in the vagina. As you approach ovulation it rises by about 2–3 cm (1 inch). After ovulation it descends again. This is because oestrogen, which is produced in greater quantities around ovulation, affects the supporting structures of the womb, causing it to rise.

Some women have a higher cervix than others, and some are not central. At the end of the day, it is very slightly lower than at the beginning, so it's best to check the position at around the same time each day.

Open/Shut — The os (opening in the cervix), opens as you approach ovulation to allow the sperm easy access. (Mother Nature is at it again.) It may be open enough to admit a fingertip. It will also widen during menstruation to allow for the flow of blood.

During early and late infertile phases, it will be closed and feel more like a dimple than a hole.

If you have had a baby (through a vaginal delivery) the os may be wider and more irregular.

Wet/Dry — Because the cervix is where your mucus is produced, it will become wetter around ovulation and drier early and late in your cycle.

If you do carry out cervical checks, you may have an earlier experience of fertile mucus than you would at the mouth of the vagina.

It's always important to check for your mucus at the same place to get a reliable pattern. Remember — the vaginal walls are always moist.

If you squeeze the cervix, some mucus will be expelled. Withdraw your finger to inspect the mucus. Some women with very little mucus find that this is the only way that they can observe their mucus changes, but if you can rely on the external mucus, it is preferable.

How to check — Adopt one of the same positions that are recommended for inserting and checking your diaphragm (see Chapter 9, 'Sexual Expression in Fertile Times') and insert your finger all the way into your vagina until you feel a lump at the top.

Cervical damage — If your cervix has been cauterised or lasered to treat abnormal cells or an erosion, mucus production should not be permanently affected; in most cases it can be fully healed through natural methods.

However, if you have had a cone biopsy to treat cervical cancer, the damage may be more extensive and can destroy the cervical crypts, causing infertility (see Chapter 12, 'Natural Remedies for Hormonal and Reproductive Health').

MITTELSCHMERZ

Mittelschmerz is the name sometimes given to pains that occur around the time of ovulation. It is a German term which literally means 'pain in the middle', and is thought to be caused by the release of follicular fluid as the egg leaves the ovary.

You may or may not experience this pain. For some women it is only a discomfort, for others quite a sharp pain. It can be experienced as a single shooting pain, or protracted over several hours, even for a few days.

Although the pain is not really a reliable indicator of the exact time of ovulation, it can be a guide as to whether or not both ovaries are working and alternately releasing an egg. You will also notice the groin lymph node swelling on the same side as that on which ovulation has occurred.

If you always experience pain on the same side, it may be that only one ovary is functional (they normally take turns, but can compensate for each other), or that there may be a problem (such as a cyst). If pain is severe, continual or occurs with sex, have a medical check.

MID-CYCLE SPOTTING

This may show as pink, brown or red streaked mucus or could even be a light flow of blood. It is caused by the high level of oestrogen at this time acting on the endometrium. If it occurs at other times in the cycle it may be due to other causes, such as endometriosis, polyps or fibroids, and should be checked medically.

SEXUAL DESIRE

Mother Nature is irrepressible in her campaign to aid reproduction. Nearly all women experience some heightening of desire at times when they can conceive (you may mark with interest whether or not this also peaks at your lunar time). Your hormones will change your mood to make you feel sexy — and the way you smell — so that your partner finds you sexy, too.

Some women also experience strong sexual feelings as they approach their period. This is due to a mixed message: as the womb suffuses with blood, it is simulating what happens at orgasm.

It is also quite interesting to note from your daily records, whether or not sexual desire and intercourse have occurred on the same day. You may discover if you are following your own desires or your partner's.

ENERGY/EMOTIONS

Energy often peaks around ovulation, with some women experiencing an almost PMT-like agitation along with a sharper appreciation of the external senses of vision, smell and taste. As you notice the patterns that emerge for you, it will help you become clear about your natural highs and lows. Then you can cease blaming external circumstances and seek treatment. Excessive fatigue at menstruation can be due to iron deficiency, and premenstrual tension increased if calcium and magnesium are low.

GREASY SKIN AND HAIR

As ovulation approaches, there is less oil secreted by the body's glands. So you may experience a clearer complexion at this time, followed by more pimples closer to menstruation.

SORE BREASTS, FLUID RETENTION, DIGESTIVE PROBLEMS, PAIN, HEADACHES, NAUSEA

Many premenstrual and menstrual symptoms can, in severe cases, start fairly soon after ovulation, and continue through until the period. Alternatively, they may be experienced at ovulation and return in the last few days of your cycle. Most of these conditions are due to imbalances of hormones, minerals or prostaglandins and will respond to natural remedies (see the next chapter). If symptoms become too distressing, seek professional help.

None of these signs can pinpoint ovulation exactly or give you a precise indication of whether you are fertile or not, but they will help you become aware of your cycle's typical pattern.

You may or may not feel like charting all of these changes, but I suggest that you start off writing down as much as possible and only cease recording a particular observation when you are sure that it is no longer being of help to you.

Charting

On the next page you can see a chart for recording most, if not all, of your fertility signs. (Blank charts are sent to you with a Natural Fertility Management kit; see Appendix 1.)

There is room to mark in all the essential identifying signs and some of the more subtle changes. Keep one chart per cycle, that way it is easy to compare one cycle with the next and see your patterns.

◆ Starting on the first day of bleeding (flow, not spotting), which is Day 1 of your cycle, mark in the day, date and month. You can then complete the rows 'Day of the Week', 'Date' and 'Month'.

◆ Then consult your personal lunar calculations and mark in the times and days of your lunar peak fertility.

◆ Your should mark in your temperature daily after the first 4 days (or from the beginning if you prefer). Put the dot in the centre of the box. You may need to adjust the reading for an early or late rising (see the rule in Chapter 5). If so, make the same mark as usual (maybe a dot) for the temperature you have read on the thermometer. Then calculate the adjustment (one box up or down for each half hour earlier or later than usual, if you use the chart illustrated here), and use a different mark (maybe a cross) for the adjusted temperature. That way you can always see what you've done, as the adjustment is not always entirely accurate (see Chapter 5 again).

◆ 'Conditions Affecting Temperature' is where you note if you have a fever, had to leave bed to answer the phone or go to the toilet, became overheated in bed, had a hangover or a disturbed night, or adjusted for an early or late rising. (Mark in the time of day you woke, for example, '9.00 am'.)

SYMTO-THERMAL CHART FOR ONE CYCLE

MONTH																				
DATE																				
DAY (WEEK)																				
DAY (CYCLE)	2	4	6	8	10	12	14	16	18	20	22	24	26	28	30	32	34	36	38	40
LUNAR PEAK																				

TEMPERATURE

37.3
37.2
37.1
37.0
36.9
36.8
36.7
36.6
36.5
36.4
36.3
36.2
36.1
36.0

CONDITIONS AFFECTING TEMPERATURE

MUCUS CHANGES
- TEXTURE
- COLOUR
- AMOUNT
- EXTERNAL SENSATION

CERVIX CHANGES
PAIN (PERIOD OR MID-CYCLE)
HEADACHES
NAUSEA/VOMITNG
BOWEL
SKIN
BREASTS
FLUID RETENTION
FATIGUE/ ENERGY LEVELS
EMOTIONAL STATE/PMT
FOOD CRAVINGS
SEXUAL DESIRE
INTERCOURSE
BLEEDING

◆ 'Mucus Changes' is a row you may have some difficulty with at the beginning. Instead of trying to make clear decisions about which type of mucus you are experiencing (especially when a novice), simply write down *one descriptive word or symbol* for each category. 'Amount' and 'Texture' are essential observations, 'Colour' and 'External Sensation' are optional extras. See Chapter 4, 'Cervical Mucus Changes', for ideas. By the time you get to the end of your first cycle you will be pleasantly surprised by the pattern that has started to emerge. You may also find that, as you look back at the words you used at the beginning, that they are no longer the right choices.

It really doesn't matter what words you use as long as they are used consistently, are specific and meaningful to you and describe what happens in your cycle.

It's your unique cycle that you are interested in, not Ms Classic Textbook's cycle. After experimenting for a few cycles with different words or symbols, try to describe each distinct type of mucus consistently. Words such as 'wet' are better used to describe texture than amount, and try to avoid relative words such as 'more' or 'decreasing'. If there is no mucus, draw a line through the space or write 'none' or 'dry' — don't leave it blank; later you won't remember if you checked or not. The colour may be helpful but does not determine fertility. The amount may be better described graphically (see below). After a while, refine the words and symbols you use to a small, consistent, precise and meaningful vocabulary, and clearly identify your BIP.

If you experience different mucus symptoms during the day, always record the most fertile condition.

◆ 'Cervix Changes' is a row you can mark in one of two ways.

- SHOW, which stands for *Soft, High, Open and Wet*.

- HLSD, which stands for *Hard, Low, Shut and Dry*.

  Or, you can describe cervix changes graphically with a series of circles rising and opening. Then you would need to record each day H or S for 'hard' or 'soft', and W or D for 'wet' or 'dry' (though this may be adequately reflected in the 'Mucus' row).

Recording Cervix Changes and Amount of Mucus Graphically

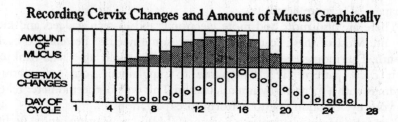

◆ Pain (period or mid-cycle) can be marked with an 'L' for left or 'R' for right at mid-cycle and with a descriptive code at menstruation.

◆ The next few rows can be filled in as you please, if you find the information useful. In 'Bowel' note constipation or diarrhoea, in 'Breasts', note if breasts are swollen, lumpy or tender.

◆ 'Intercourse' may be marked in according to whether you have used mechanical contraception (particularly if this was in conjunction with a spermicide). Sometimes I also find it interesting to see if there is a tick or a cross here, and how this ties up with the marks in the 'Sexual Desire' row!

◆ 'Bleeding' will of course start on Day 1, and you can also record any mid-cycle or premenstrual spotting. Spotting will need a different mark.

) *Charting is important. Don't just write figures in your diary; you won't be able to see patterns emerge.*

As you match your different symptoms together, you will learn more and more about your cycle (for example, your temperature graph will help you refine your understanding of your mucus changes).

As you gain more experience, you may find you need to record less. For the first 3 months you need to write down as much as possible. This need may diminish over the next 6 months or so. After a year, some women — especially those fully confident in, and relying on, mucus observations — hardly need to chart at all.

Your body awareness will become heightened to such a degree that knowing if you are fertile will become automatic.

Gadgets

Fertility thermometers are useful but can be difficult to find and may cost more than fever thermometers. They also tend to come with inadequate instructions and charts. A well-calibrated fever thermometer is quite adequate. However, if your thermometer is marked in 0.05°C (0.1°F) gradations (as are most fertility thermometers) and if you use the chart illustrated here (which is provided with all Natural Fertility Management kits), you will be able to match one division on the thermometer to one square on the graph. You'll also find mercury thermometers more reliable than most of the digital variety (see Chapter 5, 'Basal Body Temperature Changes', for more details.)

There are also more and more electronic and hi-tech gadgets and kits around. Most of these cost a fair amount; some need to be replaced each month. Thermometers with computers attached build up a data bank of your cycle pattern, which they use to supplement your temperature readings with a form of rhythm calculation. This type of thermometer relies on your cycle continuing to perform to expectations.

Kits for detecting leutenising hormone (LH) in your urine can be useful to confirm the timing of ovulation, if this is confusing you, but they are quite expensive and cannot be recycled.

Special little lipstick-sized microscopes, which allow you to view the ferning pattern of mucus, can be of interest, and since saliva ferns at the same time as cervical mucus, these can simply be licked, cleaned and re-used.

Although some of these gadgets can save you time initially, as soon as you are proficient in the use of the methods described in this book, the time required to monitor your body changes will be insignificant.

The advantages of the methods in this book are that none of them rely on any technology that is likely to be difficult to purchase or replace, or to cost you much money (a mercury thermometer only costs you a few dollars and will last forever if properly treated).

If you have a basic understanding of your body, the rewards are great and you will be able to apply your knowledge in all circumstances.

Hypnocontraception

One method, which has not been mentioned in this book so far because I have some reservations about it, but which some people feel is the ultimate in natural fertility control, is hypnocontraception.

By establishing a more intimate relationship with your body, you are perhaps laying the ground for a greater degree of influence over it. Some women feel so in tune with their bodies that they claim that they can influence their ability to conceive.

Whether this is the ultimate outcome of the familiarisation processes we are outlining here or a freak circumstance is difficult to establish. However, some hypnotherapists claim to be able to help a woman control her fertility through suggestion.

If you can use suggestion to synchronise your cycles, why not use it to affect your fertility in other ways? Might it not be possible to suggest to yourself that you don't conceive? Well, yes, but it depends a lot on what suggestions are put and, possibly, on the woman's subconscious, as well as her perhaps unacknowledged desire to conceive.

Hypnocontraception, or the ability to prevent conception through hypnosis, has been given a 99 per cent effective rating by some Italian researchers, scientists and doctors.

The method, as used in this research, is as follows.

Originally, six to eight sessions are held with the patient to make sure she can reach a deep level of hypnosis. In the last session, the therapist gives the suggestions that will make her infertile for the next 4 months.

Hypnotherapy works by deeply relaxing the patient to the *hypnoidal point*, which is like that moment just before you slip off to sleep, when everything feels fine. If you are taken to that point through deepening relaxation techniques and held there (these techniques can be very similar to those described in this book to help you achieve synchronisation of your lunar and hormonal cycles), then the subconscious mind is available to receive information.

It is the subconscious mind that does all our programming for us. It is by changing subconscious expectations that patterns of behaviour really alter. All the time you are receiving the suggestions, though, your conscious mind is fully alert and able to reject anything that makes you feel uncomfortable.

You are not in the hypnotherapist's control.

If you truly want to be infertile for the next 4 months, then your conscious mind will not reject the idea and your subconscious will accept the suggestion. The main possible problem with this is that you may have very strong subconscious reasons for not wanting to be infertile, which you may not be acknowledging.

The reproductive urge goes very deep, and maternal instincts may lurk in all sorts of dusty corners of the mind of the most determined, child-free woman. The skill of the therapist would very much determine how effectively this was dealt with. The trouble with contraception is — there are no trial runs.

Perhaps hypnotherapy is only a useful method for those who have complete faith in their hypnotherapist (and their own ability to respond), or for those who don't mind too much if it doesn't work.

Just before the initial 4-month suggestion runs out, the suggestions are put again, for a fixed period (say, 6 months) and reinforced at regular intervals. The time-span the suggestion puts in place can't be too long, or you can't change your mind.

Sessions are begun at menstruation to ensure that there is no pregnancy.

The people practising this form of contraception seem to very happy with it, stating even that their sexual relationships have become more enjoyable and that they make love more often. But, according to the Italian researchers, the way it works is by stopping ovulation. This is not necessarily a good thing, and not natural to the body, so that could be another strong reason not to use it.

CHAPTER 11

Times of Change

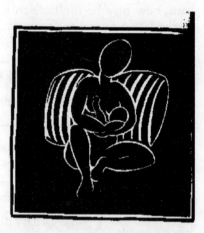

Just when you thought you had it all under control, life comes along and alters everything again. There are times when external circumstances can bring about a change in pattern. Using the sympto-thermal approach means that you can move through these times with relative ease.

Although rhythm calculations are of little help in times of uncertainty, observing your mucus and temperature (and possibly your cervix changes) should enable you to continue to have an accurate picture of what is going on.

Once you are familiar with mucus changes and can interpret your temperature graph, changing patterns of fertility become manageable.

Times of change may include

◆ coming off the contraceptive pill

◆ after childbirth or miscarriage

◆ menopause and the perimenopause

◆ menstrual irregularity

◆ amenorrhoea

◆ starting out.

During times of change, it is still possible to chart your symptoms and come to conclusions about the state of your fertility. You may need more patience, so be prepared to take things day by day.

Certainly, times of change can be more difficult to deal with, although the more experienced you are, the less they will confuse you.

There is really little difference in your approach at these times. Basic rules still apply. It's just that you need to be aware of how the patterns are likely to change: make no assumptions. The risks may be greater due to the level of uncertainty involved; these situations are often the least appropriate times for a conception to occur.

If you have been used to making your assessments on a fairly intuitive basis, now may be the time to resume full charting, double up on your methods (e.g. mucus and temperature), and start to apply the rules carefully. Of extra use in these situations are the

EARLY DAYS RULE

Dry day, safe night, skip a day,

with room for experienced mucus observers, who feel that their vaginas drain promptly, to change this to the

SIMPLIFIED EARLY DAYS RULE

Dry day, safe night,

and the

MUCUS PATCH RULE

Any change in the mucus from the BIP must be followed by abstinence or protection until the BIP has returned for 3 clear days.

With experience, this can also be altered. *If your BIP is basically one of dry days and the change you experience is to increasing levels of infertile-type mucus, you could safely reduce the 3-day wait to 2 days.*

In some of these times of change you may find that you actually have a BIP of unchanging levels of wet mucus. This can be regarded as a BIP if it seems to continue for a lengthy period of time, say 2 weeks, and the change you would be watching for would be an increase in quantity or a change to *spinn*. Observing these changes would really require some experience.

EARLY DAYS RULE FOR THE EXPERIENCED

BIP day, safe night.

If you have a long period of wet mucus (for instance, 2 weeks), then you can consider this (for this cycle, at any rate) to be your BIP.

This might occur, for example, when you are coming off the Pill, as it can be caused by the residual oestrogen stored in the fatty tissue of the body. Natural remedies can help to eliminate residual chemicals (see next chapter).

Another time when this rather unusual BIP might be expected could be during breastfeeding.

The *Mucus Patch Rule* is particularly important when dealing with the now-you-see-me-now-you-don't ovulations that are characteristic of many times of change.

You will probably find that the most useful approach to all these uncertain fertility patterns is to use mucus observations for the beginning of any possible return of fertility (with special care and use of the *Mucus Patch* and *Early Days Rules*), and temperature readings to confirm ovulation and the end of fertility.

You may find it too tedious to continue to take your temperature every day, when there are long periods of time with no change. If you generally have several days warning of ovulation through your mucus observations, you may prefer to leave taking your temperature until you have a change from your BIP.

Continual temperature-taking can, on the other hand, be extremely reassuring in the absence of periods in that they confirm that no ovulation has taken place so you cannot be pregnant.

Although there may be long stretches of time with no menstrual periods in some of these situations, it's also true that your cycles may be unexpectedly short (this is especially true during the perimenopause).

You should always consider your menstrual period as a potentially fertile time if you are uncertain about the regularity of your cycles: you cannot check your mucus while you are bleeding.

At these times, you can always choose to use barrier techniques continually until you have returned to a recognisable pattern of fertility. However, since most times of change involve lengthy periods of infertility, contraception may be entirely unnecessary much of the time. If you patiently continue to make your observations, you could have a chance for risk-free love-making.

Rhythm method is of no use in times of uncertainty and change. Remember, too, that your lunar fertile times carry on with complete regularity at all times (unless the moon changes course!) so *always consider your lunar peak to be fertile*, whatever is happening to your body (except after menopause is finally complete).

SUMMARY OF THE STEPS TO TAKE AT TIMES OF CHANGE

◆ Consider your menstrual period to be a danger time.

◆ Identify the BIP.

◆ Take extreme caution with any change from the BIP.

◆ Apply the *Early Days Rule* — this may need to be adapted if your BIP is not 'dry' (see Chapter 10, 'Charting and Coordinating').

◆ Apply *Peak Symptom* and *Mucus Patch Rules* (with only a 2-day wait necessary if the change has only been to 'probably infertile' mucus).

◆ To confirm ovulation has occurred, start taking your temperature as your mucus changes (if not before) and wait for the three higher readings.

◆ Be confident that any changes in the mucus after the temperature rise do not indicate a fertile time (except if it's your lunar peak).

◆ Always observe your lunar cycle fertile times.

◆ Do not rely on rhythm calculations.

Coming off the Pill

You've decided to come off the Pill. Whether it's because the side-effects are getting to you, the risks are too great, or you just feel bad about living life unnaturally, you will find things change quite a lot.

◆ If you have felt resentful of the health burdens placed on you for the sake of your relationship, now is the time to change all that into cooperation and mutual respect.

◆ If you have had Pill-connected health problems, now is a chance to take care of yourself. Even if you've had an apparently trouble-free time on the Pill, the chances are you will experience an increase in levels of vitality and well-being.

However, there is an inevitable time-gap between the protection of the Pill and your confident use of natural methods.

Unfortunately, you can't learn your fertility patterns on the Pill. Because of the way the Pill works (see Chapter 2, 'The Unnatural Way'), mucus patterns will not be evident, and in many cases, temperature rises will not occur. Also, when you start charting, there will be no rhythm calculations to back you up.

Rhythm calculations cannot be made without at least 6 months to 1 year of reliable records.

While you are on the Pill, your cycle is artificially induced. It has no relationship to your natural cycle, although on the Mini-pill you still ovulate.

WHEN TO STOP TAKING THE PILL

You can stop taking the combination Pill at any point in the 'cycle'.

Because it's not a real cycle, it doesn't have to come to a conclusion. If you decide to stop taking the combination Pill, you can do so straight away (this is not so for the Mini-pill). Whatever time you stop, withdrawal bleeding (not a true period) will usually start a few days later.

Your first bleeding is not a true period, but can be called the first day of your first natural cycle, for the purposes of charting.

In order to cut down on the number of days when you will have to practise contraception or abstinence, you may prefer to time your first bleeding so that your first ovulation has a good chance of synchronising with your lunar fertile time.

This may or may not work, since your first natural cycle may not be typical of your regular pattern, which is still being affected by residual synthetic hormones.

RECOVERY FROM THE PILL

The residue of the Pill can take up to 6 months to be eliminated from your body.
This is because it is stored in the fatty tissue and in the liver. The elimination process can be sped up by the use of natural remedies to detoxify the system and stimulate the normal functioning of the endocrine glands.

As the Pill depletes the body of all sorts of vitamins and minerals (see Chapter 2, 'The Unnatural Approach'), supplementation can also be important at this time. Homoeopathy, acupuncture and herbal remedies can all be very effective in expediting recovery. See the next chapter for some herbal, acupressure and nutrient advice.

Your recovery from the Pill will normally be completed by the fourth natural cycle, however, this will depend on, among other things, the type of Pill you have been taking.

Combination/sequential/triphasic pill — Recovery from this type of pill is extended as it inhibits ovulation, and your hormonal system has to get back into gear. You can normally expect your first ovulation to be delayed an average of 3–4 weeks. You may find ovulation comes right on time or you may have to wait several months; there is a very small chance it may never resume.

Temporary and even (apparently) permanent sterility from the after-effects of the Pill is usually reversible.
Don't worry too much. Although not less than 1 per cent of women fail to ovulate after ceasing to take the Pill, there are both orthodox and natural remedies available to treat this condition.

If you go to your doctor for treatment, you can expect to be given hormone therapy, which is about 50 per cent successful. Natural remedies would be similar to the usual coming-off-the-pill approaches outlined above and in the next chapter, although more intensive and extensive.

Difficulties with the resumption of a normal fertility cycle seem to be worse if you are young or were irregular when you started taking the Pill. Some difficulties also seem to occur in lightweight women.

Mini-pill — Even if you have only been taking the Mini-pill, are not young or underweight, and were not irregular, you can still anticipate some irregularity and delay in experiencing your first true period. (Remember, if you are taking the Mini-pill while breastfeeding, ovulation may still be suppressed by the high levels of prolactin for some time to come.) In normal circumstances

◆ 30 per cent of women bleed within 30 days

◆ 60 per cent of women bleed within 60 days

◆ 8 per cent of women bleed within 2–6 months

◆ 2 per cent of women bleed after 6 months.

Don't forget that this refers to your first natural period, not the withdrawal bleed you experience within a few days of taking your last pill.

HOW YOUR CYCLE RESUMES

Your first natural period may not be the only event for which you're waiting. You will need to confirm that it is a true period, that it has followed an ovulation and that normal, regular functioning has resumed for menstruation, ovulation and mucus production. You should also aim for symptom-free periods, as this indicates good hormonal and nutrient balance.

Even when your periods seem to be occurring regularly, you will need to rely on your temperature and mucus observations to confirm several important pieces of information. They will enable you to be sure that you are ovulating regularly, that the length of your pre- and post-ovulatory phases are within normal limits, and that your mucus changes in quantity and quality as you approach ovulation.

The different characteristics of your hormonal cycle may resume normal functioning at different times.

Your ovulation and mucus patterns may be affected in some of the following ways.

◆ You may have a residual discharge as a result of a cervical erosion or candida (thrush) infection, both of which are much more common in Pill users.

◆ Your BIP may be wet as a result of residual chemicals stored in your body.

◆ You may have some anovular cycles.

◆ You may have some now-you-see-me-now-you-don't ovulations, which will necessitate the use of the *Mucus Patch Rule*.

Obviously, you will need to be a lot more cautious in your first cycle. You will be gaining confidence by your second and, by the time your cycle has settled down to its normal pattern, you should be fairly familiar with the changes you need to observe.

BACK-UP CONTRACEPTION

This delay in the resumption of 'normal' cycles may necessitate a greater reliance on abstinence or protection to begin with. Bear in mind that *the more you abstain now, the less you abstain later.*

A little patience and a lot of abstinence to begin with can pay off in the long run, as you will learn your mucus pattern a lot faster without the complicating factors of residual semen, spermicide or lubrication. For this reason, if you do need to use contraception, a condom (preferably without impregnated chemicals) is less interruptive to the learning process than a diaphragm (see Chapter 9, 'Sexual Expression in Fertile Times').

If your cycle refuses to settle down, you can, if you choose, decide to use barrier methods continuously until at least a regular menstrual pattern emerges.

HOW TO START CHARTING

If you decide to start with symptom observations straight away, here are some things you can do.

◆ Count the first day of your withdrawal bleeding as Day 1 of your first cycle (even though it is not a true period).

◆ Consider yourself safe until you would normally resume taking the Pill (unless you have stopped taking it in the middle of a pill cycle, in which case, take precautions immediately).

◆ Start temperature readings from Day 4.

◆ Start mucus observations as soon as you stop bleeding.

You will definitely need to record your temperature readings daily, at least until you have confirmed and learnt your normal mucus pattern. Your temperature graph will also confirm whether or not you are ovulating.

For the first cycle off the Pill, you must consider yourself fertile from the day on which you would have resumed taking the Pill until your temperature graph shows the thermal shift as confirmed by the Three-Over-Six Rule *(always remembering your lunar days).*

You certainly can't rely on mucus observations for at least the first cycle, and you have no record of natural cycles in order to make a rhythm calculation.

As a result of the synthetic hormone residue, the temperature readings may be higher than normal at the beginning of your cycle, and in the first few cycles you may find that

◆ your post-ovulatory phase is less than 12 days long (or even less than 10)

◆ you have some spotting and breakthrough bleeding (if your temperature is still low you know that you are not experiencing a true period).

Take care if you experience breakthrough bleeding as you will find it hard to recognise mucus changes.

The first few cycles after you come off the Pill are not the easiest time to learn to recognise your signs of fertility, but a little patience will see you through.

EXTRA CAUTION REQUIRED

If you decide to start observing your fertility signs straight away rather than using mechanical contraception, you must be extremely careful to avoid conception.

You should not conceive within 6 months of taking the Pill as

◆ pregnancies that occur shortly after its usage are more subject to difficulties

◆ miscarriages are more likely to occur

◆ abnormalities of the foetus are possible, especially if conception occurs very soon after Pill use

◆ your nutritional status is very low; nutrient status needs to be restored.

See Chapter 2, 'The Unnatural Approach', and 'Chapter 12, 'Natural Remedies for Hormonal and Reproductive Health', for details on vitamin and mineral deficiencies and what to do about them.

An additional reason for those who go off the Pill in order to have a child to delay conception is that a little practice in mucus and temperature charting will come in extremely useful after childbirth.

After childbirth

Your experiences after childbirth will depend on whether or not you are breastfeeding. Fortunately, breastfeeding is fashionable again. It is by far the best food for your baby, having superior nutrients to bottle formulas. Also, breast milk changes its composition to suit your child's needs at different times of day, and provides immunity from all sorts of conditions.

Breastfeeding is also far easier for both mother and child, convenient, always ready, requires no preparation (a Godsend in the middle of the night) and provides both mother and child with a much deeper bonding experience.

Although there are some women who have difficulties with breastfeeding, they often find that these problems are responsive to remedies, rest and relaxation. Even if you have to return to work, you can express milk and store it in the freezer to be fed to your baby later by bottle.

Most countries have associations that advise and help with breastfeeding. The Nursing Mothers' Association is very helpful. Natural remedies can be very useful with such problems as too great or too small a flow of milk (see the next chapter).

BREASTFEEDING IS NATURE'S WAY OF SPACING YOUR CHILDREN
Breastfeeding is an advantage when it comes to contraception, too. This is important, because evidence shows that second (or subsequent) children, born less than 2 years after the previous baby, are often nutritionally compromised, the mother not having had time to recover her full nutritional status since the depletion of pregnancy.

The longer and more frequently you feed your baby, the longer it will take your fertility to return.

Although other factors will also have an influence on the duration of your post-birth infertility, breastfeeding is critical because ovulation is inhibited during breastfeeding by prolactin, the hormone which controls the production of milk. The production of prolactin is stimulated by your baby sucking on the breast, and 'sterilises' the ovaries by its action on the pituitary gland.

Another factor that seems to have a role to play in influencing the return of your cycles is the frequency of sexual activity.

There is a strong link (as was mentioned in the last chapter) between sexuality and fertility. During breastfeeding, a full and active sex life will tend to hasten the return of your menstrual cycle.

Interestingly enough, many women feel relatively sexually uninterested during this period — perhaps this is another part of Mother Nature's way of spacing children.

The majority of women feel most highly sexually motivated when they are fertile, at ovulation, and also (we have found at our clinic) during their lunar fertile time.

With the absence of ovulation, sexual feelings may be reduced, this in turn reducing the chances of ovulation. Many women feel physically focused on their child to such a degree during the breastfeeding period, that their need for physical sexual activity can be diminished. Depending on their experience of childbirth, they may also feel that their reproductive organs could do with a rest.

Don't worry if your sexuality seems reduced after childbirth and during breastfeeding. This is quite a natural experience — it will pass.

The third factor which can affect the return of your cycles is stress. Stress experienced during breastfeeding can reduce prolactin, which results in the milk drying up and ovulation returning. This is in contrast to a 'normal' non-feeding situation, when stress can tend to increase prolactin and delay ovulation.

Finally, good nutrition seems to have a role to play, with studies showing that well-nourished women tend to experience a faster return to a fertile state.

FULLY BREASTFEEDING
You can reasonably confidently consider yourself infertile for the first 10 weeks (even 12) after childbirth *if*

◆ you have experienced no bleeding since the end of the blood-stained discharge (called lochia) that follows childbirth

◆ you are fully breastfeeding; this means
  • no supplementary bottles of formula
  • no solids
  • the breast is used as a pacifier
  • you feed during the night (at least every 4 hours).

If you fully breastfeed during the first 6 months and then partially breastfeed but use the breast as a pacifier, you are unlikely to ovulate before 9–12 months, although you may bleed and have anovular cycles.

Although I have known of one conception occurring within 3 weeks of birth (a lunar conception in a fully breastfeeding situation) and am therefore cautious when giving the following advice, you can generally consider

◆ the first 10 weeks safe and

◆ the first 16 weeks low risk.

Then the risk starts to increase, with a 6–9 per cent chance of conception before the first menstruation, because *the first ovulation will usually precede the first menstruation*, especially if the periods resume after 9 months.

NO BREASTFEEDING (BOTTLE-FED)
You can generally consider yourself infertile for the first 2–3 weeks, although, given the case mentioned above, you can't be 100 per cent sure. You will probably experience your first menstrual period within 6–12 weeks.

FACTORS IN RESTORING FERTILITY

◆ Less sucking.

◆ Using a pacifier in place of the breast.

◆ Cutting out night feeds.

◆ Feeds spaced more than 4 hours apart.

◆ Introducing solids.

◆ Introducing supplementary formula bottles.

◆ Weaning.

◆ Frequent sexual activity.

Given the (slight) uncertainty of the guidelines given above, you may prefer to consider yourself fertile immediately after childbirth.

If you have had children before, it is very likely that your fertility will restore in the same pattern., that is, it will be affected in the same way by the activities described above.

NATURAL BIRTH CONTROL WHILE BREASTFEEDING

While you are experiencing unchanging mucus — either dry, sticky, or even unchanging amounts of wet mucus — you can consider this your *Basic Infertile Pattern* (BIP). *You may need to use the Early Days Rule to continue to monitor your mucus, modified to 'BIP day, safe night'.*

Throughout your pregnancy your ovaries are naturally sterilised and ovulation is suppressed for at least some of the time that you are breastfeeding. As a result of this, you may experience some changes from the BIP as ovulation goes through a series of 'I think I will, I think I will ... No, I won't' hiccoughs before reasserting itself with 'Yes, I will!'

Use the Mucus Patch Rule to deal with these false alarms and, if you like, double check by monitoring your cervix changes.

Don't be alarmed if your first few cycles are irregular. (Herbal remedies can help; see the next chapter.)

Your pattern may also be quite different from how it was before conception. It will be a lot easier to use natural methods to anticipate your returning fertility if you have had some prior experience. This is not the easiest time to learn mucus and temperature methods. However, your mucus, if patiently watched, will give you warning of your first ovulation, while your temperature readings will confirm if ovulation took place at or after the peak symptom.

You may prefer to only take your temperature if and when your mucus pattern changes from your BIP, or you may feel more confident that you haven't missed anything if you continue to take it and see that it hasn't risen.

Previous experience will help you to recognise a lower and higher range of temperatures, but your readings may be slightly higher when breastfeeding and you may need to compensate for disturbed nights and different rising times.

In your first few cycles, you may have a longer pre-ovulatory phase and a shorter post-ovulatory phase.

If the post-ovulatory phase is less than 10 days, the cycle is infertile, with the endometrium breaking down before the fertilised egg has a chance to implant.

You must consider your lunar days fertile from 2–6 weeks after childbirth, depending on whether you breastfeed or not.

This is because of the chance of a spontaneous ovulation occurring, triggered by sexual activity, with no advance warning of mucus changes. Given the additional cautions covered in the last few pages, you may prefer not to wait even these few weeks before taking precautions.

BREAST MILK QUALITY

While you are breastfeeding, you need to have adequate rest and nutrition. The demands on the nutrients in your body are even greater than during pregnancy; the quality of your breast milk will reflect your state of health. *Eat well and avoid drugs of any kind. Continue to supplement with essential nutrients* (see Chapters 12 and 13). Essential fatty acids have been found to protect against sudden infant death syndrome (SIDS — or cot death).

Stress has a notoriously deleterious effect on breastfeeding. Even cows have problems letting down their milk if they are upset by being in a different stall than usual, if milked from the wrong side, or if Buttercup is milked before Daisy instead of after her.

Nearly everything that you eat or drink and the state of your mind and body will affect your breast milk. If your baby seems upset, look at what is happening for you.

As your cycle returns you may find your child less eager to suck around the time of ovulation and menstruation, as the changing hormones affect the milk.

Do not use the Mini-pill while breastfeeding.

◆ The synthetic hormones affect the quantity and the quality of the milk.

◆ The protein quality is affected.

◆ The levels of fats and many minerals are affected.

◆ There is a higher chance of neonatal jaundice.

◆ The synthetic progesterone can masculinise a female infant.

Miscarriage

If you have a miscarriage early in your pregnancy, after-childbirth rules do not apply. Treat any problems as irregularity.

The average time for the return of ovulation is 50 days for first trimester (3 months) and second trimester miscarriages. The range, however, is wide: from 12–104 days (first trimester), and from 10–96 days (second trimester). After a termination, it can be as early as Day 10, with an average of 22 days.

Menopause

The menopause, sometimes called the *change of life* or *climacteric*, used to be considered to have arrived after you had experienced no periods (or ovulation) for 1 year. Recently, this has been updated to 2 years, as patterns seem to be changing.

Stress, poor nutrition, use of the Pill or tubal ligation can create a higher risk of an early menopause, but normally it will take place some time between 45 and 55 years of age. At the completion of menopause, you can consider yourself infertile, although fertility declines dramatically after 45 even if you are still cycling.

After 45 years of age, one in 700 women conceive. After 50 years of age, one in 25 000 women conceive.

The perimenopause refers to the time when you are experiencing changes in your fertility patterns as your ovaries change from egg-bearing organs to hormone-secreting glands. This phase can last several (often rather confusing) years, as the cycle rarely just stops without warning.

Natural fertility awareness techniques can help enormously to get you through this somewhat chaotic and possibly confusing time. A little patience helps, too!

First signs of perimenopause

◆ Loss of libido (not inevitable, and certainly reversible, although it may help you to solve your contraception problems!).

◆ Erratic cycle lengths (very short or very long).

◆ Anovular cycles.

◆ Post-ovulatory (luteal) phase of less than 12 days, or more than 16 (these cycles may be infertile).

◆ Less mucus production. This is a result of lower levels of oestrogen (as is vaginal dryness). Less mucus may mean you need to check at the cervix for changes in both the cervix and mucus (see Chapter 10, 'Charting and Coordinating the Methods for Contraception'). It may also mean that you are infertile (if there is no mucus), even if you still ovulate.

◆ Breakthrough bleeding (use the *True Menses Rule*).

◆ Breast tenderness. You may have greatly increased and quite distressing breast tenderness or, if you previously had this problem, you may find that it goes away. This is a result of low oestrogen and could be an indication of infertility.

◆ Hot flushes. These are sudden feelings of intense heat that last for a minute or two (if they last longer, they have a different cause), strong enough that they may cause perspiration. Hot flushes are another result of decreasing levels of oestrogen, in fact, they indicate such a low level that a day on which you experience them will be infertile. Hot flushes are also associated with sudden releases of LH that occur at this time, and fluctuations in corticosteroids and other adrenal hormones.

◆ Different bleeding pattern. You may experience lighter, shorter periods with browner, darker blood, or heavier periods with clotting.

◆ Different ovulation pattern. You'll be more likely to have now-you-see-me-now-you-don't ovulations. Use the *Mucus Patch Rule*.

◆ Emotional upsets. You may experience irritability, tearfulness, depression, anxiety attacks, temper tantrums or excitability, sometimes compounded by events occurring in midlife, and an increased tendency to the mood swings and emotional tension associated with PMT. Some women experience headaches, dizziness and insomnia.

◆ Weight gain and bloating. These are due partially to hormonal changes and may also be partially caused by increased eating due to depression.

All these conditions can be helped by natural remedies; see the next chapter.

CONTRACEPTION DURING THE PERIMENOPAUSE

◆ Mucus observations are most important as they will warn you of irregular ovulations.

◆ Temperature readings will help enormously to confirm whether or not ovulation has taken place and stop you worrying about pregnancy when you experience delayed periods.

◆ Since your cycles may suddenly be extremely short, you should not consider the bleeding days infertile but wait until you can check your mucus.

◆ Beware of spotting — it may be ovulation. Wait 3 days (you could think of this as the *Blood Patch Rule*).

◆ You cannot rely on rhythm calculations.

◆ You should continue to avoid unprotected intercourse on lunar peak fertile days.

◆ If you have had no periods for 1 year, you are probably not fertile any more. If you have had no periods for 2 years, you are definitely not fertile any more.

Irregularity

Hormone imbalance is one probable cause of irregular cycles. Your mucus and temperature readings may provide you with some clues. Irregularity needs treatment. See your natural health practitioner (or the next chapter).
Temporary irregularity can be brought on by

◆ polycystic ovarian syndrome, ovarian cysts or other pathology of the ovaries (try natural remedies unless a crisis requires surgery)

◆ stress (try relaxation therapy, meditation, hypnotherapy, herbs, dietary changes, vitamins and minerals, exercise, or change your lifestyle)

◆ fever (watch for where the temperature readings resume — you may have ovulated while in a fever, although it's more likely that ovulation will be delayed)

◆ thyroid disease (see your natural health practitioner or doctor)

◆ abnormal pituitary function or growth (see your doctor for diagnosis and your natural health practitioner or doctor for treatment)

◆ diabetes

◆ travel

◆ illness

◆ excessive exercise

◆ diet changes

◆ sudden, dramatic weight changes

◆ drugs (prescription or otherwise)

See Chapter 4, 'Cervical Mucus Changes', for details.

Irregularities in your mucus pattern can be brought on by abnormalities of the cervix or nutritional deficiencies, as well as by hormonal imbalance (see Cervix Changes in Chapter 10, 'Charting and Coordinating the Methods for Contraception').

◆ *Don't use rhythm calculations if you are irregular or in a situation likely to cause irregularity.*

◆ Use mucus readings to confirm pre-ovulatory infertility (with special care and use of *Early Days* and *Mucus Patch Rule*).

◆ Use temperature readings to confirm post-ovulatory infertility.

◆ Always consider your lunar peak and bleeding days as potentially fertile.

◆ If you feel *really* confused, use a barrier method until the situation resolves.

Amenorrhoea

It's the lack of change that is a worry here. This term denotes a total lack of periods for 6 months or more. For treatment, see the next chapter. For contraception, see Breastfeeding section.

Natural Remedies for Hormonal and Reproductive Health

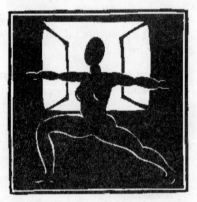

Do you enjoy your periods? Or does that sound like a contradiction in terms to you? Have you become so inured to menstrual and premenstrual distress that you have begun to think of it as normal? Well, it isn't.

It is neither normal nor natural to suffer distressing symptoms before or during your periods. In fact, believe it or not, for some women menstruation is a welcome event, and not just because it means the end of a week or so of PMS. You can learn (if you don't already know how) to experience menstruation as a private, inward time of affirmation of your femininity and fertility.

You will undoubtedly have different feelings at this time, but there is no need for them to be traumatic or uncomfortable.

For everything there is a season,
and a time for every purpose under Heaven.

In Chapter 2, 'The Unnatural Approach', we looked at some of the patriarchal attitudes that have developed towards the menstruating woman — seeing her as unclean and dangerous — and some of the more woman-celebrating ideas that acknowledge feminine power at this time, when the senses are more inwardly directed.

If we accept our cyclical natures and give ourselves a chance to express ourselves differently at varying times of the lunar month and provide for our needs — physical, psychological and psychic — we can experience our cycles in the same way as Mother Nature experiences the seasons, thus giving us richly varied monthly experiences.

Of course, it'll be difficult for you to develop a positive approach if you suffer from pain, tension, bloating, headaches, fatigue and pimples. So here is where we look at what can be done to bring you back to health.

There's another good reason to balance your hormones, prostaglandins and nutrients apart from your well-being. Good hormonal and nutritional health will result in regular cycles, with obvious mucus and temperature changes that will help you to apply the timing methods in this book with greater ease and success.

Orthodox medical approaches

While some of you may grit your teeth and battle on, others may resort to pain-killers and even synthetic hormones in an attempt to cope. The drugs do not deal with the origins of the problem. If you take pain-killers, they may enable you to keep going, but you'll feel just as bad next time. If you take synthetic hormones, your body is likely to make less of its own and you'll feel worse next time.

Natural remedies

There is much that you can do to help yourself back to real hormonal health. Diet, exercise, vitamins, minerals, herbs and other natural remedies, massage, osteopathy, acupressure, relaxation therapy, yoga — there are lots of possibilities. It's best if you experiment and find out what works for you. Be patient. The results may take a while to become apparent. Natural remedies, because they are affecting you on a fundamental level, can act more slowly than some of the more drastic drugs of orthodox medicine.

Herbal medicine (my own particular love), has much to offer. Most of the herbs used for 'women's complaints' have wonderful names, evoking fertility, mythology and the feminine: *False Unicorn Root, True Unicorn Root, Chastetree, Squaw Vine, Cramp Bark, Poke Root* (a little crude, maybe!) — to name a few.

If you are thinking of using herbs, you can either start by yourself or go to an experienced medical herbalist. If you see a herbalist, you will probably be treated with fluid extracts and tinctures, a liquid form of herbal medicine which makes it easier to make up individually relevant formulae.

For the do-it-yourself approach, there are a number of commercially available encapsulated dried-herb formulae; some of which are also used by practitioners. Or, you can make up herb teas (infusions) from the loose, dried or fresh herb. Since quality control is variable in herbs available though retail outlets, you may be more confident if you purchase these loose herbs through your herbalist.

How to make an infusion

◆ For every 30 g (1 oz or 2 tablespoons) of herb, pour on 600 mL (1 pint) of boiling water.

◆ Let it steep (infuse) for at least 15 minutes, to get the full benefit of the active ingredients of the herb.

◆ Strain, and drink a teacupful three times daily.

◆ Make a fresh brew every day and use it within 24 hours or refrigerate.

While infusions are not as strongly active in most cases as the herbal preparations you will receive from a herbalist, they can still be very effective, and in some cases are the preferred form. Although you will find you can treat yourself easily in instances of mild conditions, any severe or continuing problem requires professional diagnosis and treatment.

The physiological basis of menstrual distress is complex and varies with different women, but most menstrual problems are to do with some form of hormone imbalance, or with infection.

While ingesting synthetic hormones is not helpful in the long term (see the section on menopause for more on so-called 'natural' progesterone), herbal remedies work quite differently. Herbs do not contain hormones as such, but they do have precursor or plant hormone-like substances which can be utilised by your body to re-establish normal hormonal levels.

It is also important to have healthy liver function so that the old hormonal waste is efficiently and effectively eliminated. Here again, we can look to herbal medicine for help.

Diet and nutrition

Hormone imbalance and poor reproductive health can often be due to nutrient deficiencies. Diet and supplements are an indispensable part of caring for your hormonal health.

Vegetarians take care

The body makes hormones from proteins. Although most vegetarians are very health-conscious and very aware of what they eat, it is also quite common for them to neglect their protein levels.

In spite of the claims by some that too much protein is harmful, it's also true that too little protein is problematic, especially if combined with high levels of carbohydrate, as this can adversely affect your hormonal balance. If you are a vegetarian, you need to find a suitable way of sustaining your protein intake.

Plant proteins are called 'secondary' proteins, as they do not contain the full range of amino acids. In order to provide yourself with complete proteins each day, you will need to eat foods from *two* of the following groups:

◆ nuts

◆ grains and seeds

◆ legumes or pulses

if you do not eat any animal foods (which contain 'primary' proteins).

Even if you prefer not to eat much — or any — red meat, you may still find fish, poultry or eggs acceptable. Fish is a wonderful way to get your protein, especially if you need to watch how much saturated fat you eat.

PROSTAGLANDINS

In the second half of your cycle, saturated fats are a particular problem because their consumption, as well as that of alcohol, blocks the production in your body of certain prostaglandins.

Prostaglandins are divided into several types, or families, which, for simplicity, we shall call PG1, PG2 and PG3. An imbalance in their production can lead to PMS and spasmodic dysmenorrhoea, eczema, hypertension, and benign breast disease, as well as hyperactivity in children,.

The goodies among the prostaglandins, the PG1 and PG3 types, are necessary for the control of hormonal activity. A deficiency is related not only to the saturated (animal and heated) fats and alcohol, but also to stress (increased adrenal output), viral infections, ageing, high cholesterol levels, preservatives and flavourings, and pesticide residue in foods.

An excess of the baddies (sounds like a soap opera, doesn't it?), the prostaglandin PG2 family, overstimulates the contractions of the uterus, causing cramping; it can also result in diarrhoea.

To avoid this imbalance, it is best to cut down on the animal and heated fats in your diet and look carefully at your protein sources (you'll find more information on which foods to avoid and which to eat further on). Cold-pressed oils on salads are beneficial, as they contain essential fatty acids (EFAs) which will help to restore balance.

All fats (saturated or not) should come from an organic source, as fat is the reservoir for most pollutants and toxins.

THE CHICKEN AND THE EGG

Your egg must come before the chicken. If you eat poultry as a protein source, you will need to eat it without the skin, the main source of fats. Unfortunately, most chickens available these days are commercially and intensively raised in batteries.

Quite apart from any concerns you may justifiably have about the treatment of these animals, the threat to your health is quite serious. These birds are usually fed large amounts of antibiotics and steroids. These concerns also relate equally to red meat from non-organically fed animals. Once they get into your body, the synthetic hormones will interfere with your own hormonal production. The antibiotics will create problems in your immune system and can contribute greatly towards another big problem — candida.

Part of the treatment for a candida infection will be a very strict diet, without which there is little chance of any medication having any success. We'll discuss this later on in this chapter. Even if you aren't a candida sufferer, there are quite a few recommendations you would do well to heed for your hormonal and reproductive health.

MORE CARE WITH YOUR DIET

Your optimum weight will serve your hormonal interests best, and this should be easy to maintain on a healthy diet. Fat women tend to produce too little progesterone in relation to their oestrogen, thin women too little oestrogen.

The need to avoid saturated fats, pollutants and chemical hormones extends beyond the replacement of red meat with fish and poultry. Here is a list of easy-to-achieve recommendations for this and other dietary concerns.

◆ *Less red meat.* Trim the fat. Glandular meats, such as liver, are full of nutrients. These must only be eaten if they come from organically fed animals, otherwise they will be full of toxins. All meats should be organic. Avoid sausage, mince and delicatessen meats which are usually made from offal, unless they are lean and made from organic meats.

◆ *Poultry must be free-range and organically fed.* These are not always the same thing. Unless the food is certified as organic, you may need to ask specific questions about hormones, antibiotics and other chemicals. Don't assume that labels such as 'grain-fed' or 'vegetarian-fed' mean that the animal's feed is free from these toxic substances. This advice also applies to eggs, which are a useful source of protein, as long as you are not allergic or otherwise sensitive to them (many people are). Don't eat the fat-laden chicken skin.

◆ *More fish and seafood (including seaweed).* Choose ocean and deep-sea fish in preference to coastal or river fish to avoid pollution and to increase EFAs. Avoid large fish (tuna, swordfish, shark, etc.); being high in the feeding chain, they may also be high in mercury. Fresh fish is preferable to tinned or frozen.

◆ *Protein every day.* If no animal food is eaten, combine two of the following groups:
  • nuts
  • (whole) grains and seeds
  • pulses and legumes (this includes tofu and tempeh, made from soya beans) as single plant proteins have incomplete amino acids. You should eat a portion of protein — providing food that is the same size as the palm of your hand — at least twice a day.

◆ *More nuts and seeds.* Not only for vegetarians, who need these as a protein source, but for everyone, to benefit from their rich store of nutrients. These are best eaten raw and unsalted, without dried fruit, which is very high in sugar. Nuts go rancid very quickly and should be fresh and eaten before they get a bitter taste. Store them in the refrigerator.

◆ *Fewer dairy products*. Don't rely on dairy products for protein if you are vegetarian. If you are sensitive to cow's milk (most people are), substitute with goat's, sheep's, soya or rice milk. Even if you are dairy-sensitive, you may be able to tolerate yoghurt, which is a helpful food if free of sugar and additives. Choose the 'acidophilus' variety. Butter (in moderation) is preferable to margarine. Avocado, hummus, nut spreads and banana are better still. (Keep nut spreads in the fridge.)

◆ *Lots of fresh vegetables every day*. Use a wide variety of vegetables, especially dark green leafy, red or yellow vegetables, and avocados. Eat some raw and some cooked vegetables on a regular basis. Buy organic if possible, otherwise peel.

◆ *Limit fruit to 2–3 pieces daily*. This includes fruit that is juiced, so it's better to eat your fruit whole (a glass of juice uses more than 3 pieces). Fruit is high in sugar, which destroys other nutrients when eaten in excess. It can also cause insulin resistance, resulting in hormone imbalances. Use your 2–3 pieces to fill the gaps left by other sugary foods that you may be used to eating. Avoid the peel if not organically grown.

◆ *Use chopped fresh herbs such as parsley and watercress in green salads*. These are a good source of minerals, and minerals feed glands.

◆ *Use a variety of vegetables* in your salads (organic if possible). Don't rely on the lettuce and tomato stand by. The darker the lettuce the more minerals it contains.

◆ *Cook vegetables lightly*. Steam, stir-fry or dry bake. If you don't get enough vegetables in your meals (a minimum of 40 per cent of your total food intake), top up with vegetable juices.

◆ *Olive oil for salads and cooking*. Use cold-pressed olive oil (or flaxseed, safflower or sunflower), 2 tablespoons daily, on salads. They're full of EFAs when cold-pressed and never heated. Use olive (or canola) oil for cooking. They're monounsaturated and won't become saturated when they're heated or affect prostaglandin balance (or cholesterol).

◆ *No fried foods*, except the occasional stir-fry with a little olive oil.

◆ *Whole grains only*. Bread, pasta, rice and cereals should be brown, not white, though being brown is not always a guarantee that the product is made from the whole grain, so check this out. Use organically grown products where possible to avoid chemical residues, and check labels for sugars and preservatives.

◆ *Little, if any, sugar.* This includes honey, artificial sweeteners and undiluted juices. All forms of sugar destroy nutrients.

◆ *Little, if any, salt.* You get plenty naturally through your food. If you need some extra occasionally, use rock or sea salt.

◆ *Limit alcohol*, especially when you are premenstrual. Red wine is full of bioflavonoids, which at least makes it partially beneficial (that's my excuse, anyway!).

◆ *Limit tea, coffee, cola and soft drinks.* Coffee is better avoided (even decaffeinated). If you must drink it, limit yourself to 1 cup a day. Ideally, try *Dandelion Root* or cereal substitutes instead. Limit tea to 2–3 cups daily, preferably the varieties that are naturally low in caffeine (toxic chemicals are widely used in decaffeinating process). Even better, drink green or herb teas. Soft drinks are all high in sugar and chemicals, and mineral waters often have a high salt content; cola drinks are high in caffeine.

◆ *Drink lots of fresh water.* Eight to 12 glasses daily. If it comes from the tap, use a purifier to filter out toxins. Purify water, even if it is going to be boiled; boiling only kills bacteria, it doesn't destroy toxins.

Diet is a very personal matter. There are two common misconceptions about diet.

◆ The same diet works for everyone.

◆ The same diet works all the time.

Each individual has different dietary needs and intolerances which will vary according to health and lifestyle. The important thing is to find out what works for you and when. Trust your body's response (except when you have a craving — this may be the 'rush' you initially get with an allergic response).

Apart from the guidelines above, there are basically three golden rules.

◆ *Eat food that is as fresh and as recently prepared as possible.*

◆ *Eat food that is organically grown or fed whenever possible.*

◆ *Eat as wide a range of foods as your diet allows.* (If you suffer from food allergies which restrict the foods available to you, consult a natural health practitioner or doctor trained in nutrition to treat your immune system and strengthen your digestion so that you can gradually reintroduce these foods.)

A LITTLE OF WHAT YOU FANCY DOES YOU GOOD!

There is a fourth golden rule — avoid junk food or previously prepared foods (especially those with additives). Although the fourth golden rule is a natural consequence of the three, let us put a strong rider on this and on your general approach to diet: Don't beat yourself up!

Having done what you can to fulfil your need for a healthy lifestyle, remember that there are constraints on you, especially if you lead a busy, urban existence. The occasional lapse won't do you nearly as much harm as the guilt and feelings of inadequacy which can follow hard on the heels of idealism.

Hopefully, if you re-educate your tastebuds and learn how much better you feel when you eat well, what you fancy will be mainly healthy. When it isn't, a little will go a long way.

Nutritional supplements

Although it would be nice to think that we could get all our nutrients from our food, unfortunately, this is not often the case. The reality is that many of our foods are robbed of their nutrients through chemical-laden growing methods, toxic environments, lengthy transit times and long shelf-life.

All of these pollutants, and those found in our air and water, constitute what are known as anti-nutrients, which destroy the body's ability to make use of the goodness in our foods. It's difficult to avoid the pollutants in the air, although some locations are much worse than others, but water pollutants can be filtered out with a water purifier, and those in food by eating organically grown items whenever possible.

If we could all live in splendid isolation from the twenty-first century and grow organic produce in pollution-free gardens, then — maybe — we could rely on our diet for the necessary nutrients. However, we make our choices about our lifestyles and not all of us will choose this. Those of you reliant on supermarkets for much of your food cannot rely on its nutrient content.

Fruits recently analysed from the shelves of Sydney greengrocers showed that some had adequate levels of vitamin C, some virtually none at all. In order to be sure that you are getting adequate levels of certain nutrients, you may need to take nutritional supplements.

HOW MUCH?

There is a great difference between the amounts of vitamins, minerals and other nutrients required to maintain health (recommended daily requirements), the levels used by therapists as medicine (therapeutic doses), or that required by people who have specific deficiencies.

The following levels are a guide only. If you feel that your symptoms are extreme, it would be better to consult a natural health practitioner or doctor trained in nutrition.

Calcium — Serum calcium levels drop about 10 days before menstruation. Calcium has a big role to play in muscle contractions and nerve transmissions and in the production of fertile mucus. Low levels contribute to fluid retention (by causing the production of cortisone and aldosterone in the adrenal cortex), cramping, headaches and nervous tension. Loss of calcium after menopause is the main reason (along with reduced magnesium) for osteoporosis.

Just because you have an adequate intake of calcium, doesn't mean you absorb it properly. Magnesium, vitamin D and oestrogen are essential for you to retain calcium, with magnesium levels best at about half those of calcium.

If you are taking adequate amounts of these nutrients, you may find a marked decrease in some of your symptoms both before and during menstruation. If cramping still occurs, calcium and magnesium (in a 2:1 ratio) can be taken hourly. The tissue salts, calcium phosphate and magnesium phosphate are easily and immediately absorbed. Reduce the amounts if you get diarrhoea.

Recommended daily intake — 400–800 mg (the higher levels in the post-ovulatory phase and during menopause).

Food sources — Dairy and soya products, nuts (especially brazil nuts, walnuts and almonds), sunflower and sesame seeds, tahini, sardines, salmon, dark green, leafy vegetables, parsley, watercress, kelp, carob, wheatgerm and wheat bran.

Magnesium — Women with PMS generally have low serum magnesium levels. Because magnesium is so important for the nervous system, this deficiency leads to nervous tension and irritability which in its turn (as with low calcium levels) leads to overproduction of adrenal hormones, then more magnesium is excreted and its absorption inhibited.

As magnesium levels drop further, aldosterone causes fluid retention. Another effect is to inactivate the body's natural pain killers. Magnesium is necessary for correct muscle function; a deficiency can cause menstrual cramps.

It is also necessary for the production of oestrogen and progesterone, the utilisation of vitamin B6 and to activate enzymes, especially those related to energy production. It's essential for hormonal health, and for strong bones in old age. Saturated fats interfere with magnesium absorption. Women taking the oral contraceptive pill are commonly deficient.

Magnesium levels should generally be about half those of calcium. Alcohol consumption increases your needs. The cell salt magnesium phosphate is also very useful.

Recommended daily intake — 200–400 mg

Food sources — Whole grains, dry beans (especially soya), nuts, bananas, kelp, wheat bran and germ and dark green leafy vegetables. Chocolate is a rich source of magnesium. While this isn't the best way to take it, chocolate cravings can indicate a magnesium deficiency. (And vice versa — sufficient dietary magnesium may stop the cravings.)

Zinc — Premenstrually, copper levels rise and as a consequence, zinc levels drop. Zinc is perhaps the most important nutrient for female and male fertility and hormonal health. It has been shown to enhance the metabolic efficiency of the essential fatty acids, which are required by the body to produce the PG1 and PG3 type prostaglandins — the goodies. (Magnesium has a role to play here, too.)

It is also vital for the prevention of premenstrual pimples, and is needed for proper pituitary functioning, normal growth, cell division and tissue repair. It is an important antioxidant: it protects you from toxins, strengthens your immune system and reduces ageing problems.

Zinc can be particularly lacking in users of copper IUDs and those who take the Pill. A deficiency is often indicated by white banding in the nails. Absorption of this mineral is problematic, as it has an antagonistic relationship with many other nutrients and foods (including dairy produce and legumes). Zinc supplements should be taken on an empty stomach, away from food and other supplements (last thing at night may be the easiest time).

Recommended daily intake — 20–60 mg

Food sources — Whole grains, wheatgerm, nuts, seafood (especially oysters), meat, milk, green vegetables, mushrooms, onions, root ginger, egg yolks, seeds and herbs. However, even these foods (with the exception of oysters) are not particularly rich in zinc, and refined foods, alcohol, sugar and caffeine will strip zinc from your body's reserves. Supplementation is required for most people to ensure adequate levels.

Iron — You can lose too much iron if you bleed excessively. If you have marginal levels of iron, as many women do, this can, paradoxically, lead to heavier periods and clotting, or it can inhibit menstrual flow. As iron is required for the proper function of the mucous membranes, a deficiency can affect mucus production.

Iron absorption is helped by taking the homoeopathic cell salt ferrum phos(phate), and vitamin C. Tea, coffee and soft drinks, especially if consumed at the same time as iron-rich foods, will hinder absorption. A deficiency may cause the nails to have ridges or to separate.

Recommended daily intake — 15 mg (must be organic and chelated. Only take in proven need (a blood test will show this) and in conjunction with a comprehensive range of other nutrients. In excess it's toxic and carcinogenic; if not organic it may cause constipation.)

Food sources — Kelp, lean meat, glandular meats (only from organically fed animals), dried fruits, dried beans, wheatgerm and bran, nuts, seeds, herbs, yeast, parsley, Nettle and Red Raspberry teas. Green leafy vegetables contain iron, but in a form which is poorly absorbed.

Manganese — In combination with chromium and the B vitamins, manganese is one of the minerals that assists greatly in relieving the sugar cravings some women experience premenstrually. A deficiency can affect fertility. This important mineral is extremely deficient in foods grown with chemical fertilisers.

Recommended daily intake — 10 mg

Food sources — Nuts, whole grains (especially buckwheat, barley and rye), green leafy vegetables, cloves, ginger, thyme, bay leaves, tea, parsley, eggs and liver (from organically fed meat).

Potassium — This is another mineral that works for glandular health in combination with the others. It is crucial for water balance and nerve function, muscle contraction and blood-sugar levels. It is particularly important if you use diuretics to relieve fluid retention as pharmaceutical diuretics can cause potassium depletion. Avoid salt as it contributes to a sodium/potassium imbalance. The cell salt potassium chloride is also very useful.

Recommended daily intake — 50 mg

Food sources — Kelp, bananas, nuts, dried fruits, potatoes, carrots, mushrooms, green leafy vegetables, beans, avocados, sunflower seeds and wheatgerm.

Iodine — This is an essential mineral for the healthy functioning of the thyroid, which is crucial for healthy endocrine activity and hormonal balance. An underactive thyroid, which can result in anovulatory cycles, will result in the temperature readings on your graph being lower than normal. Iodine is needed in cases of excessive bleeding.

Recommended daily intake — 75 mcg

Food sources — Kelp, seafood, eggs.

Selenium — This is an extremely important antioxidant, which is also essential for healthy breasts and male fertility. Unfortunately, the soil in Australia is very low in selenium, a problem which is compounded by the fact that only small amounts are available in non-prescription supplements. High doses (especially of the forms sodium selenite or selenate) can be toxic, so keep to the levels recommended here. Some forms of selenium are rendered ineffective if taken at the same time as zinc or vitamin C. Selenomethionine is the preferred, most effective, form which is stable and can be taken with other nutrients.

Recommended daily intake — 100–200 mcg

Food sources — Garlic, onions, butter, wheatgerm, brazil nuts, seafoods (but not present in large amounts, even in these foods).

Chromium — This mineral is a part of glucose tolerance factor (GTF) and works with manganese and the B vitamins to control sugar cravings and low blood-sugar levels, which can be a problem premenstrually. Chromium is not easily absorbed, and is also leached from your body's stores when you eat refined grains or sugar, or drink alcohol.

Recommended daily intake — 100–500 mcg

Food sources — Brewer's yeast (not for candida sufferers), liver (organic only), beef, chicken, haddock, whole grains, milk.

Boron — This mineral is essential for normal oestrogen levels in postmenopausal women. A diet high in boron can double the oestrogen content in the blood. There is normally no need for supplements if you eat well.

Recommended daily intake (at menopause) — 3 g

Food sources — Boron is found in most plant foods, fresh vegetables and fruit, and in other foods in the following proportions:

♦ vegetables   13 mcg per gram

♦ dairy   1.1 mcg per gram

♦ cereals   0.92 mcg per gram

♦ meat   0.16 mcg per gram.

All minerals are found extensively in nuts, seeds and herbs. Chop parsley, watercress and other green herbs into your salads; sprinkle seeds and chopped nuts on your cereals.

If you take mineral supplements, they should be in chelated form (as this enables you to assimilate them), and if possible from an organic, natural source.

Essential fatty acids — These nutrients are indeed essential, so that you can produce the healthy prostaglandins that are the precursors of hormonal balance. They help reduce period pain, PMS (especially tender, swollen and lumpy breasts), menopausal discomfort and a host of other complaints. They are also essential for male fertility and have been shown to be very effective in the treatment of endometriosis and skin problems. They have an anti-inflammatory effect. The best sources are Evening Primrose oil and fish oils.

Essential fatty acids are destroyed by heat and compete in your body with the saturated fats. You should avoid dairy products, fat meat, margarine, chicken skin, fried foods and foods such as biscuits and cakes which contain a lot of fat.

Recommended daily intake — 500–1000 mg 3 x daily (of Evening Primrose oil and deep-sea fish oils—or flaxseed oil)

Food sources — Deep-dwelling or cold-water fish, soya beans, cold-pressed vegetable oils such as olive, flaxseed, safflower and sunflower, blackcurrant oil, wheatgerm, walnuts, raw safflower and sunflower seeds, meat, prawns, dairy produce (yoghurt is helpful), green leafy vegetables. Take care if using supplements made in the form of encapsulated oils. If they are too old, they may have become rancid, and this will raise the serum level of free radicals. In hot weather, keep all oil-based supplements in the refrigerator.

Vitamin A — This vitamin is essential for healthy mucous membranes and for the formation and utilisation of amino acids in the protein chain. Useful for premenstrual depression. Enhances metabolic efficiency of the essential fatty acids. Also helpful for heavy periods, fibrocystic breast disease, male and female fertility, and the health of the fallopian tubes. Due to vitamin A's potential toxicity, it is best taken as mixed carotenoids (or, if unavailable, Beta-carotene), which your body will convert to vitamin A as required. It is an important antioxidant.

Recommended daily intake — 10 000 iu, 6 mg mixed carotenoids or Beta-carotene

Food sources — Liver, carrots, chillies, green leafy vegetables, dried apricots and peaches, sweet potatoes, oily fish, egg yolk, dairy produce.

Vitamin B-complex — The B-complex vitamins are crucial to reduce PMS and dysmenorrhoea and play an essential role in the hormonal response to stress. They are essential for the regulation of homocysteine (which can lead to miscarriage and cardiovascular problems), and in the metabolism of many nutrients (including EFAs, which help to correct oestrogen and progesterone levels).

Certain of the B vitamins are indicated separately, but are best taken together, which is how they occur in nature. If one is taken alone, a deficiency in another may arise. B6 is particularly important to relieve premenstrual fluid retention and sore breasts. It may increase progesterone levels, it inhibits excessive prolactin production by a dysfunctional pituitary gland, furthers the absorption of zinc, and is crucial to normal brain function and a stable mood.

Oral contraceptives, coffee, alcohol, smoking and stress all increase your need for the B vitamins, and sugar leaches them from your body, as do all refined carbohydrates.

Recommended daily intake —

B_1 (thiamin) 30–50 mg (50–100 mg for PMS)

B_2 (riboflavin) 25–50 mg

B_3 (niacinamide) 50 mg (100–200 for PMS)

B_5 (pantothenic acid) 25–50 mg

B_6 (pyridoxin) 50–200 mg (200 mg for PMS, lower levels if breastfeeding)

B_9 (folic acid) 200–400 mcg

B_{12} (cobalamin) 50–400 mcg (vegetarians may be deficient in this vitamin)

Biotin 65 mcg

Inositol 25 mg

Para-amino-benzoic acid (PABA) 25 mg

Folic acid and PABA taken in larger doses may aggravate fluid retention and breast tenderness.

Dosage of B_6 remains controversial. Numbness or tingling (in lips, tongue, legs and feet), and an impaired sense of touch are symptoms experienced if too much has been taken. Up to 200 mg is generally considered very safe, although individuals can tolerate much higher doses. One way to determine dosage is to set it at the level required to ease PMS symptoms. This can occasionally be up to 800 mg. If it is taken in combination with the other B vitamins (which should always be the case) and zinc, the side-effects may be eliminated. It is best to consult a health professional and not to try doses over 200 mg on your own. (The recommended daily allowance — RDA — of B_6 is only 2 mg.)

Food sources — Yeast (if you do not suffer from candida), seeds, glandular meats (organic only), beans, nuts, seafood, dairy products (if not sensitive to them), wheatgerm, whole grains, oily fish, avocados, mushrooms.

Vitamin C — This vitamin helps to strengthen blood capillaries and to alleviate heavy periods and premenstrual depression. Needed for iron absorption, the metabolism of EFAs, and production of sex hormones, particularly after menopause when the adrenals take over this role. Vitamin C has also been shown to promote ovulation in women whose cycles are anovular. It is an important antioxidant. The levels of vitamin C in the body are decreased by stress, infections and smoking.

Recommended daily intake — 1500 mg minimum + bioflavonoids 300 mg

Try to choose a vitamin C supplement that contains bioflavonoids, such as those from a natural source. Ascorbic acid is preferable to calcium ascorbate, as the latter can affect magnesium levels.

Food sources — All fresh fruits and vegetables, most of which also contain the bioflavonoids.

Vitamin D — This vitamin is needed for calcium absorption. You will form your own vitamin D if you receive enough sunshine on a daily basis.

Recommended daily intake — 200 iu

Food sources — Sardines, salmon, tuna, dairy, sunflower seeds, liver, eggs.

Vitamin E — This nutrient has been called 'the fertility vitamin' because of its important role in reproductive health. It is of great help with fibrocystic breast disease, headache, sweet cravings, increased appetite, fatigue, dizziness and palpitations, all of which tend to occur premenstrually. It is also helpful for the relief of menopausal symptoms. Used by the body in the metabolism of EFAs and selenium and to normalise oestrogen levels. Vitamin E is also an important antioxidant. Use with caution if you are hypertensive.

Recommended daily intake — 100–500 iu

Food sources — Wheatgerm, seeds, cold-pressed vegetable oils, nuts, whole grains, avocados, egg yolk, whole milk, green leafy vegetables.

All the vitamins and minerals work together to help the liver break down oestrogen and sugar, lessening the chances of hormonal, sugar and brain chemical imbalance. See Chapter 2, 'The Unnatural Approach', and Chapter 13, 'Conscious Conception' for more information on nutritional effects on reproductive and foetal health.

If you have difficulty swallowing pills, the water-miscible (able to be mixed with water) liquid preparations, micelles, can be taken in fruit juice and are, in fact, more readily absorbed by the body.

Obviously, it is impossible to take all these supplements separately. If you feel that your diet is inadequate, look around for a good multivitamin and mineral formula which contains approximately the dosages recommended. There are several 'women's formula' or 'PMS' products on the market which will be similar in their doses to these amounts, or at least reduce the number of extra tablets you need to take.

♦ Digestive enzymes will help you to absorb nutrients.

♦ Take vitamins and minerals with a meal (except zinc).

♦ Take them daily throughout your cycle.

♦ Some vitamins and minerals may be required in extra dosage premenstrually.

♦ They will work better if you eat well and exercise regularly.

♦ Needs will vary according to circumstance. It's important to experiment.

Exercise

Far from lying down in bed when you're suffering from hormonally based problems, as our Victorian forebears had to do whether they felt bad or not, one of the best ways to alleviate distressing symptoms is regular exercise, although, during menstruation, this may need to be a little gentler than usual.

All exercise is hormonally beneficial, except if it's taken to extremes. Excessive training can reduce oestrogen levels by cutting back too far on body fat. Exercises which strengthen abdominal muscles and increase circulation and lymphatic drainage are most helpful.

Swimming (avoid chlorine-treated pools) and brisk walking are good, as are non-violent forms of aerobic exercise, which increase cardiovascular activity.

Yoga is very helpful in building muscle strength and flexibility, and stimulates digestive, respiratory, circulatory and endocrine systems.

EXERCISE FOR LAZY OR BUSY PEOPLE

It's difficult sometimes to fit regular exercise into busy lifestyles. Most forms of exercise require travelling, changing clothes, buying special equipment, joining clubs and all sorts of other extras about which you may have the best intentions — at least for the first 3 enthusiastic months.

There is one form of exercise that is easy to fit into busy days, doesn't require you to go anywhere or change your clothes. You can even do it while you watch television — and it's not knitting! It's rebounding.

Rebounding

This gentle form of exercise, done on a mini-trampoline, happens to be one of the most thorough, and it gently exercises every cell in your body.

Even though your body virtually propels itself upwards on the rebound, it satisfies the principle that exercise means working against resistance.

If you're swimming, the resistance is in the water (in some forms of exercise it's all in the mind!); in rebounding, the natural resistance of gravity is increased by the acceleration and deceleration of the upward and downward movements and changes in direction.

This increases circulation and encourages lymphatic drainage, and it tones the organs, including the endocrine and reproductive systems because the lower body gets a thorough workout, unlike in many other forms of exercise.

Although it is effective aerobic exercise, it is gentle on the body — no violent jerks or strains, no jolting or jarring to the skeleton. Best of all, you can do it at home in front of the late-night movie.

Pelvic congestion is greatly relieved by this kind of exercise. I recommend it heartily to all those suffering from hormonal disturbances or infertility.

There are some extremely good (if rather expensive) rebounders available. If these are beyond your means, it is possible to buy a cheaper version that will work well for you if you take care to check that your rebounder has a *good, firm bounce*. Not so soggy that you dip down to the floor, and not so sharp that you hit the ceiling. This good, firm bounce will only stay this way if the rebounder has the *correct spring construction*.

If the springs are arranged *radially*, all the strain is taken through the middle of the mat and it will sag very quickly (see the first diagram). If they are arranged as shown in the second diagram, your bounce will stay firm, your rebounder should remain serviceable, and all you will need to worry about (in the cheaper versions), is taping over splits in the plastic cover and screwing the legs back on.

Other ways to relieve congestion include the following.

Trampoline Spring Construction to Avoid

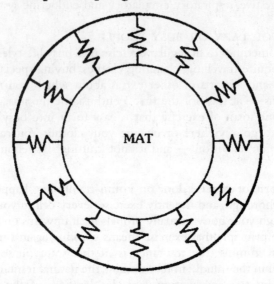

Trampoline Spring Construction to Choose

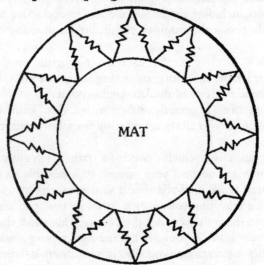

Massage and osteopathy

Deep-tissue massage and the soft-tissue stretching techniques and skeletal adjustments of osteopathy can relieve pain and congestion enormously, help to drain and detoxify the pelvic area, and increase blood and nerve supply to the ovaries. This should be carried out by professionals, but massage is helpful even when it is done by complete novices (your family and friends, for example). Yoga will help to stretch tight muscles.

Homoeopathy

Homoeopathic remedies can be very deeply effective in nearly all physical and emotional conditions. It's almost impossible to use self-help homoeopathy as the exact, single remedy needs to be found for each individual case, taking all aspects of health into consideration.

Acupuncture

Nor am I going to suggest that you put needles into yourself! However, acupressure, where finger pressure is used instead of needles, is easily adapted to home use. Hand-held machines which give a small electric buzz are also available. Some of these machines will even find the right spot for you.

The principle behind acupuncture is that health-giving energy — *chi*, or life force — flows through the body on certain pathways. It is the blocking of this energy which causes disease and distress.

When the energy is blocked at particular points, it affects specific organs and systems. Puncturing, pressing, using electrical charges, laser or ultrasound on these points can liberate the flow of energy and restore health. Some helpful tips will be given for specific conditions.

Relaxation

Whether you use creative imagery, affirmations, meditation or hypnotherapy, relaxation and stress management are essential for any health program. Using autosuggestion (self-hypnosis) can effectively regulate the body's responses.

Use the full body relaxation outlined in Chapter 8 and add to the visualisation of a healthy reproductive system the specific needs that you feel you have to fulfil. Then affirm, verbally, that this will be the case. Your belief systems affect your body and the way it works, and your capacity to change bad habits for good.

Affirmations can be most effective if said out loud to yourself while you look in a mirror and make eye contact with yourself. Then, if you don't believe what you're saying, you'll feel really silly!

Good nutrition and exercise also help to reduce stress, though stress in itself is not necessarily a bad thing. It's just a problem when there is too much of it around and/or you're not dealing with it very well. Stress affects your use and absorption of nutrients, and too much activity in the adrenal glands will interfere with the normal balance of your hormones.

It's natural to be healthy

It is difficult to believe that women could have evolved in such a way as to be endlessly plagued by our hormones. I can only suppose that we should change the common response 'It's your hormones', to 'It's your lifestyle'.

Although severe conditions and disease must be referred to your health practitioner, there is a great deal that you can do to help yourself. Indeed, for many conditions, there won't be a great deal that can be done for you by anyone else unless you are prepared to take responsibility for making a few changes.

In whatever ways you choose to look after your hormonal and reproductive health, don't forget to include regular Pap smears and breast examinations.

Once you find out how wonderful you feel without the supposedly inevitable ups and downs in your health and well-being, the changes will become permanent.

Premenstrual syndrome (PMS)

Perhaps the most insidious condition of all, PMS is a term that covers a multitude of sins. The emotional swings (premenstrual tension, or PMT) and the physical discomforts can be extreme. Sometimes the woman herself doesn't even realise how bad it is.

Often, when in consultation with a couple, after asking a woman about her symptoms, I will turn to her partner. 'Bit cranky, is she?' This question releases a veritable flood of acknowledgment. The woman herself is often quite surprised.

The trouble is, when we are cranky, irritable and tense, it's often the external things that we get irritated with, that we blame. This is where regular charting and growing awareness of patterns come in useful. Your relationship doesn't have to fall apart once a month any longer because you realise what is happening and do something about it.

PMT is only part of the whole syndrome. You may suffer from any or all of the following symptoms during the week or so prior to your period, usually with substantial and immediate relief as you start to bleed. However, for some women, the problems continue into the first days of the next cycle.

Tension	Abdominal bloating
Anxiety	Swelling of hands, feet, legs and face
Reduced concentration	Sore, swollen or lumpy breasts
Tearfulness	Backache
Aggression and anger	Pelvic pain
Depression	Aching legs
Listlessness	Ovarian pain
Confusion	Sweating
Fatigue	Hot flushes
Insomnia	Bladder problems
Headache, seeing spots	Constipation

Excessive weight gain	Diarrhoea
Fluid retention	Nausea
Low blood–sugar	Bruising
Sugar and chocolate cravings	Muscular tenderness
Food cravings	Joint tenderness
Increased appetite	Blood spotting
Thirst	Increased allergic response
Itchiness	Increased tendency to arthritis
Greasy skin and hair	Increased tendency to epilepsy
Pimples	Increased tendency to schizophrenia
Heart pounding, palpitations	Increased tendency to infections
Dizziness, fainting	Increased tendency to herpes
Sore eyes	Increased tendency to candida
Decreased libido	Increased tendency to asthma
Highly increased libido (this can be a problem!)	Increased tendency to eczema
Hives	Increased tendency to hay fever

This (incomplete) list covers over fifty symptoms! Their only common feature is that they all get worse cyclically.

If you are practising natural methods of contraception, all of this is doubly bad news, as it comes during the post-ovulatory phase when you can be much more certain of your infertility and could be practising protection-free love-making. Suffering from a range of these symptoms is unlikely to make you feel very sexy.

The range of symptoms experienced varies from woman to woman: the individual hormonal imbalances interact with unique personalities, metabolisms and circumstances.

The imbalance is usually of too little progesterone, and is critically linked with the production of prostaglandins, which, in its turn, is linked with the availability of certain nutrients.

Your efforts to overcome PMS need to reflect this. As well as using self-help techniques to relieve the symptoms, you need to address the underlying cause, which is not, as Hippocrates thought, a wandering uterus, somehow disturbing the brain on its journey around the body. So you don't need to burn incense at your vaginal opening to entice it back! (He suggested you did.)

Hormone Levels in a PMS Sufferer

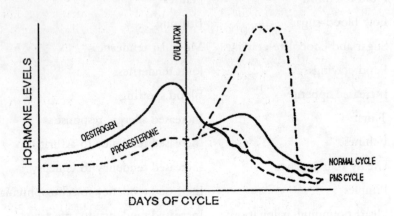

Self-help for PMS

◆ Take a good multivitamin and mineral supplement which fulfils the guidelines laid down earlier.

◆ Vitamin B6 (taken in conjunction with the other B-complex vitamins) is specific for PMS. For dosage guidelines, see the earlier section in this chapter.

◆ Vitamins A, C, and E are also helpful for a number of PMS symptoms.

◆ Calcium and magnesium levels drop premenstrually, but they may be required in greater amounts at this time as deficiencies can result in a broad range of symptoms.

◆ Potassium has also been shown to be effective in preventing PMS symptoms.

◆ Take *Evening Primrose* oil supplements (some come with marine fish oil which is also helpful).

◆ *Kelp* and *Garlic* supplements can be useful (candida sufferers will need plenty; take care with *Garlic* if you are hypoglycaemic).

◆ Eat well throughout your cycle, but pay special attention to your diet as soon as ovulation is over. Focus particularly on green leafy vegetables, lentils, nuts, seeds and fish.

◆ Avoid all saturated fats, cut out sugar and all its substitutes, alcohol, white flour and salt. Salt increases water retention, alcohol increases your need for vitamins B1 and D, calcium, magnesium and zinc, white flour leaches nutrients.

◆ Don't smoke, and keep tea and coffee to a minimum. Tea restricts iron and zinc absorption; coffee does too, and is linked with all inflammatory conditions and breast problems. Both also act as diuretics, and with increased urination you lose minerals. This is not a problem with herbal diuretics, which contain minerals. Water retention is not helped as you will want to drink more. Add to this their disturbing effect on anxiety states (coffee and tea are both stimulants) and you'll be better off drinking herbal teas and *Dandelion* coffee (see list of helpful herbs at the end of this section).

◆ Exercise daily for at least 20 minutes to get circulation to the ovaries and womb. Try rebounding.

◆ If you suffer from premenstrual headaches, this may be because your liver is under stress as a result of having a load of oestrogen to remove. If you have other liverish symptoms such as nausea or diarrhoea, try the herb *Fringetree*, a herb. If fluid retention seems to be the problem, vitamin B$_6$ and the diuretic herbs may be more helpful. If it's simply related to stress, nervine herbs such as *Wood Betony* are specific remedies.

◆ Tender, swollen or lumpy breasts will respond to the hormone balancing and diuretic herbs listed at the end of this section, as well as to the essential fatty acids, vitamins B$_6$ and E, magnesium and selenium. Another useful herb is *Poke Root*, but only take this in dosages recommended by your herbalist as it can be toxic if you overdose. Caffeine increases breast problems and should be avoided. Persistent breast problems can be the result of a hypothyroid condition. This can be alleviated by making organic seaweed a regular addition to your diet.

◆ If you have bowel problems during or before menstruation, it may be your liver again, or it could be prostaglandin disturbance (see the list at end of this section for herbal remedies).

◆ If you are really tense, anxious and irritable or can't sleep, try the nervine or hormone balancing herbs listed or calcium and magnesium in hourly doses (the cell salts calcium phosphate and magnesium phosphate are best for this). These minerals will also help to relieve pelvic pain or headache.

◆ If calcium and magnesium aren't sufficient for pain relief, try increasing your doses of essential fatty acids (*Evening Primrose* and deep-sea fish oils).

◆ If nausea bothers you, the liver herbs may help (see the list at end of this section), or you can try *Ginger* tea.

◆ If you suffer low blood-sugar levels at this time, with fatigue and a desire for food (particularly sweets), try eating small amounts of nutritious, high-energy foods fairly frequently. Almonds and other nuts, proteins and complex carbohydrates are the best. Chromium, manganese, magnesium and zinc are important nutrients for this condition. You will know if your magnesium levels are low as you will tend to crave chocolate. However, though magnesium is plentiful in chocolate, it's not a recommended source!

◆ Also, avoid sugar completely as it increases your excretion of chromium (thus reducing your tolerance for sugar); it also uses up your zinc and B vitamins.

◆ Since lowered blood-sugar levels lead to allergenic activity and lowered resistance to infection, take extra care at this time not to expose yourself to allergens and pathogens (substances of which you are intolerant — allergens, and viral or bacterial organisms — pathogens).

◆ All PMS sufferers would do well to check on their allergy status. The most common allergies are to cow's milk, wheat, gluten, yeast and house-dust mites. Try removing these from your diet or environment and see how much difference it makes.

◆ Yeast is thought to stimulate oestrogenic activity and may make PMS worse (and you may easily have an allergic reaction to it).

◆ If oestrogen is excessive, eat plants containing phyto-oestrogens (see Menopause section later in this chapter) for their balancing effect and avoid non-organic animal foods. If hypothyroid, avoid the cabbage family and soya foods.

◆ Practise massage, yoga, relaxation, meditation or self-hypnosis to encourage helpful habits and a peaceful mind.

◆ Seek therapy or help for any underlying emotional problems which may only surface at this time.

◆ Give yourself a break. If it is possible for you, use this time for the less strenuous, less externally demanding activities. Allow your energies to become more inward, and quieter. Don't have expectations of yourself that are unrealistic and unconnected to your cyclical nature.

◆ Acupressure can be useful for many symptoms of PMS. The following points can be used as self-help as often as you need. Press with thumbs or fingers. Breathe easily and hold while you become used to the pressure, then increase it. If you increase the pressure about three times, you will find you can press fairly hard without tensing up and resisting.

SOME USEFUL ACUPRESSURE POINTS
Kidney 27 — this is a specific pressure point for PMS which is situated in the hollows just below the collar bone, in line with the outer edges of the neck.

Finding Kidney 27

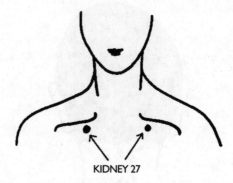

Good headache points are

Colon 4 — on the outside of the hand, at the joint between the thumb and the first finger, right down in the V, between the bones. This point is often very sore, so increase the pressure slowly. It will also relax the uterus.

Finding Colon 4

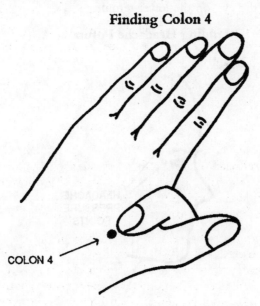

Bladder 10 — right under the base of your skull, on either side of your spine, pressing up.

Finding Bladder 10

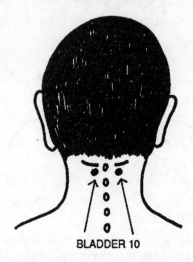

BLADDER 10

Two more — on the upper temple, in the slight depression, and next to the outer corner of the eye, on the lower temple.

Finding Headache Points

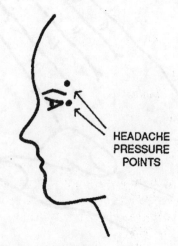

HEADACHE
PRESSURE
POINTS

SOME USEFUL HERBAL REMEDIES

Herbal remedies can also be extremely useful at this time. The herbal remedy of choice is *Chastetree* (botanical name *Vitex agnus castus*). The berries of this plant can be made into an infusion (see earlier instructions). This herb is a tonic for the pituitary gland and the ovaries and helps to balance the hormones, particularly in favour of progesterone. It can be extremely effective.

A more comprehensive herbal formula might include a liver drainage and detoxifying herb to help remove waste oestrogen, and various herbs to address specific symptoms, such as fluid retention and nervousness. Here is a list of herbs you may find useful.

Hormone balancing herbs
Chastetree, Peony, Sarsaparilla, Wild Yam.

Liver herbs
Dandelion Root, Fringetree.

Diuretic herbs
Dandelion Leaf, Juniper Berries, Uva Ursi (Bearberry), Parsley, Horseradish, Buchu.

Nervine herbs (for anxiety and irritability)
Kava, Chamomile, Skullcap, Valerian.

Nervine herbs (for sleeplessness)
Passiflora, Hops, Chamomile.

Herbs for depression and fatigue
Damiana, Oats, Gotu Kola, Ginseng, St John's Wort, Withania.

Herbs for headaches
Fringetree, Wood Betony, Valerian, Pulsatilla, Feverfew, Skullcap.

Herbs for nausea
Ginger, Black Horehound.

Herbs for sore breasts
Blue Flag, Poke Root (use only under professional supervision), Thuja (pronounced thoo-yah).

Anti-prostaglandin herbs
Feverfew, Ginger, Evening Primrose.

Herbs for pelvic congestion
(see Dysmenorrhoea)

Dysmenorrhoea

This disorder, whose name means 'painful periods', is often thought of as normal and part and parcel of being a woman. Most women are much too ready to accept that view, even though the extent and frequency of the problem may be quite disabling.

Although it may be quite *usual* to have to take a day off work and retire to bed with a hot water bottle and a packet of prescription drugs, it is not *normal*. If your period pain does not respond to the suggestions outlined in this section, it may be due to some underlying disease state and should be investigated.

Dysmenorrhoea can be divided into two distinct types. Congestive dysmenorrhoea tends to be associated with the premenstrual syndrome, and is often worse before menstruation. The pain is a dull, heavy and dragging ache, and is usually associated with other congestive symptoms such as fluid retention.

Spasmodic dysmenorrhoea refers to the sharp, cramping pains that start with bleeding. This is often also associated with hormonal, prostaglandin and nutrient imbalances or, occasionally, can be to do with a tight or obstructed cervix, especially in younger or childless women or adolescents, who are the typical sufferers of this type of period pain.

It is quite possible to suffer from both types of dysmenorrhoea. If you experience the congestive type, use the suggestions in the previous section, 'Premenstrual Syndrome'. In this section, we will be looking at remedies for the spasmodic type.

First, you should establish that you are not miscarrying. Then you need to rule out any underlying condition that may be causing or exacerbating the pain and distress.

POSSIBLE ASSOCIATED DISEASES

Endometriosis — In this condition, parts of the endometrium (lining of the womb) migrate into the pelvic cavity, where they may attach to the outside of the womb or other organs and bleed when you are menstruating. This blood cannot escape and results in adhesions to the various organs. A variation on this condition is called *adenomyosis*, in which the endometrial tissue starts to grow within the muscular uterine wall.

PID — Pelvic inflammatory disease (PID) results from infections in the reproductive system caused by genito-urinary infections (GUIs) which can include sexually transmitted diseases (STDs), an IUD, a termination or other abdominal operation.

Ovarian cysts — There are a lot of different types of ovarian cysts; some are more serious than others. Some are formed as the follicle expands at ovulation; this kind will resolve quite naturally. If pain occurs at times other than at ovulation or menstruation, is one-sided or severe, treatment may be necessary.

Uterine fibroids — These can grow very large, but are usually not too serious unless they are in a certain spot which prevents embryo implantation, or are causing severe dysmenorrhoea or excessive bleeding.

If there is an underlying condition such as one of these, then the dysmenorrhoea is called 'secondary'. It will not improve until you have dealt with the associated disease. Natural remedies can be successful, although it's best to consult your practitioner rather than attempt self-help.

Secondary dysmenorrhoea is characterised by pain that often occurs at other times in the cycle, starts before bleeding begins, or worsens towards the end of the period. It may also continually worsen from cycle to cycle. There may be pain on intercourse, fever and other symptoms. However, the pain is not necessarily extreme, and can often be less intense than that caused by hormonal, nutrient and prostaglandin imbalances.

If the dysmenorrhoea is 'primary' (that is, not a result of some other condition), then the cause is usually a result of nutrient deficiencies leading to the familiar imbalances in essential fatty acids and saturated fats, prostaglandins and hormones.

Potassium, magnesium and calcium are all minerals which are needed in good supply for the contraction of muscles. A lack of any of these will cause irritability of the muscles and cause problems once the uterus starts to contract to dispel the blood.

Evening Primrose oil or other sources of the essential fatty acids will help to alleviate the imbalance of prostaglandins commonly found in those who suffer severe cramping.

Vitamins A, B-complex (especially B$_6$), C and E levels should be maintained (see the earlier section on diet).

All of these supplements, if they are not being taken on a regular basis, should be used for at least 1 and preferably 2 weeks before menstruation. It may be preferable to take them throughout the cycle.

Herbal remedies should also be taken *before your period starts* and, in the case of hormonally balancing herbs, may have a progressive effect over several cycles.

SOME USEFUL HERBAL REMEDIES
Antispasmodic herbs
Black Cohosh, Blue Cohosh (especially for cervical pain with scanty flow), Tansy, Black Haw, Cramp Bark, Wild Yam, Dong Quai, Peony.

Pain-relieving herbs
Pulsatilla, Corydalis.

Anti-prostaglandin herbs
Ginger, Feverfew, Turmeric, Tansy.

Circulatory stimulants (for easy release of blood)
Ginger, Cayenne, Mugwort, Yarrow, Ginkgo, Cinnamon, Tansy (these herbs are also warming).

Organ remedy herbs (to tone uterus)
Raspberry, False Unicorn Root, True Unicorn Root, Blue Cohosh, Squaw Vine, Dong Quai (this herb may be contraindicated if flow already profuse).

Hormone balancing herbs
Chastetree, False Unicorn Root, Saw Palmetto, Sarsaparilla, Dong Quai, Peony.

Relaxing herbs (nervines)
Valerian, Vervain, Skullcap, Motherwort.

Astringent herbs (for heavy flow or pelvic congestion)
Squaw Vine, Raspberry, Ladies' Mantle, Witch Hazel.

Laxative herbs (not for regular use)
Rhubarb, Cascara, Senna.

Some of the herbs mentioned here (for example, *Ginger* and *Feverfew*) counteract the troublesome prostaglandins. Others, such as *White Willow Bark* and *White Poplar*, contain high levels of natural salicylates which, in their pharmaceutical form (aspirin), also have this effect. Although these herbs are often sold as natural pain killers, they are not usually sufficiently concentrated to have much effect.

SELF-HELP PAIN RELIEVERS

If you do experience cramping in spite of preventative measures, there are several self-help techniques to alleviate pain.

◆ You can try taking calcium and magnesium supplements (twice as much calcium as magnesium), every hour or two as soon as cramping starts. The most easily absorbed and fastest-acting supplements are the cell or tissue salts, calcium phosphate and magnesium phosphate.

◆ Avoid saturated (animal and heated) fats, coffee, alcohol and added salt. Eat fish, cold-pressed oils (for essential fatty acids) and plenty of fibre. If your pain responds to heat treatments, avoid too much cold food. Fruits high in bioflavonoids, such as berries, can help reduce pelvic congestion or a heavy flow.

◆ You can try heat — a hot-water bottle on your tummy or back, or a hot bath. There is a brand of briefs called 'Warm-ease' which have heat-retaining inserts for use through the day; they are sold through some pharmacies. Some of the herbs listed above are also warming in their action.

◆ Get adequate aerobic exercise.

◆ You can try having osteopathic treatment of the lower back to ease congestion.

◆ Any local massage will relieve pain and stimulate circulation and easy blood flow, particularly massage over the womb itself, over the lower back and down the legs. Head, neck and shoulders are good areas to massage for relieving headaches, particularly if you concentrate on the base of the skull and areas on the scalp where there are sore spots. If you can't find a willing masseur, do it yourself.

◆ Make sure you are not constipated around the time of your period; this will increase your symptoms. Eat 2–3 pieces of fruit daily and drink plenty of fluids. Half a lemon squeezed into a glass of warm water and drunk before breakfast is an effective remedy. Fibre supplements, such as psyllium husks, may be helpful, and *Slippery Elm* or acidophilus powders will keep the gut healthy. Bitter herbs and those which affect the liver can be useful, though laxative herbs (see above) should not be used too frequently.

◆ Switch from tampons to pads (the reusable cotton variety if synthetic give you thrush; see Appendix 2, 'Contacts and Resources') and wear loose clothing.

◆ Aromatherapy can be very helpful. Essential oils such as *Clary Sage* and *Lavender*, can be added to your bath or massage oil.

◆ Try relaxation therapy with specific affirmations or visualisations, or soothing music.

◆ Pressure points can be included in a massage. For cramping, try these points. Increase pressure gradually to reduce your tensing reaction. Breathe gently and rhythmically.

SOME USEFUL ACUPRESSURE POINTS

Spleen 6 — four finger widths (the fourth finger finds the spot) above the interior ankle bone, behind the leg bone.

Colon 4 — (see PMS) is also helpful for headaches.
  Do not use these two points if you are, or may be, pregnant.

Finding Spleen 6

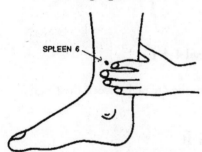

SPLEEN 6

Finding Spleen 10

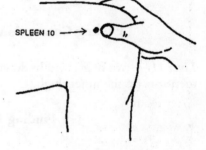

SPLEEN 10

Spleen 10 — bend your leg at a 90° angle. Place the fingers of your opposite hand along the front of the kneecap, and stretch the thumb backwards towards your groin. The tip of your thumb will be on Spleen 10, three finger widths above your knee.

Conception Vessel 4 — on the midline, slightly below the halfway mark between your navel and your pubic bone.

Conception Vessel 6 — halfway between Conception Vessel 4 and your navel.
  Do not use conception vessel points if you are, or may be, pregnant.

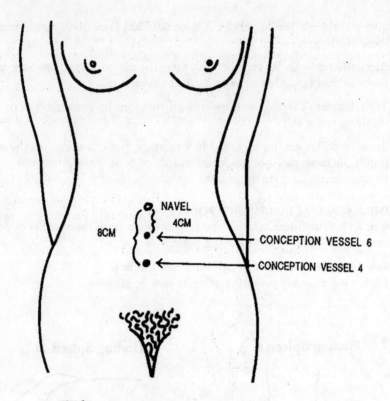

NAVEL

4CM

8CM

CONCEPTION VESSEL 6

CONCEPTION VESSEL 4

Finding Conception Vessel 4 + 6

Liver 11 — two finger widths down from the crease between the thigh and the torso, on the inner thigh.

Finding Liver 11

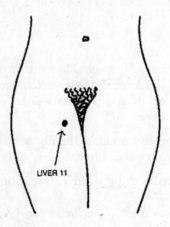

LIVER 11

The points on the bladder meridian, which runs down either side of the spine, can be pressed all down the lower-back region while you lie on your front as some (kind) person gives you a massage. The best way to persuade someone to massage you is to massage them first. Then, while they are glowing with pleasure, you undertake to do this for them regularly, *as long as they return the treat(ment)*.

Acupuncture (from a qualified practitioner) can often succeed if self-help fails.

SOME USEFUL YOGA POSITIONS

Yoga is a tried-and-true method for relieving period pain. Lie on your back, bring your knees to your chest, grab them with your arms and raise the head; both legs separately and then together. Hold for a count of ten each time and then release.

Yoga Position for Period Pain

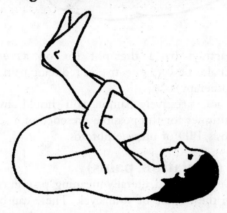

Cobra (to stretch the muscles in the lower back) — Lie face down, with your hands flat on the floor next to your shoulders, and gradually raise your head and chest without using your arms. Then, pressing on the floor with your hands, continue to arch your back and bend your head back as far as possible. You should be aware of your shoulders moving down and back.

Cobra

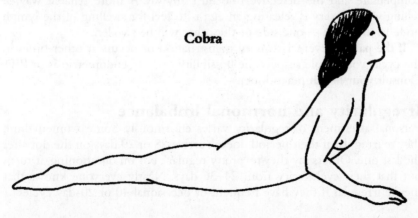

Bow *(to relieve uterine cramps)* — Still lying face down, bend your knees, grab your ankles with your hands, pull your legs towards your head, then release and relax. It's important to be aware of extending and arching your spine while in this position. While holding your breath in this pose, you can try rocking backwards and forwards.

Bow

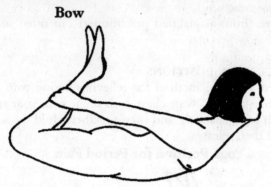

Hypnotherapy practised by a therapist (or on a recording, or by autosuggestion) can also be very effective in reducing pain (see Chapter 10 for more on hypnotherapy).

If your periods are excessively painful, you should always check with your medical practitioner for the possible presence of a serious condition such as endometriosis, PID or uterine fibroids.

Mittelschmerz (ovulation pains)

Mittleschmerz is a German word, literally meaning 'pain in the middle' — in *your* middle, and in the middle of your cycle. These can be sharp, twangy pains felt over a short time such as a few minutes, but they can also last longer and be quite severe.

The pain is usually felt on one side or the other, often alternating because the ovaries generally take turns to release an egg. It can be one way of telling which ovary is active, although if one is defective, the other may compensate and the defective one hurt anyway. A more reliable way of telling which ovary is releasing an egg is to feel for swelling of the lymph node in the groin —one side or the other will be swollen.

If the pain is severe, lasts until menstruation or occurs at other times in the cycle, you should suspect the possibility of cysts, endometriosis or PID. Consult your health practitioner.

Irregularity and hormonal imbalance

Personal assessment of regularity varies enormously. Some women think they're irregular if their period doesn't arrive 28 or 29 days on the dot after the last one. Others say they're 'pretty regular', but on questioning, it turns out that their cycles vary from 24–36 days. Nearly everyone knows that they're irregular if they have frequent or occasional 40 or 20-day cycles.

So, let's define irregularity.

The 'norm' is a cycle of 29 and a half days duration, the length of a lunar month. This is an average-length cycle, as opposed to the 28 days (4 weeks, or a lunar orbit) that is generally accepted.

Variations of a few days either side of this are really not a huge problem, although it may make it difficult for your lunar and hormonal cycles to synchronise.

Irregularity due to external circumstances such as stress, travel across time zones, ill health, diet and dramatic weight changes, fasting or drugs (medical or recreational) is something you should be able to assess easily enough.

External stimuli will usually extend your cycle (that is, delay ovulation) rather than shorten it (with the exception of breastfeeding).

If your cycle varies by more than a few days each month, or you occasionally have very long or very short cycles which do not coincide with any of the abovementioned circumstances, it may well be due to hormonal imbalance.

This can result from past use of the Pill (see the appropriate sections in Chapters 2 and 11, and later in this chapter). Hormonal imbalance can also result from eating disorders, malnutrition (you don't have to be starving to suffer from malnutrition; see nutrition advice in the previous chapter), low levels of healthy gut flora, fasting, diseases of the endocrine system, excessive exercise, toxic overload (especially from heavy metals or chemicals with hormonal effects) and medication, among other possibilities.

It can result in lack of ovulation, amenorrhoea, irregularity, problems with the length of the pre-ovulatory and post-ovulatory phases, problems maintaining a pregnancy, lack of cervical mucus and more.

The problem may lie with

♦ the corpus luteum

♦ the ovaries (which may be cystic, or suffering from polycystic ovarian syndrome, premature failure or menopause)

♦ the pituitary (which may be overactive, producing prolactin and inhibiting ovulation, and also inappropriately stimulating milk supply, a condition which can be a result of vitamin B6 deficiency).

♦ the thyroid (which may be underactive and cause amenorrhoea)

♦ the hypothalamus (which can become underactive, commonly as a result of eating disorders, obesity or underweight, excessive exercise, use of the Pill, some drugs and depression).

Medical treatment is with drugs and/or surgery (for example, in the case of ovarian cysts). Some of the drugs can have quite severe side-effects and their tendency is not to cure the problem, merely to stimulate temporary activity, often resulting in your own body's manufacture of hormones being further disrupted. If you conceive while on these medications, any pregnancy that ensues may then progress with the disorder intact (or aggravated).

Natural and holistic therapies are designed to improve the natural functioning of the glands themselves, rather than relying on the drug for the effect. If the cause is known, the treatment used may be more specific.

Let's get rid of one myth. *It's not possible to miss a period.* Your menstrual bleeding is a direct result of having ovulated, and should occur about 2 weeks later. If you have a cycle that appears to be twice as long as usual, your ovulation has, for some reason, been delayed by approximately the same length of time that your whole cycle normally takes.

In order to treat irregularity, the ovarian and pituitary functions are the ones that need to be stimulated and corrected, allowing for the whole endocrine system and the factors which affect it.

It is really no good inducing a period if you're overdue (*always have a pregnancy test first*); it's more likely the ovulation that was late. You should be aware of this if you have been charting your temperature. Occasionally, the bleeding may be delayed, but we'll look at that shortly, in a section on amenorrhoea (lack of menstruation), below.

Once again, diet, supplements and exercise are of key importance; you can also use acupuncture, homoeopathy and herbal remedies to bring some correction.

Remedies that are useful here include:

Hormone balancing herbs

Chastetree, Peony (to increase progesterone relative to oestrogen), *False Unicorn Root, Dong Quai, Shatavari* (to increase oestrogen relative to progesterone), *Saw Palmetto* (if ovaries are underfunctioning, and hormone levels generally low), and *Pulsatilla* (which can shorten an overlong pre-ovulatory phase if taken from menstruation to ovulation). *Squaw Vine, Liquorice* and *Sarsaparilla* may also be helpful, as may the phyto-oestrogenic herbs and foods (see Menopause section) which balance excessive or deficient oestrogen levels.

Liver herbs

Herbs such as *Dandelion* and *St Mary's Thistle* will help if a delayed ovulation is due to a build-up of old oestrogen.

Herbs to help the endocrine system

Chastetree for the pituitary, *Blue Flag, Bladderwrack (Kelp)* and *Poke Root* (not to be taken except under professional supervision) for the thyroid.

Nutrients for hormone balance

These include

◆ zinc, magnesium and vitamin C for general hormone production

◆ vitamin B_6 (with B-complex) to boost progesterone (up to 200 mg is very safe) or reduce excessive prolactin levels (up to 500 mg may be required, but only with professional supervision)

◆ vitamin E to regulate oestrogen production.

To get a clearer diagnosis of the relative balance of oestrogen and progesterone and possible deficiencies, your mucus (governed by oestrogen) and temperature (governed by progesterone) readings should be most helpful. A trained Natural Fertility Management practitioner would be able to help you interpret the charts more accurately. Excessive oestrogen levels are often the result of oestrogen-like substances in the food and water supply and the environment. Hormonally treated animal foods, the urine from these animals and from women on the oral contraceptive pill (which contaminates the water supply), plastics, plastic food wraps are all a problem — the list is endless.

Acupressure

Conception vessel 4 and *Spleen 6* are useful acupressure points. If your cycles tend to be short, add *Spleen 10* (see 'Dysmenorrhoea', above, for these three points). If your cycles tend to be long, add *Stomach 36*.

Stomach 36 — measure four finger widths below the knee, on the outside of the tibia.

Finding Stomach 36

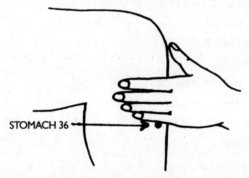

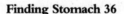

STOMACH 36

It is also possible to influence the regularity of your cycle through suggestion, just as, in Chapter 8, we looked at how you can bring it into synchronisation with your lunar cycle. This, if it works for you, will automatically make your cycles regular on an average 29 and a half day interval.

If your irregularity involves short cycles, it's important to find out (through charting your temperature) if it's the pre-ovulatory or post-ovulatory phase that is contracted. If the defect is after ovulation and the luteal phase is less than 12 days, there is not enough progesterone being produced. If it is less than 10 days, the cycle is infertile. This can often be corrected by nutritional supplementation, especially with high doses of vitamin B_6, and the herb *Chastetree*. If the defect is before ovulation, you need to boost your oestrogen levels. This may show as reduced amounts of cervical mucus.

If irregularity involves long cycles and this extends into several months, you can now consider yourself to be suffering from amenorrhoea.

Amenorrhoea

This term means a lack of menstruation (for more than 6 months). If you haven't had a period for that long, you are also suffering from a lack of ovulation, which is more to the point.

Amenorrhoea is called 'primary' if you have never had a period and are over 17, or 2 years past the time when other signs of puberty manifested. It is called 'secondary' if you previously had a (fairly) regular cycle. Occasionally, amenorrhoea is a result of blockage of the cervix, uterus or vagina, which could result from adhesions caused by infections or surgery, congenital abnormalities or other disorders of the uterus. Usually, the cause will be a lack of ovulation (you can check if you have ovulated or not by taking your temperature). Once the underlying cause is determined, it can be treated accordingly. Once in a while the emmenagogue herbs (which promote menstrual flow) may be helpful to kick-start the cycle.

First, you must have a pregnancy test. Then, you need to assess whether you could be menopausal (presumably you're not on the Pill). All of these could be reasons why you are not ovulating or menstruating.

Other reasons could include

    post–Pill sterility

    excessive exercise

    low body fat

    dramatic weight loss/gain

    fasting

    anorexia

    malnutrition

    anaemia

    too much raw food (not enough cooked food)

    breastfeeding

    premature menopause

    stress

    drugs (such as tranquillisers and narcotics)

    disorders of the circulation

    illness

    severe infection

    PID/GUIs/STDs

    chronic kidney or liver disease

    endocrine dysfunction (in pituitary, adrenal and hypothalamus)

    hyperprolactinaemia (raised prolactin levels)

hypothyroidism (underactive thyroid)

polycystic ovarian syndrome

ovarian cysts (including endometriomas)

endometriosis

ovarian cancer

some autoimmune disease

Remember — nutrition, supplements and exercise again! See the earlier section for dosages of nutrients.

Levels of vitamin B$_6$ may need to be higher if the reason for lack of ovulation is high levels of prolactin generated by a dysfunctional (overactive) pituitary gland. (This is how ovulation is suppressed during breastfeeding.) The dosage can be determined by the level required to alleviate PMS symptoms. Useful herbs are *Chastetree*, *Liquorice* and *Peony*.

Weight can be crucial. Too little body fat can lead to low levels of oestrogen, too much can contribute to polycystic ovarian syndrome (PCOS), another major cause of ovarian dysfunction and hormone imbalance.

Other useful remedies include the following.

Hormone balancers/uterine tonics
Chastetree, False Unicorn Root, Blue Cohosh, Dong Quai, Wild Yam, Sarsaparilla, Saw Palmetto, Liquorice, Peony.

Emmenagogues/circulatory normalisers
Mugwort, Ginger, Yarrow, Prickly Ash.

For emotional trauma
Pulsatilla, Valerian.

Acupressure points include *Spleen 6* and *Spleen 10*.

If your periods have not actually ceased but are so light as to be virtually non-existent, treat similarly, with the accent on herbs that boost oestrogen, such as *Dong Quai, False Unicorn Root* and the circulatory stimulant herbs. Sometimes light bleeds are not true periods, and no ovulation has occurred. This will show on your temperature graphs.

If amenorrhoea does not respond to treatment, you should see a health practitioner.

If your periods are *too profuse*, you are suffering from menorrhagia.

Menorrhagia
Menorrhagia, or dysfunctional menstrual bleeding, is a term which refers to periods that are too profuse, or occur excessively often.
The causes could be

miscarriage

uterine cancer

uterine fibroids

polyps

endometriosis

PID

IUD

cervical abnormalities

ovarian cysts

underactive thyroid

liver dysfunction

ectopic pregnancy

spontaneous abortion

pelvic circulatory congestion

capillary fragility

blood disorders

severe hormonal imbalance

malnutrition

Whatever the cause, excessive bleeding can lead to anaemia. Ironically, low iron status can itself be a cause of excessive bleeding and clotting (although it can also inhibit the menstrual flow). Other nutritional deficiencies which can contribute to this condition are low levels of vitamin A and the bioflavonoids.

If the cause is any of the more severe of these conditions, follow the guidance of your health practitioner. However, before you accept any drastic solution to this problem (and some medical 'solutions' include long-term hormone therapy and hysterectomy), make sure that your bleeding pattern is excessive. Subjective assessments vary enormously.

It would be best to first attempt the methods outlined in this book. If your dietary habits have been such as to create a severe hormonal imbalance, it may be necessary to give yourself a head start by going on a fast before commencing healthier eating habits.

If you fast, it must be under the guidance of a qualified practitioner.

The hormone-balancing herbs (especially those favouring progesterone — see the section on 'Irregularity'), and phyto-oestrogenic herbs and foods (see Menopause section) would be indicated here, and acupuncture can be helpful.

OTHER HELPFUL HERBS

If you suspect anaemia, capillary fragility and associated vascular deficiencies, then take vitamin C and the bioflavonoids in large doses, and

◆ *Parsley*

◆ *Lime Flowers*

◆ *Buckwheat*

◆ *Yarrow.*

If it's due to pelvic congestion, try rebounding, massage, osteopathic adjustments and

◆ *Cayenne*

◆ *Blue Cohosh*

◆ *Ginger*

◆ *Ginkgo.*

For underactive thyroid, try *Kelp* (a good source of iodine) and

◆ *Coleus*

◆ *Poke Root* (see warning below).

For liver problems, fast on juices 1 day a week, stay off all alcohol and drugs, and try

◆ *Dandelion*

◆ *Celandine*

◆ *St Mary's Thistle*

◆ *Bupleurum.*

In order to check the bleeding, use haemostatic and astringent herbs. Try

◆ *Shepherd's Purse*

◆ *Raspberry*

◆ *Beth Root*

◆ *Periwinkle*

◆ *Ladies' Mantle*

◆ *Black Haw*

◆ *Cranesbill*

◆ *Squaw Vine.*

And to tone the uterus, try the organ remedies, such as

◆ *Cramp Bark*

◆ *Blue Cohosh*

◆ *False Unicorn Root*

◆ *True Unicorn Root.*

Normalise the circulation with

◆ *Ginger*

◆ *Yarrow.*

And, if you suspect that the cause is hormonal, as well as the usual balancing herbs, a very effective herb to use is *Poke Root* for excessive or frequent bleeding, but be careful. *Use of this herb needs to be supervised by a practitioner; it can be toxic if you overdose.*

Menopause

Menopause is the complete cessation of menstrual periods, which is experienced by most women these days between the ages of 45 and 55, with an average age being 50. Most women are going through menopause later now (which seems to be connected to an earlier menarche), although there is also an increasing number of women experiencing a premature menopause. Completion of menopause is confirmed after 2 full years of no menstrual activity rather than one, which was the previous standard.

The years leading up to and occurring shortly after the menopause are called the perimenopausal years, during which many of the symptoms described below can start to become apparent. These symptoms can be very distressing, and are really best treated in advance by following the guidelines for hormonal health previously set out.

If you are one of the lucky 25 per cent of women who experience no problems, the likelihood is that you have had the benefit of a healthy lifestyle for some time prior to the onset of menopause.

Many of the problems are associated with low oestrogen levels, which is why many women take oestrogen replacements, known as hormone replacement therapy (HRT). These hormonal drugs also contain chemical progesterone substitutes, as this hormone will also usually be deficient. These hormone supplements are, however, not without their problems, some of them serious and possibly related to some cancers. The problems associated with menopause can also be serious, but there may be better and more natural ways of dealing with them than HRT.

The glands, such as the adrenals, which take over much of the oestrogen production from the less-active ovaries, will not activate to the same extent if your body is already full of artificial hormones.

This means that, having started HRT, there will be problems with stopping. If you are taking it to prevent osteoporosis, you will need to continue forever as, once you stop, there's a reaction period when the bones rapidly lose all the artificially sustained tissue.

Although it is the lack of oestrogen which is the main reason for menopausal problems, oestrogen replacement on its own has been shown to contribute to cancer, particularly of the endometrium. These days, the HRT that's prescribed is usually a mixture of oestrogen and progesterone supplements (except in the cases where there has been a hysterectomy).

Unfortunately, progesterone supplements (progestogens) tend to have some rather unpleasant side-effects, such as bloating, weight gain, breast swelling and tenderness, depression, PMS and bleeding. That's right! You get your periods back! Just when you were ready to move on. Combined HRT may also increase the risk of cardiovascular problems, although it's too early yet to be sure.

HRT is *not* for sufferers of

> diabetes
>
> endometriosis
>
> hyperlipidaemia (high blood fats)
>
> epilepsy
>
> high blood pressure
>
> uterine fibroids
>
> migraine headaches
>
> gallbladder disease
>
> multiple sclerosis
>
> liver disease, *or*
>
> cigarette smokers, *or*
>
> those at risk of breast cancer, which includes anyone who has already had it, or comes into two or more of the following categories:
>
> • close relatives suffering from breast cancer
>
> • periods starting before 12 years of age
>
> • use of the Pill starting in the teens, or for 5 or more years
>
> • no full-term pregnancies
>
> • overweight

Breast cancer risk may increase by up to 50 per cent when HRT is used for more than 10 years, as it does with delayed menopause, but it is really too early to tell what the likely effects will be. Cancer can remain dormant for a long time after the trigger experience, and hormone treatments have been associated with cancers of all the organs in the reproductive system.

Other hormonal imbalances which come with menopause include huge surges of LH and FSH, as the pituitary tries to wake up the increasingly dormant ovaries and stimulate them into action. These surges are associated with hot flushes and other symptoms. Progesterone levels also change, drastically declining.

In order to ease yourself through menopause and to keep producing sufficient amounts of hormones, your diet must be adequate. Hormones, and the substances required to transport them around the body, are made from nutrients. Unless you eat well, you can't expect to create a healthy hormonal environment.

The importance of stress reduction cannot be overemphasised, as the adrenals, if exhausted, will make this time much worse, being less able to take over oestrogen production from the ovaries.

Oestrogen

Oestrogen is important for calcium absorption, and to prevent hot flushes and other symptoms. If your serum levels are low, try supplementing with phyto-oestrogenic foods such as soya beans or soya products such as tofu and tempeh, and herbs such as Red Clover. See the list coming up for more sources.

Progesterone

This hormone may also be deficient during perimenopause and is thought by some authorities to be of equal (or greater) importance to oestrogen. See list of useful remedies coming up.

Calcium

Deficiencies of this mineral contribute to many of the symptoms experienced:

◆ insomnia

◆ nervousness

◆ depression

◆ headaches

◆ irritability

◆ osteoporosis (thinning of bones).

You can see that it is important to eat the calcium-rich foods mentioned earlier (not too much of dairy products if you are sensitive to them), and to take calcium supplements.

Magnesium

This mineral is perhaps even more important than calcium for problems of the skeleton. It's also important for your nervous system. It should be supplemented at half the dose for calcium. See earlier for food sources and supplementation levels.

Vitamin E

This vitamin has proven very helpful in alleviating the hot flushes that beset many at this time, as have vitamin C, selenium and the herbs *Sage*, *Blue Cohosh* and *Motherwort*.

A deficiency in vitamin E has been associated with low bone density. Marked benefits should be seen on a dose of 100–1000 iu daily (depending on need). Vitamin E combined with vitamin C and the bioflavonoids will also help circulation problems. Take care if you have high blood pressure.

Aluminium
This heavy metal contributes to dementia and interferes with mineral absorption, causing bone damage. Avoid aluminium cookware, anti-perspirant sprays and antacids containing aluminium. Use a water purifier.

Evening Primrose oil
Essential fatty acids are important during perimenopause. EPO, fish oils, flaxseed oil and appropriate food sources (see earlier) may help to reduce many symptoms.

Cigarette smoking
Smoking will contribute to osteoporosis, and tends to bring on an early menopause (as can excessive alcohol). IUD and Pill users also tend to cease ovulating earlier. Other causes may be an underactive thyroid or pernicious anaemia (vitamin B_{12} deficiency).

Fats
Because fat cells are instrumental in converting hormones from the adrenal glands into oestrogen, it's important not to be underweight. Avoid saturated fats and keep to the dietary and supplement recommendations previously described. Your needs at this time in your life are very similar to those at any other.

Garlic
Supplements will help to alleviate circulatory disorders, although a high dose is needed — 5000mg daily is recommended.

B vitamins
The B-complex will help to keep energy high; B_6 especially will keep progesterone levels stable.

Boron
A diet high in boron can reduce excretion of calcium, phosphorus and magnesium, thus protecting both the bones and the cardiovascular system. It increases levels of oestrogen (a high-boron diet can double the serum levels) and testosterone (which governs your sex drive), and reduces arthritis and rheumatism. See earlier section for food sources.

Water
Drink 8–12 glasses of purified water daily.

Depression
Depression is a very common menopausal symptom. It can often be relieved by the herbs *St John's Wort* and *Damiana*. Depression may be exacerbated by the events that occur in many women's lives around this time. Children leaving home and the death of parents can bring significant changes to self-image.

Counselling is important here, to help make sure that physiological changes aren't the trigger for wrong decisions and self-defeating attitudes. A positive attitude to life at this time can be all-important.

Welcome the chance to bring to the fore those gifts of yours appropriate to later life. So much time is spent in childbearing and rearing; now you can rejoice in the opportunity to celebrate other aspects of your life.

It's also important to become aware of how to manage your energy, and emotional peaks and troughs, just as you needed to when your body was more cyclic. This should have been good practice for you and helped you to have become more adaptable, a quality that will serve you well during and after menopause.

Learning to do without cycles is one of the changes you will need to make. Learn to tune in to other cycles in your environment — the seasons and the lunar month — to satisfy these needs. Your personal lunar cycle may continue to be relevant for you.

Accepting your age, rejoicing in your accumulated experience and wisdom, and finding an appropriate and useful role to play in society can prove vital for a successful transition at menopause. In China, where until recent times older women were revered, menopausal problems were virtually unknown.

Exercise regularly, especially favouring weight-bearing exercise. Steady exercise, such as walking, is ideal. Rebounding and yoga are also excellent.

A full list of the possible symptoms of menopause may be a little daunting, but given that you have many ways of dealing with them, here goes.

> Menstrual irregularity
>
> Flushing and sweats
>
> Chills
>
> Pins and needles
>
> Lethargy
>
> Nervous problems (anxiety, depression, irritability)
>
> Palpitations
>
> Dizziness
>
> Insomnia
>
> Poor memory
>
> Lack of concentration
>
> Headaches
>
> Joint pains
>
> Osteoporosis
>
> Atherosclerosis
>
> Hair and skin changes
>
> Weight gain
>
> Bloating
>
> Sore breasts

Urinary problems

Vaginal discharge

Dry vagina (due to lack of oestrogen)

Pain on intercourse (due to dry vagina)

Reduced sex drive (due to pain on intercourse)

Loss of femininity

Loss of confidence

Loss of appetite

Allergic responses and food sensitivities

Of course, after middle age, most men will also have less energy, a lower sex drive and sleep less — it's not just a female problem!

HELPFUL HERBS
Plants that contain or boost oestrogen

◆ *Alfalfa* (the sprouts may contain toxins, but the tea is good).

◆ *Aniseed* (crush the seeds or chop the leaves and infuse, or use in cooking or salad dressings).

◆ *Black Cohosh* (helpful for rheumatism and neuralgia).

◆ *Carrots* (also for carotenoids, important antioxidants).

◆ *Cucumbers* (now's the time for those ladylike sandwiches; use rye bread).

◆ *Dong Quai* (also a good heart tonic).

◆ *False Unicorn Root* (will also help to tone the reproductive system).

◆ *Fennel* (seeds and finely chopped fresh leaves).

◆ *Ginseng* (take for short intervals only).

◆ *Hops* (not in times of depression, but useful for insomnia).

◆ *Liquorice* (don't use if you suffer from fluid retention or hypertension).

◆ *Maca* (a root vegetable from Peru; it tonifies the whole endocrine system).

◆ *Parsley* (a handful a day, at most).

◆ *Passionflower* (will also get you to sleep).

◆ *Red Clover* (sprouts or tea).

◆ *Sage* (particularly for hot flushes and sweating).

◆ *Sarsaparilla* (also for skin problems).

◆ *Soya beans* (and by-products such as soya milk, tofu and tempeh).

◆ *Tribulus* (also helps to boost testosterone, which is deficient postmenopausally, and restore libido).

◆ *Yeast* (not if you tend to suffer from candida).

Be careful if you are sprouting seeds not to get those intended for commercial agriculture as they will have been chemically treated. Check on the back of the packet. Similarly, ready-to-eat sprouts should only be eaten if they are certified organic.

Plants that boost progesterone
During the perimenopause, you may well become deficient in progesterone as well as oestrogen, and this may be equally, if not even more, significant. Only one herb has been shown clearly to boost progesterone levels, and that is *Chastetree*. Other herbs which have traditionally been used to support progesterone production are *Fenugreek*, *Sarsaparilla* and *Peony*, as these herbs often alleviate symptoms associated with progesterone deficiency. However, there is no proof that they actually increase progesterone levels.

Although *Wild Yam* also has been used in this way and contains precursors of progesterone, there is no evidence to suggest that the body can use these substances to form the hormone (although this can be performed in a laboratory). Creams containing *Wild Yam* may have many therapeutic properties, but they have not been demonstrated to raise progesterone levels. *Wild Yam* does contain phyto-oestrogens, and these may have a therapeutic effect.

Creams containing progesterone which has been synthesised from natural sources (such as Wild Yam) will not help the body to return to a state of balanced production of its own hormones. These creams are just another form of hormone replacement.

Herbal formula
A helpful formula could be made up from some of the following herbs, depending upon the symptoms experienced.

◆ *Red Clover* (for phyto-oestrogens)

◆ *False Unicorn Root* (for oestrogenic effect and as an uterine tone)

◆ *Dong Quai* (as above)

◆ *Chastetree* (to support progesterone)

◆ *Black Cohosh* (oestrogenic, and for hot flushes)

◆ *Sage* (as above)

◆ *St John's Wort* (for anxiety, depression)

♦ *Damiana* (for flagging sexual energy, depression)

♦ *Motherwort* (for palpitations, insomnia)

ACUPRESSURE POINTS
Spleen 6 and *10* (see Dysmenorrhoea).

Hysterectomy

Avoid it if you can. Women who have had this operation tend to have a much higher rate of illness and depression, especially if the ovaries are removed which will lead to premature menopause unless this has already occurred. Even if the ovaries remain intact, there is often damage to their nerve and blood supply, with the same result (see Chapter 2, 'The Unnatural Way'). Use the ideas in this book, see your natural health practitioner, and try to solve the problem naturally before opting for such drastic measures.

Some gynaecologists (mostly male) are all too willing to whip it out. One wonders if their attitude might be different if it were a part of male anatomy involved. This is not to say that you might not be better off having this operation if all else fails.

Mucus production

Problems with mucus production are usually the result of low hormonal output, specifically oestrogen, so, apart from healthy eating and good exercise habits, the herbs to use would be hormone balancing and ovarian tonic herbs, plus mucous membrane tonics.

Hormone balancers
False Unicorn Root, Saw Palmetto, Shatavari.

Mucous membrane tonics
Saw Palmetto, Golden Seal, Bayberry (since the last two herbs are also astringents, this may counter the tonic effect and dry up the mucus while they are in use).

Phyto–oestrogenic herbs can also help (see Menopause section) if given in the first half of the cycle, although these may not stimulate you to produce your own oestrogen in the long term. In order to achieve a lasting effect, you need to use the hormone-balancing herbs.

Calcium and magnesium are required to make the mucus stretchy; zinc is another essential nutrient for healthy mucus. Iron is needed for mucous membrane function, as is vitamin A. Vitamin C is required to make the hormones that are responsible for mucus production, while too much manganese can cause the mucus to become thick, dry and infertile. These considerations are not only of concern if you are trying to observe your mucus pattern with the aim of avoiding conception, but also for proper fertility once you decide the time has come to become pregnant.

Sperm Penetrating Mucus

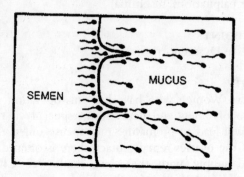

If the mucus is too acidic, the sperm are immobilised. This can be detected in a post-coital test, which examines the mucus after intercourse to see if the sperm are surviving and swimming well. Overacidity is usually responsive to dietary remedies.

You will need to avoid eating too many acid-producing foods (not to be confused with foods that are acidic that become alkaline once digested, such as tomatoes, pineapples, grapefruit and lemons). This is a good diet strategy for your general health as well as your fertility.

Acid-forming foods
Meat, fish, eggs, all animal products, sugar (all forms), coffee and tea, alcohol, most grains and seeds, oranges, plums, prunes and cranberries, vinegar and legumes (except soya and lima beans).

Alkali-forming foods
Nuts (especially almonds, brazil and hazelnuts), most fruit (especially cherries), all vegetables, apple cider vinegar, millet and buckwheat, soya and lima beans.

If you juice your vegetables, you will get greater benefit from them, though you will still need to eat whole vegetables for their fibre content. A good juice base is carrot, beetroot and celery, to which you can add whatever else you have available. *Alfalfa* and *Red Clover* sprouts are strong alkali-forming agents, and both these herbs can also be taken as teas or herbal extracts. Protein (especially from a plant source) buffers acidity, fish is less acid-forming than meat, and milk is neutral (though cheese is acid-forming).

Until your mucus is no longer acidic, you should continue to eat a balanced diet (see also Chapter 13 if you are trying to conceive), using foods from both groups but with the emphasis on the alkali-forming foods.

You can test this with pH sticks (available from your pharmacy), or have a test carried out at a pathology laboratory. Your vagina should be slightly acidic (pH 5.5), your mucus should not.

Chemical douches and lubricants may also kill sperm.

Cervical damage or infection

If the cervix has been damaged, it may not be able to produce sufficient fertile mucus, which can create difficulties with observation of mucus patterns. It can also create fertility problems if there is insufficient mucus to enable the sperm to survive in the female reproductive tract.

It is common for the cervix to be damaged after a cervical cone biopsy for precancerous or cancerous conditions, when the crypts may be damaged or removed. Severe cauterisation, freezing or laser treatments (the common treatments for cervical erosions) can also have this effect. Other possible causes of damage include birth, termination, IUD insertion, D&C, tampons and the Pill. If the cervix is sufficiently damaged, it will become 'incompetent' and have to be sewn together during the pregnancy to avoid losing the foetus.

A course of treatment should be undertaken as soon as possible after the damage occurs. Natural remedies can sometimes reverse damage to tissue. Try taking the herbs *Golden Seal, Calendula* and *False Unicorn Root* internally, as well as douching with *Golden Seal, Calendula, White Pond Lily* and *Tea-tree* oil in a base of glycerine and water. See the next section for how to douche, and don't use glycerine if there is any candida. *Aloe Vera* or vitamin E oil can also be applied directly to the cervix.

Take vitamins A, C, E and B-complex with extra folic acid, and selenium, zinc, calcium and magnesium in adequate doses.

Cervicitis, an infection or inflammation of the cervix (or cervical erosion), can usually be treated similarly. A *Garlic* clove used as a suppository (see next section) and the herbs *Echinacea* and *Thuja* taken internally can be an additional support to combat viral and bacterial infection.

Candida, vaginal thrush and other discharges

Vaginal discharges can be due to yeast infestation which is also known as *thrush, Candida albicans* or *monilia*. This infection can also become systemic if the digestive system is affected.

Systemic candida infection is certainly the 'in' condition. Although it's very easy to blame candidiasis as the root cause of all evil (and some practitioners are perhaps a little over-zealous in their diagnoses), there is no doubt that extensive use of antibiotics and our old friend the contraceptive pill, have encouraged massive yeast infestations in many women.

Candida albicans is a harmless fungus that is always present in the body. It only becomes a problem when the immune system fails to function correctly. Normally held in check by the lactic acid produced by certain healthy bacteria that are also usually present in the body, it can proliferate alarmingly if the balance of bacteria is disturbed.

This is not the place to go into a long treatise on systemic candida infection, and there are certainly many excellent books and articles on the subject, but some of the conditions we discuss in this chapter are definitely exacerbated, even caused by, this pernicious disorder.

The most obvious result of the gynaecological–candida link is vaginal thrush, and those alarming and antisocial itches, especially the chronic, recurring type that worsens premenstrually, are one of the first signs that candida has spread from the external surfaces of the body and is infesting the gut. It's also a sign that your immune system is not functioning optimally, and that the level of lymphocyte activity required in the mucosa, especially at times of low oestrogen, is deficient.

There are quite a few other chronic menstrual disturbances — PMS in particular — which can be traced back to this underlying condition.

If you suspect that you are suffering from a systemic candida infection, it will need to be remedied before you are able to have much success with treating vaginal thrush. Treatment will involve measures to accomplish the following.

◆ *Starve the yeast.* This means completely avoiding all refined carbohydrates, such as sugar, sweeteners, white grains and flour products (including white rice, bread and pasta), and alcohol.

◆ *Kill the yeast.* This can be achieved through natural agents such as *Garlic, Capryllic Acid, Citrus Seed* extract, herbs such as *Pau D'Arco, Golden Seal, Calendula* or medical drugs such as Nystatin.

◆ *Boost the immune system.* Good nutrition and herbs such as *Echinacea* can help achieve this.

◆ *Avoid foods to which you are allergic,* as they affect the immune system and the health of the gut adversely. As well as the common allergens, such as dairy products (except acidophilus yoghurt), and possibly wheat, you may have become allergic to yeast-containing, fermented and mouldy foods (such as leftovers).

◆ *Reline the gut* with friendly bacteria. This can be achieved through the use of lactobacilli, such as acidophilus and bifidus, natural, unsweetened yoghurt, and bitter tonic herbs such as *Dandelion Root* and *Golden Seal.*

Systemic candidiasis treatment may need professional supervision, but vaginal thrush, especially if not recurring (which is an indication that the gut is infested) can be treated through self-help. It can be triggered by

> hot weather
> tight trousers
> synthetic underwear
> constant douching
> vaginal deodorants
> excess sugar consumption
> antibiotics
> the contraceptive pill

intercourse (semen is alkaline)

hormonal imbalance, *or*

any other health condition or medication that disrupts the normal balance of yeast cells and healthy bacteria

The number of healthy, protective bacteria are reduced through any of these circumstances, causing the yeast to proliferate, which will lead to an infestation. You may experience intense itching, burning and a white curdy discharge that smells yeasty. It is not usually an offensive odour, but different from your normal smell.

Try this natural remedy — mix

◆ 4 drops of *Tea-tree* oil (a natural antifungal and antiseptic agent) with

◆ 2 tablespoons of white vinegar (this contains no sugar and is used to re-acidify the vagina) in

◆ 1 litre (2 pints) of warm, purified water.

You can douche, bathe (in a sitz bath, basin or bath) or insert an impregnated tampon, depending on whether the infection is internal or external. *Never leave a tampon in place for longer than 8 hours, or you could suffer toxic shock syndrome.*

The amount of solution required will vary according to the method used. Keep the proportions the same — you obviously don't need as much to dunk your tampon in as you do to sit in.

Use two or three times a day, depending on the severity of the condition, until the symptoms have subsided for several days, otherwise they will reappear.

Do not douche during pregnancy or for 10 weeks after childbirth.

Creams and lotions containing Tea-tree oil will soothe external itching and irritation. *Tea-tree* pessaries, if available, will help the internal symptoms. Acidophilus yoghurt (live culture), which you can purchase from health-food shops, can also work well, as can Citrus Seed extract used as a douche.

If the discharge is profuse, yellow-green, slightly foamy, smells bad (fishy) and causes itching and soreness, it may be caused by the protozoa trichomonas. If it doesn't itch, isn't sore, but smells offensive and is grey in colour, it may be a bacterial infection such as gardnerella.

Trichomonas or bacterial infections may respond to herbal douches and internal medicine.

Remedies to take internally

Citrus Seed extract, acidophilus and bifidus, *Golden Seal, Echinacea, Wild Indigo, Calendula, Pau D'Arco* and *Capryllic Acid*. These activate your immune system and help fight the bacteria or fungi.

Garlic is strongly antibacterial, antifungal, a good immune stimulant and can even be inserted into the vagina. A *Garlic* oil capsule, or a clove carefully peeled so that it isn't nicked, wrapped in gauze with a tail you can pull on, and dipped in vegetable oil, can be inserted as a pessary (change every 8 hours). Or you can douche with the following herbs:

◆ *Golden Seal* (antibacterial)

◆ *White Pond Lily* (astringent to repel pathogens)

◆ *Uva Ursi* (disinfectant)

◆ *Witch Hazel* (astringent)

◆ *Calendula* (antibacterial).

Glycerine makes a good base for a douche (except if the infection is candida, in which case only purified water should be used), and you can add a few drops of *Tea-tree* oil for the strong antifungal and antibacterial properties.

Always add white vinegar to help re-acidify the vagina.

Intercourse should be avoided, as it spreads the infection back and forth between partners (you should both be treated), or you can use a condom. Semen is alkaline, so will encourage infections.

If your partner needs treatment, he can use the same herbs and treatments as you. Instead of douching, he can dunk.

If the condition does not respond to treatment, you should have a diagnosis carried out by a health practitioner. If you are having recurrent candida infections, you will need to investigate the possibility that you are suffering from systemic candida (in the gut).

Other possible causes of discharge are

◆ a retained tampon

◆ vaginal deodorants and spermicides

◆ cervical erosion

◆ cervical infection such as chlamydia.

A damaged cervix may respond to vitamin E oil which you can dab on with a cotton swab, or the juice from an *Aloe Vera* plant. An infected cervix may respond to the douches or *Garlic*.

To avoid vaginal infections, practise the following preventative measures.

◆ Avoid recurrent antibiotics.

◆ Avoid the contraceptive Pill.

◆ Treat your sexual partner at the same time as yourself to avoid re-infection.

◆ Don't use soap, vaginal deodorants or bath preparations.

◆ Don't use detergents to wash underwear.

◆ Eat wisely, and include acidophilus yoghurt in your diet.

◆ Avoid tight trousers, synthetic underwear and tights.

◆ Wipe from front to back (from the vagina to the anus).

◆ Keep your vagina acidic (you can measure this with a pH stick available from your pharmacy), and douche with white vinegar or yoghurt.

◆ Keep your vulva clean using water only.

How to douche

A douche has a rubber bulb attached to a plastic nozzle and can be bought from a pharmacy. Suck up the solution by squeezing the bulb, then squirt it into the vagina. Using an empty bath tub allows you to raise your hips and keep the solution in the vagina for 2–3 minutes.

Never douche if you are pregnant or have given birth in the last 10 weeks.

Characteristics of discharge for vaginal infections

Condition	Smell	Colour	pH	Consistency	Effect
Candida albicans	Yeasty	White	4	Curdy, thick	Itching, burning
Trichomonas	Bad (fishy)	Yellow/green	5–6	Foamy, profuse	Itching, soreness
Gardnerella	Bad (fishy)	Grey	5–6	Foamy, profuse	–

Herpes

Herpes blisters usually occur on the external genitalia, but occasionally on the buttocks and thighs or inside the vagina. The risk is greatest to pregnant women; risk of miscarriage increases if a woman contracts the disease while she is pregnant. If there is an active outbreak present at the time of birth, delivery by caesarean section is necessary to avoid possible brain damage, blindness or even death of the new-born.

The herpes virus is impossible to eliminate from the body completely, but a lot can be done to keep it dormant and treat the blisters.

To keep it dormant, you need to boost your immune system. Here's how.

◆ (Surprise, surprise) eat properly, avoiding nuts and increasing fish.

◆ Deal with your stress levels and PMT.

◆ Cut out smoking, excessive alcohol and drugs.

◆ Use the antioxidants zinc, selenium, vitamins A, B_1, B_6, E and C (with bioflavonoids), and manganese, magnesium, vitamins B_1 and B_6.

◆ Try the amino acid lysine (1200 mg daily), and avoid arginine.

◆ Take *Evening Primrose* oil and eat lots of raw seeds, fish, fish oils, cold-pressed vegetable oils.

◆ Use *Garlic, St John's Wort, Lemon Balm, Echinacea* and other herbal immune stimulants such as *Reiishi* and *Shiitake* mushrooms.

To treat the lesions, use the following.

◆ *Garlic*, before the lesions develop. At the first sign of tingling, take a high dose (up to 5000 mg) supplement, and repeat every 6 hours for 3 days.

◆ Ice, applied to the site at first appearance of symptoms.

◆ The homoeopathic remedy *Rhus Tox* 3x–6x potency, 5–10 drops as lesions start to develop.

◆ *Calendula* or *Witch Hazel* extract or ointment, applied topically.

◆ *Aloe Vera* applied topically.

If you are sexually active during an outbreak, cover the blister with a sticking plaster if the blister is in a position where you are able to do so, and ask your partner to wear a condom.

Genital warts

Medical treatment for warts is harsh. Freezing or acid-burning treatments can leave scar tissue. Laser, electric and chemical treatments are not without problems, and may not be successful in the long term. Holistic treatment includes dietary and stress-control approaches, with the accent on improving the immune system, as for herpes.

Thuja is the wonder herb for all wart virus complaints. Taken internally, it can be extremely effective, especially given the support of antiviral herbs such as *St John's Wort* and immune-stimulant herbs such as *Echinacea*. *Thuja* can also be used homoeopathically, although classical homoeopaths will want to treat the whole person and not just the symptom.

Tea-tree oil applied topically, with the support of *Thuja* ointment, can complete the cure.

Hypnotherapy can be very effective. 'Magic' or suggestion has traditionally been used for eliminating all forms of warts, with such 'spells' as tying a string around them, or telling them to go away.

Coming off the Pill

I treat all my patients who are coming off the contraceptive pill in such a way as to make sure that everything returns to normal as soon as possible.

As well as the dietary and exercise recommendations, supplementation is particularly important here, as the vitamin and mineral deficiencies that result from taking the artificial hormones need to be addressed. Otherwise, you may suffer from the results of the imbalance: PMS, irregularity, lack of ovulation and lack of mucus production (See Chapter 2, 'The Unnatural Approach', for suggestions).

A good herbal formula to eliminate the residual chemicals from the system and to stimulate normal hormonal activity, is

◆ *Chastetree* — to stimulate the ovarian/ pituitary axis

◆ *Golden Seal* — to tonify the mucous membranes

◆ *Schisandra* — to detoxify through the liver and kidneys

◆ *Ginger* — to encourage pelvic circulation

◆ *False Unicorn Root* — as a general reproductive tonic

◆ *Wild Yam* — to reduce inflammation

But other herbs that have been mentioned with similar functions could be substituted.

Herbal birth control

Don't use it! There are several herbs which have a traditional or new-found reputation for having a contraceptive action. Some of these are known to act through a toxic effect: they are unsafe to use in this context. Also the contraceptive effect may be insufficient to ensure infertility.

Neem oil seems to hold the most promise, and is currently under investigation for its efficacy and safety. In Chapter 9, 'Sexual Expression in Fertile Times', there is more information on topical (not internal) use of this oil. Cottonseed oil has been used traditionally as a contraceptive, has been shown to reduce sperm count and is present in many processed foods and salad dressings. Men might need to be aware of this, especially if their sperm count is of concern.

Herbs used for termination are more dangerous than surgical extraction, which you may need anyway if the termination is incomplete. If they don't work, they could damage the embryo.

Use herbs instead to recover from a termination, and be more careful to conceive only when you want to do so (see the next section and Chapter 2, 'The Unnatural Approach', for more on termination).

Miscarriage and termination

Recovery after a miscarriage or termination can be sped up enormously by the use of natural medicines, good nutrition and exercise. Counselling is often also an important component. Recovery should be complete before another conception is attempted, so natural birth control methods should be used. The following herbs might be useful.

Rebalancing hormones
Chastetree, False Unicorn Root, Sarsaparilla, Saw Palmetto.

Womb recovery
Raspberry, Beth Root, Squaw Vine, True Unicorn Root, Blue Cohosh.

To stop bleeding
Shepherd's Purse, Beth Root, Ladies' Mantle.

For infection
Golden Seal, Myrrh, Echinacea, Calendula.

For stress
Chamomile, Oats, Vervain, Kava.

To normalise circulation
Ginger, Yarrow.

Vitamins A and E are especially important for the recovery of the womb, and the B complex and C vitamins are needed to cope with stress. Vitamin C will also help combat infection, calcium, magnesium and zinc will help muscular and hormonal recovery and iron may be needed if much blood was lost.

Lactation
There is a great need for you to be well-nourished at this time as you will be recovering from the depletion of pregnancy, during which the baby gets first pick of all the nutrients.

While you are lactating, you get first preference, so for the baby to get any nutrients (through the milk) there must be plenty there. Take a comprehensive vitamin and mineral supplement and eat well.

You can refer back to Chapter 11, 'Times of Change', for more on breastfeeding. If you feel your milk diminish, get lots of rest, practise relaxation, and get your baby to suck as much as possible.

Useful herb teas
Chastetree, Blessed Thistle, Fenugreek, Alfalfa, Aniseed, Fennel, Nettle, Dill.

If you have too much milk, *Sage* and the higher doses of vitamin B_6 will help to diminish the supply (be careful that you don't take too much), and dry it up when you (or your baby) decide to wean.

Breast lumps
Not all breast lumps are cancerous, although if you do find one it is important to have it investigated. You may find you have a tendency to benign lumpiness in the post-ovulatory phase. This is called fibrocystic breast disease, although there is some doubt about whether it really is a disease. Cysts filled with fluid develop in the breasts, causing lumps, pain and swelling.

Fibroadenomas are lumps that do not fluctuate with the menstrual period. They can be removed surgically, although there is much you can do before resorting to this measure.

Hypothyroidism can result in persistent breast disorders; it is also associated with excess oestrogen relative to progesterone. A low temperature recorded in the pre-ovulatory phase of your cycle can alert you to this condition.

Useful supplements
Vitamins A, B–complex (especially, B_1, B_3, B_6), C and E. Selenium, zinc, manganese, calcium and magnesium. *Garlic* supplements with allicin (high dose, 5000 mg, three times daily). *Evening Primrose* and fish oils. Iodine (as potassium iodide) may be useful if thyroid function is low.

Useful herbs
Diuretic herbs (see other lists). Liver herbs may be useful to help eliminate excess oestrogen, which exacerbates the problem, and to deal with fats. Try *St Mary's Thistle* or *Dandelion Root. Bladderwrack* may increase thyroid activity if this is a problem (or add organic seaweed to your diet).

Violet Leaves, Blue Flag and *Poke Root* are specific for lumps of any kind. Take care with *Poke Root*, it can be toxic; the dosage is critical. *Do not take Poke Root during pregnancy.* In fact, don't take anything during your pregnancy that is not absolutely necessary and that has not been recommended as being completely safe. However, *Poke Root* is also very useful as an ointment, as is *St John's Wort*; steamed cabbage leaves make a good poultice. Massaging the breasts can also help.

Avoid coffee, saturated fats, refined carbohydrates, dairy produce, alcohol, salt and cigarettes; these are often part of the problem. Make sure that all chicken and other meats are organically fed to avoid artificial hormones and trim off all the fat.

Drink 3–4 glasses of raw vegetable juice daily. Carrot, beetroot and celery is a good base — throw in anything else you have.

Eat lots of fish, salads, seeds and nuts, fruit, cold-pressed oils and whole grains.

Postnatal depression
Include under this title, post-miscarriage and post-termination depression. Although anyone is likely to feel depressed after a termination or a miscarriage and may need grief counselling, the huge drop in progesterone production that accompanies the end of a pregnancy is part of the problem (this drop will be greater the further the pregnancy is advanced).

It can be treated in much the same way as PMS, which is also, according to most accepted opinion, a result of a drop in hormone levels.

Other conditions
There are plenty of other gynaecological conditions that respond to natural remedies, but the more serious should be referred to a therapist for specialist care. Some that have responded well include:

◆ ovarian cysts

◆ abnormal cervical cells

◆ PID (pelvic inflammatory disease)

◆ polycystic ovarian syndrome (PCOS)

◆ blocked fallopian tubes

◆ endometriosis

◆ fibroids

◆ male fertility problems

◆ mutual infertility.

Some of these (and other conditions) can lead to fertility problems, and are further explored in my book *The Natural Way to Better Babies*, co-authoured by Janette Roberts, the Australian representative of the British organisation Foresight, and published by Random House. In this book we further explore treatments to promote fertility and overcome fertility problems, and give comprehensive guidelines for preconception care for a healthy conception, pregnancy, birth and baby, the subject of the next chapter.

CHAPTER 13

Conscious Conception

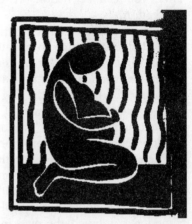

For most of you during your active sexual lives, the issue you primarily concern yourselves with is *contra*ception. Even if you decide to have children, the occasions on which conception is actually sought are few and far between, unless there are problems of low fertility.

Quite reasonably, you tend to develop a contraceptive attitude to sex. However, there is a natural outcome to the sex act; it's called babies, and each time you approach sex with a contraceptive attitude means you are holding back from this extra dimension. All the more reason to plan and consciously enjoy the few times in your life when you can embrace the sexual act in its entirety, fully experiencing the moment when you can share your life with another being.

A child consciously conceived and welcomed in this way can only benefit from the parents' positive experiences that surround its beginnings. So often, pregnancies, even when welcomed, are only confirmed after several weeks have elapsed, during which time the baby has been developing extremely fast, without the conscious participation of either parent. Many more are mistakes, to which the parents later (hopefully) become reconciled.

With unplanned conceptions, there is often a panic reaction when the mother (and the father) realise what has happened. Many women have a deeply ingrained fear of pregnancy, which can be difficult to overcome even when a pregnancy is planned and desired.

The baby's psychic and psychological connections with its mother and, to a lesser extent perhaps, with its father, are of enormous importance in its emotional development.

To conceive consciously and optimistically, and be aware of and loving towards the child from the very beginning, can provide the best possible environment for healthy emotional growth. Anyway, it's nice! You might as well enjoy your pregnancy as much as possible.

In order to recognise that moment of conception, you need to know that your reproductive system is healthy and when your fertility peaks. Then you can be reasonably confident that intercourse will result in conception.

Of course, your baby's health concerns are not only emotional; the physical side of things is vital too. And here we have to go back even further. *In the instant that the sperm and egg combine, an irreversible genetic blueprint is formed for the future development of the baby.*

Clearly, the health of the egg and the sperm is of crucial importance. After conception, the growth of the embryo is so rapid that, unless all the nutrient building blocks are there, ready and waiting, vital stages of development can be compromised.

There is growing evidence that the first few days, even hours, of the embryo's life are critically important. In the first trimester (3 months) the foetal mass increases over 2 500 000 times; a phenomenal rate of growth that has exceptional nutritional requirements. In the second and third trimesters combined, the mass increases (only!) 230 times. Also, in the first trimester, vital events such as cell differentiation and organisation, and organogenesis (the making of the organs), take place.

After this time, your baby is formed, including any anomalies. For example, if there is insufficient folic acid and zinc available on day 27 or 28 of your pregnancy, when the neural tubes close, your baby could suffer from a neural tube defect, such as spina bifida.

Of course folic acid isn't the only nutrient required to create a healthy baby. All of the nutrients have a role to play in a sequence of events that proceeds whether they are present in adequate supply or not. Nutrient X needs to be present on day Y to make part Z; if it is not, then that process will not have an optimum outcome.

You can only ensure that your body is fit to reproduce successfully if you have prepared it well for several months before conception.

Luckily, the human body is hardy and most pregnancies and babies are without major problems. But why take chances when a little care could mean so much? Every woman (and her partner) wants a successful pregnancy and a healthy child — they're not that difficult to achieve.

Preconception health care for *both* parents can not only reduce the incidence of infertility, miscarriage, malformation and perinatal death, but also of asthma, allergy, learning and behaviour problems. No one wants to spend the first years of their child's life dealing with colic, chronic upper-respiratory and middle-ear infections, eating disorders and wakeful nights. No one wants their child to go through school unable to take advantage of their learning opportunities, or grow into an adult with a lowered immune system and greater risk of degenerative disease. Your child deserves the best possible start in life — the one Mother Nature intended for it.

A little planning, and you can not only minimise the risks of fertility and foetal health problems, but maximise the chances of your children being beautiful, well-formed, intelligent and well-balanced, and of your experience of conception and pregnancy being one of confidence and joy.

Consider how much time, money and other resources went into planning your wedding (if you had one), your first home, or other important milestones in your life. Your children deserve at least the same level of concern. *Your preparation for conception should ensure an adequate supply of all those factors essential to the health of the sperm, ova and foetal development, and an absence of all those which have been shown to be harmful.*

Many of you reading this book may be prospective mothers — but babies have fathers too! And more and more studies are showing the vital role that the health of the sperm plays in the future health of the child. While it may not be possible to tempt the father with promises of an easy pregnancy, no stretch marks, a short and successful labour with no perineal tearing and a relaxed breastfeeding experience — yes! — all this and more! — his role in caring for a child with or without health problems will depend to a great extent on his involvement before conception takes place.

Many men are unaware of how critical their contribution is. It's easy to feel that the mother, who provides two out of the three factors (egg, sperm and nurturing environment, including the womb) is largely responsible for the health of the pregnancy and foetus. But just as we now understand that fertility problems are equally shared between both partners, it is becoming quite clear that the preconception health of the father can have a significant impact on the outcome. In fact it may even be more important, in some instances, than that of the mother.

This is because sperm are more vulnerable than eggs. They are considerably smaller (see Chapter 3, 'Your Bodies') and their development takes place wholly within the present existing environment which, especially for men in certain occupations, may contain a high level of exposure to toxins. Spermatogenesis takes up to 116 days; this is the amount of time for which there is a requirement for as high a level of nutritional support and as low an exposure to toxins as possible. This is equally true for the mother, as ova are susceptible to damage during their period of maturation, which is approximately 100 days before ovulation.

So, preconception health care needs to be in place for both partners for a minimum of 4 months before the pregnancy begins. For maximum benefit, certain processes, such as detoxification and establishment of adequate nutritional status, should have been achieved before the start of this 4-month period, so that the sperm and egg develop in the healthiest possible environment.

At my health clinic, the Jocelyn Centre in Sydney, we help couples achieve this preparation. Some of these couples are using the program to plan their 'better baby' and others to overcome a history of fertility problems, as this approach also has a high degree of success in the treatment of infertility. We also train health practitioners in many countries in the requirements of preconception health care. Although our success rate is reflected in the profusion of smiling baby faces that adorn our walls, we have yet to complete the formal study we are undertaking which will give a clear statistical rate of success. However, much of our work is based on that of Foresight, the British Association for the Promotion of Preconceptual Care, which has conducted two studies in conjunction with Surrey University, one of which (with more than 1000 couples) is still being assessed. The completed study was the first to assess the outcome of a holistic approach to preconception health care.

Foresight results

These statistics are an example of the effectiveness of preconception care as practised by Foresight. The 'Better Babies' program at the Jocelyn Centre for Natural Fertility Management includes and extends the Foresight program. The study involved 367 couples and lasted 2 years.

Age of females — 22–45 years.

Age of males — 25–59 years.

Presenting with a previous history of	Percentage in sample
infertility	37 per cent
miscarriage	38 per cent
therapeutic abortion	11 per cent
still birth	3 per cent
small-for-dates or low birth weight babies	15 per cent
malformation	2 per cent

Results	
No miscarriages, perinatal deaths, malformations.	
No baby admitted to intensive care.	
Normal expectation — 70 miscarriages, 6 malformations.	

Outcome	Percentage in sample
Live births	89 per cent
Live births to those previously infertile	81 per cent
Average gestational age	38.5 weeks
Average weight of males	7 lb 4.5 oz (3299g)
Average weight of females	7 lb 2 oz (3238g)
Lightest baby	5 lb 3 oz

You can see from this table of results that this approach gives you

♦ *a greatly increased chance of a healthy pregnancy and baby*

♦ *an extremely high rate of success in overcoming fertility problems.*

We'll move on to fertility issues later and compare this success with that offered by orthodox medical approaches. We can make that same comparison when it comes to the health of future generations.

Preconception health care is the ultimate preventative approach. It has the potential to change the health of future generations for the better and enable them to grow up into children and adults with robust immune systems and constitutions, able to withstand the environmental problems which are precisely those factors adversely affecting fertility and the health of so many of our babies.

Genetic engineering also makes some of these promises. How much simpler, healthier, cheaper and more ethical to use preconception health care to achieve these aims. Not only do we avoid the potential for abuse (with sexist, racist, socio-economic overtones) but also it's a win/win situation where the least that can be achieved is a healthier outcome for the prospective parents!

In *The Natural Way to Better Babies* you will find all you need to know about preconception health care if you want to take this further. In this book, I'll summarise the areas that require attention so you can get started.

Preconception health care

There are several things to which both of you must attend if you are about to try to conceive (remember, all this applies to the prospective father as well as to the mother).

♦ Start learning, if you haven't already, the contraception techniques in this book. This will ensure that you don't conceive before you plan to, that you don't harm your body in any way through the contraception technique you employ, that you will be competent and sufficiently experienced to use natural methods of contraception while you are breastfeeding, and that you become very sure of your fertility timing so you can conceive with full awareness at the optimum time in your cycle to ensure that fresh, healthy sperm are ready and waiting for a fresh, healthy egg. The charting that you carry out during these cycles will also enable you to identify hormonal and other imbalances which should be rectified before conception.

♦ You must come off the oral contraceptive pill, well before conception (see Chapter 11, 'Times of Change', for how to use natural contraception methods when you first come off the Pill.) *Conception should not occur within 6 months of ceasing to take the oral contraceptive pill.* You are likely to be deficient in nutrients as an after-effect (see Chapter 2, 'The Unnatural Way'); there is a profound disruption to your hormonal status and reproductive health, and the chance of miscarriage and malformation is increased.

◆ The effect of the chemical hormones should be eliminated in most cases within 6 months, but you can speed this up with herbal and natural remedies (see Chapter 12, 'Natural Remedies for Hormonal and Reproductive Health'), although it could take longer to restore your nutrient status, especially if you were not eating well or supplementing at the time.

◆ You should have your IUD removed at least 4 months before conception. This is not quite as vital as withdrawal from the Pill, but it's important to let your natural cycle and hormonal levels resume. If you were using a copper IUD, your copper levels may be high, which will reduce the availability of zinc.

◆ Do not use spermicides, as they can cause malformation. At the time of conception, avoid lubricants, as all are spermicidal, even saliva. Raw egg-white is the only lubricant proven to allow the sperm passage.

◆ Where possible, both of you should take no medication of any kind for at least 4 months before conception. If you are on medical drugs for a chronic condition, consult with your natural health practitioner to see if there is an alternative treatment available. If so, enlist the cooperation of your medical doctor in making the transition. If this is not possible, research the effects of the medication on fertility and foetal health. Often there is a distinct difference in the risks involved in different drugs.

◆ Over-the-counter and prescription drugs are better avoided if possible. There's usually a natural, non-toxic (not necessarily the same thing) alternative. Seek professional advice and attempt to resolve the issue before conception. If you are sick and need treatment, you are not fit (yet) to conceive. Get yourself fit and in good health first, and then prepare to conceive. It's as well to have a few tests early on to confirm that you don't need treatment. This applies to both of you.

◆ Identify any allergic responses and sensitivities, and if there is not time to restore your ability to cope with these substances through natural remedies, reduce your exposure to a minimal level because if you have an allergic response during pregnancy, your child is very likely to inherit it. If both parents are allergic, they have a 60 per cent chance of an allergic child. A very occasional, low-level exposure gives greater protection against this transference than complete avoidance of the allergen.

◆ The most common allergens are dairy products, wheat, gluten and yeast. Milk and wheat have also been shown to affect fertility in other ways. Wheat can cause raised levels of prolactin, and milk contains galactose, a substance that is harmful to the ovaries if not converted to glucose by the liver (in some women this process is deficient). An allergic response is also often triggered or exacerbated by our old friend candida, which should be identified and dealt with before conception as the increased levels of hormones can result in the escalation of the condition, which creates an unhealthy environment for the growth of your child. Candida can also result in thrush in the newborn's mouth and digestive system, and in your breasts, making breastfeeding extremely painful (see Chapter 12, 'Natural Remedies for Hormonal and Reproductive Health').

◆ Have your urine tested to determine sugar and protein levels.

◆ Have your blood pressure checked.

◆ Have your immunity to rubella checked and be (re-)immunised, if that is your choice, at least 3 months before conception. Immunisation of any kind is controversial: it may have long-term effects on your immune system as well as immediate side-effects on your health. Naturopathic philosophy favours keeping the immune system strong and supporting it with immune-stimulant herbs such as Echinacea, and good nutrition, especially antioxidants such as zinc and vitamins A, E and C. However, this is a very personal decision and you may wish to do more research before making it. My book, *The Natural Way to Better Breastfeeding*, due out in early 2001 and co-authored with Janette Roberts, will look at this issue in detail.

◆ It is also wise to have your immunity to toxoplasmosis and cytomegalovirus (CMV) checked. If you have antibodies, you will be immune; you may also be alerted to a present infection, which can be treated with natural remedies. These infections can have devastating effects upon fertility, the healthy progress of your pregnancy and your baby's health. Toxoplasmosis can be contracted through contact with cat's excreta or contaminated soil (when you are gardening), or by eating raw meat or fish. CMV is often epidemic among small children, who are unaffected, unless their immune system is weakened. If you have contact with a pre-school, isolate yourself if there appears to be an outbreak of 'flu, as this may be CMV.

◆ Blood tests should be carried out for syphilis, HIV status, and hepatitis B and C.

◆ If you have a history of thyroid disorders or liver disease it may be as well to have blood tests for thyroid and liver function. While using the basal body temperature observations as part of your natural birth control program, you will be alerted to a hypothyroid condition (common among women) by any readings that are below 36.4°C (97.5°F) for 3 consecutive days.

◆ There are a number of other diagnostic tests which can usefully be carried out at the start of your preconception preparation. For the male, a semen analysis will give invaluable information about the quantity and the quality of the sperm, and whether treatment is required (see later in this chapter). The measures we are recommending here should significantly change any poor result, but there are additional treatments for specific problems. For the woman, if one has not been performed recently, a Pap smear for abnormal cells should be carried out. If your cycle is irregular or the charting shows imbalances, you can have blood tests for hormone levels. An internal examination will also show any obvious deformity of the uterus or damage to the cervix.

◆ Most other fertility tests for women are invasive and better avoided if possible, or only performed if indicated by a history of fertility problems.

◆ It is also advisable at this time to be checked for a whole range of GUIs, the presence of which can affect fertility and foetal health. This test can be performed for both partners by blood test and swabs or cultures. In the female, the swabs should be taken from high inside the cervix or through colposcopy, as vaginal swabs are insufficient to show if the infections are present in the upper reproductive tract. For this reason, these infections are sometimes called 'hidden', as they may not show on routine swabs. Another reason for using this term is that the individual can be asymptomatic, as many of these infections are subclinical. In the male, the test can be done through urethral swab or by a culture test on the semen. A full list of the infections to be checked is as follows, and though many medical personnel may question the need for this comprehensive approach, there is plenty of evidence that any of these infections can result in infertility, recurrent miscarriage and malformation. These infections may respond to natural remedies, but they can take a long time and are not reliable — antibiotics may be required. If so, be sure to supplement with acidophilus and bifidus to replenish the gut with healthy flora.

Gonorrhoea	Ureaplasma	Herpes	*Staph. aureus*
B. strep	Mycoplasma	*Haem. influenza*	*Strep. millerii*
Candida	Klebsiella	*Haem. strep*	*E. coli*
Anaerobic bacteria	Gardnerella	Enterococcus	Chlamydia

◆ Although nutrient status is all-important, blood (serum) levels are not the best indicators as they are transitory. Hair-trace mineral analysis is the best indicator of mineral status, as stored in the body's tissues; this can also give some information about vitamin deficiencies (by association), malabsorption, thyroid and adrenal health and the level of toxic (heavy) metals (see below). A blood test for stored iron (ferritin) levels can be informative; the woman should enter into pregnancy with adequate iron stores, since the rise in blood volume she experiences will otherwise cause problems. A ferritin level of between 55 and 65 mcg per litre is recommended.

◆ Zinc, perhaps the most important nutrient for male and female fertility, is best measured through the zinc taste test, where 5 mL of zinc sulphate solution is swished around the mouth. A prompt, strong taste indicates sufficient zinc in the body, a slight or delayed taste shows inadequate zinc, and no taste confirms a high level of depletion. Since zinc is poorly absorbed through the diet, supplementation is the best way to go.

◆ Both parents need to check for heavy metal contamination, including lead, copper, mercury, cadmium and aluminium. Copper is not, strictly speaking, a heavy metal, but it is toxic in excess and inhibits zinc and other antioxidants (as do all the heavy metals). A hair-trace mineral analysis is by far the best test for this because it can indicate if you are having trouble absorbing your nutrients. This deficiency can be corrected by taking digestive enzymes, hydrochloric acid and bitter tonic herbs. Detoxification can be achieved by eating foods such as broccoli, onions, *Garlic* and legumes, by taking vitamin C, selenium and zinc, by balancing the nutrient minerals, by using liver-drainage herbs such as *Schisandra* and, if there is a really high load, through chelation therapy.

◆ In order not to re-absorb these toxins, it may be important to identify their origin. Lead may come from lead water pipes, flaking paint or traffic exhaust, cadmium from cigarette smoking (active or passive), copper from the Pill, a copper IUD or water pipes, aluminium from cookware, aluminium foil, antacids or anti-perspirant sprays, and mercury from fish caught in contaminated river or coastal waters, or from dental fillings.

◆ Other environmental toxins to avoid are pesticides, paint and paint strippers, dry rot or woodworm treatments, glues and chemicals such as solvents. Even household cleaning agents such as oven cleaners, mould treatments and ammonia-based products have been shown to have a negative effect on the health of sperm and ova. You may need to change a few things in your lifestyle to avoid them. To be really safe, avoid anything with fumes, wear protective clothing and masks. If you can't avoid exposure, don't undertake home renovations and use environmentally friendly, non-toxic products. Also purify all water that ends up in your body, boiled or not.

◆ Both parents should take no drugs for at least 4 months before conceiving. Give up alcohol, tobacco, caffeine and any other drugs you normally use. Apart from impaired fertility, the fact that they rob your body of nutrients, and their possible contribution to birth defects, you definitely do not want to be taking any of these substances while you are pregnant — they can affect foetal growth.

❯ ◆ *Nicotine is a vasoconstrictor which stops oxygen getting through to the unborn child.* Smokers are twice as likely to miscarry, their babies are less healthy at birth, are more likely to suffer from congenital abnormalities and to die in their first year of life. Smoking fathers (we're talking preconception here) have an increased chance of having a child with asthma and a 30 per cent higher risk of having a child who develops cancer (especially leukaemia). He also has a 30 per cent higher risk of impotence, as well as an increased chance of atrophy of the testicles, low sperm count (a reduction of 20 per cent) and immotile and deformed sperm. Smoking mothers have an increased chance of irregular cycles and early menopause, and a three times higher incidence of infertility (the decline in fertility is proportional to the number of cigarettes smoked).

◆ Alcohol consumption can lead to foetal alcohol syndrome (FAS) which includes congenital defects such as mental retardation, and can affect the health of both egg and sperm. FAS also increases the chances of endometriosis by 50 per cent, raised prolactin levels and early menopause. Caffeine will affect your fertility: more than 100 mg of caffeine, or one caffeinated soft drink, per day causes a 50 per cent reduction in conception rates. Caffeine will also affect your hormone levels, your risk of miscarriage and your baby's health. Remember, caffeine is present in chocolate and soft drinks as well as coffee. Decaffeinated coffee (especially if chemically processed) has also been shown to be at least as detrimental as the normal variety.

◆ Four months is a minimum time to be sure you are safely withdrawn from the effects of these drugs and unlikely to start using them again.

◆ Both parents must avoid X-rays (including dental X-rays) for at least 4 months before conception (effects of radiation are cumulative). So, have a thorough dental check-up and any necessary repairs done well in advance. Radiation effects have been shown to contribute to abnormalities of sperm and ova, and foetal malformations such as Down syndrome, as radiation can affect DNA and cause chromosomal damage. Ionising radiation (the form present in X-rays) is also a problem when you fly: the exposure to cosmic radiation experienced when you take an international or high-altitude domestic flight is equivalent to one X-ray through your whole body. Natural remedies such as *Reiishi* mushroom, *Burdock*, *Astragalus* and *Siberian Ginseng* herbs, vitamin B5 and some homoeopathic remedies can aid recovery, but exposure should be avoided. It may be that cosmic radiation levels are higher during certain planetary configurations (see 'Heavenly

Conceptions' later in this chapter). They are also higher if you fly over the polar regions.

◆ Non-ionising radiation, such as that from computer terminals (not the LCD screens which are used for laptops), mobile phones, microwaves, lasers, TVs, radar and ultraviolet and infrared lights, is also a problem. Again, reduce exposure and put in place protection where you can.

◆ The more modern the computer monitor the less radiation it emits. You can purchase anti-radiation screens to place in front of your monitor. Turn the screen off when it's not in use rather than letting it display a screen-saver motif. Epsom salts absorb some of the radiation; a cushion cover stuffed with these and placed on your lap may afford some protection. Epsom salts can also be used when flying. Unfortunately, the hands-free devices available for mobile phones have lately been shown to increase exposure, acting as a form of aerial. The small screens placed around the aerial are effective in directing the radiation away from your body.

◆ Keep as far away from these devices as you can — 2–3 metres (6–9 feet) at least — and use them as little as possible. The back and sides of computer monitors emit at least as much radiation as the front. The least suitable place for your mobile phone is on your belt, or in your bag, hanging close to your lower body (and your reproductive system). Use the same remedies as for ionising radiation.

◆ In order to reduce the effect of electromagnetic pollution, try to sleep in a room which has no active electrical gadgets (especially water beds or electric blankets, which should be turned off at the wall). Be aware of pilot lights or fuse boxes that may be drawing current around the walls and creating an electromagnetic field. Think about moving house if you live near power lines or transmitter towers.

◆ Reduce tea drinking to a minimum (2 cups daily). Caffeine levels are lower than those in coffee but there is enough to inhibit iron and zinc absorption. Try green tea, which is high in antioxidants, or herb teas, instead. *Raspberry Leaf* tea is a good source of folic acid, and tones the cervix and the uterus.

◆ Reduce salt and sugar intake to a minimum. Sugar bingeing, especially in the third week of pregnancy, can lead to a rapid increase in insulin production in the infant, which may result in it being born obese. Like all refined carbohydrates, sugar also strips a number of essential nutrients from your body. As these are depleted, your sugar cravings increase, and on it goes. It's also important to get your blood sugar levels under control before pregnancy so as to minimise the chances of developing gestational diabetes. Remember, all sweet things contain sugar in one form or another, including honey, soft drinks, cakes and biscuits, fruit juices and even fruit (2–3 pieces a day is plenty).

◆ If under or overweight, make concerted attempts — both of you — to reduce (or gain) to your optimum weight. Healthy women have at least 10 per cent more fat than men, and their fertility depends on certain levels of fat. If you eat correctly, your weight should balance itself. If you are too fat, you may produce too little progesterone; if too thin, too little oestrogen. Overweight women may also be more likely to suffer from miscarriage and polycystic ovarian syndrome, which is associated with poor insulin metabolism and increased male hormones; it also affects fertility. The children of overweight women are more likely to suffer from congenital abnormalities.

◆ Avoid storing food in plastic containers or plastic wraps. These contain synthetic compounds that mimic oestrogen and can cause hormonal disruption. Use paper, ceramic or glass containers instead.

◆ Start to use the synchronisation autosuggestions to bring your two fertility cycles into alignment to optimise fertility.

◆ Start to use the affirmative techniques suggested later in this chapter to increase your confidence and optimism.

◆ Start on a program of exercise. Rebounding is ideal; walking and swimming are both useful as they can be continued well into pregnancy (though some swimming pools have a high level of chlorine and copper in the water). Yoga will help to get you supple (see Chapter 12, 'Natural Remedies for Hormonal and Reproductive Health'). Pelvic congestion, which can be a source of fertility problems in both men and women, is relieved by exercise. Osteophatic and massage treatments are also excellent remedies to ensure good circulation, lymphatic drainage and decongestion.

◆ Since heat and pressure kill sperm, the prospective father should avoid hot baths, saunas, tight trousers and underpants (wear boxer shorts), wetsuits, lycra sports shorts, sitting on hot engines and hard saddles, and even sitting down for long periods of time (as in an office situation). Those testicles are hanging outside the body for a good reason, as even body heat is detrimental. A radical remedy for overheating is to dunk the testicles in cold water for a few minutes several times a day! . 'Goolie-coolers', an ingenious device for keeping the testes cool, are available in the USA, though not as yet in Australia.

◆ Start paying great attention to your nutrition.

Nutrition

It was convincingly shown in data collected during the Dutch famine in the Second World War, that preconception starvation, which caused damage to the egg and the sperm, affected foetal health more profoundly than if the starvation occurred during pregnancy. Subsequent studies have confirmed this.

A healthy preconception diet followed by both parents has been shown to lead to children who have

even and beautiful features	freedom from allergic response
well-formed skulls	freedom from mental retardation
good posture	advanced development
semi-circular dental arches	well-balanced emotions

During pregnancy, because the considerable nutritional needs of a growing foetus take precedence over the mother's, you're going to need a bit more than the baby requires to have any left for yourself — the extra being required for your body to manufacture the enormous supply of necessary additional hormones.

If deficiencies arise, it's very difficult to make them up during pregnancy; you should be looking to eat for two for several months before conception.

This doesn't really mean that you need more food (though you may need to increase your intake slightly once you're pregnant), but it does mean that you need better food. You'll require a substantial stock of the nutrients that baby-building demands. Once you've conceived, you'll also need a few extra kilojoules (calories).

The quality of your food is much more important than the quantity. You won't need to double your intake, even when you are pregnant — your baby will be smaller than you! However, you will need a few extra kilojoules. Indeed, a larger weight gain and heavier baby can lead to an easier delivery, and a healthier and more intelligent child. Therefore, once you've conceived, you can — within reason — eat more.

Preconceptually, however, you want to keep your weight at normal levels. Just make sure all your food is nutritious (and organic, if possible), so you don't have to eat more to eat well. Overweight and underweight people, both men and women, tend to be less fertile.

Your food should be packed with vitamins and minerals, be rich in fibre, protein and complex carbohydrates, and low in saturated fats, sugars, salt, tea, coffee and chemical additives. All the guidelines we explored in Chapter 12, 'Natural Remedies for Hormonal and Reproductive Health', apply here.

If you eat too much junk food, there won't be enough space for the nutritious healthy stuff. Cut out the sugar and white flour — they take up valuable space! Sugar creates other problems. The possibility of obesity in the infant has already been mentioned, as has the connection between sugar and candida to which you are much more vulnerable during pregnancy. What sugar and refined carbohydrates will also do is leach nutrients, create an increased risk of insulin resistance (which can affect hormonal and reproductive health) and contribute to an overacidic environment in your body, which will immobilise the sperm (see Chapter 12 for more information on acidic mucus).

Other foods you should avoid are those to which you have an allergic reaction. These will deplete your stores of energy and nutrients, and may pass on the problem to your child.

If you have not embarked on a program to rid yourself of your allergies with the help of a natural health practitioner, simply find a way of providing yourself with sufficient nutrients while avoiding the allergenic foods. Some foods, such as green potatoes, can cause malformations. Others help to reduce the chance of malformation. Some of the best preventative foods are

◆ vegetable juices, particularly broccoli and green capsicum

◆ any other juices (especially vegetable) high in vitamin C and the other antioxidant vitamins, A and E, and selenium, zinc or magnesium

◆ milk (though only from goats or sheep unless you're sure you're not sensitive to cow's milk products).

◆ cold-pressed vegetable oils (for the essential fatty acids); use cold-pressed olive oil for cooking and salad dressings.

Because of the preventative activity of the antioxidants, it is important to have a diet high in vegetables (and some fruits), preferably at least some of these in juice form. Make sure your meats, animal products, vegetables and water are as free from chemicals and additives as possible.

Organically grown and fed foods are significantly higher in nutrients and lower in toxins. Many studies have confirmed this, and the director of the Institute of Brain Chemistry at the Queen Elizabeth Hospital for Children in London had this to say: 'Factory farm, intensively produced food is undermining public health and the nation's intelligence.'

HELPFUL HINTS FOR CHANGING YOUR FOOD HABITS

To help you make what may seem to be quite substantial changes in the way you eat with as little trauma as possible, here are some ideas.

◆ Give away all your unhealthy foods to someone else (who is not trying to conceive!)

◆ Fill your cupboards with healthy, nutritious, delicious foods for snacks, etc., so you don't find yourself down at the shops buying junk before you've had time to say 'Better Babies'!

◆ Use your daily quota of 2–3 pieces of fruit to substitute for other sugary foods you may be used to eating.

◆ Think daily of the positive step you are taking for the health of your pregnancy and your child.

NUTRIENTS FOR PROSPECTIVE PARENTS

In addition to the guidelines on diet and nutrition given in Chapter 12 and the problems of deficiencies highlighted in Chapter 2, there are some specific requirements for prospective parents, which are outlined here. Remember that this applies to both of you.

Protein

This is essential both for yourselves (for healthy eggs and sperm) and to form your baby's muscles and organs. *To ensure optimum birth weight (8–10 pounds or 3500–4500 grams), you need good-quality protein, and plenty of it.*

There are studies showing a strong link between low birthweight, infant mortality and congenital defects, and higher birthweight (not too high) and protein intake. It is better not to wait until you are pregnant to change to a higher protein intake; you need it preconceptually. Try to eat a serving of protein-providing foods, which is the size of the palm of your hand, 2–3 times daily.

Adequate protein is also vital for the number and quality of eggs produced, healthy sperm, the fertilisation process and the early development of the embryo. It acts as a buffer to excess acid present in the system, which could create a hostile environment for the sperm. A deficiency can lead to chromosomal abnormalities.

Because excessively high protein diets also seem to create problems in much the same ways as a deficiency, there's no need to go overboard. However, the implications are serious for the vegetarian or vegan, who gets little, if any, primary protein, and must combine secondary, or plant, proteins from two of the three groups daily. These groups are nuts, grains and seeds, and legumes.

Animal protein is also necessary for the optimum functioning of the testes and the amino acids present in animal protein are needed for sperm production. Therefore, preconceptually, ensure that you eat adequate protein, using milk, acidophilus yogurt and cheese (from goats or sheep if you, like the majority of people, are sensitive to cow's milk products), seeds, nuts, sprouted grains, meat, fish and eggs according to your preference.

Fish is a wonderful source of protein and other nutrients. It has no saturated fat problems and, if you eat the deep-dwelling, cold-water, ocean and deep-sea varieties, has plentiful essential fatty acids and little pollution. However, avoid the larger fish, such as tuna, shark and swordfish, which may be high in mercury. Pollution is generally more of a problem with animal products as it is stored in the fat. Organically fed meats are often more difficult to obtain than organically grown vegetables. If the meats are not organic, avoid the organs (where toxins collect) and all products made from organ meats, such as sausage, delicatessen meats and, frequently, mince.

For this reason, as well as the need to avoid fats for their effect on your hormonal balance, trim all meats, use only free-range, organically fed eggs and chickens (trimmed of skin), avoid dyed, smoked or irradiated fish or meat products, and any prepared meats which may contain mutagenic substances.

Once you have conceived, you should increase your protein intake by about 20 per cent.

Vitamin A

A lack of this vitamin can result in either a lack of conception or a tendency to miscarry. When the pregnancy does run to term, there may be an increased risk of birth defects such as cleft palates and even the absence of eyes. Due to potential toxicity, it is best taken as mixed carotenoids (or, if these are unavailable, as Beta-carotene) as this avoids the potential risk of birth defects associated with high dosages of vitamin A, though dosages of up to 10000 iu daily have been shown to be very safe.

It is the vitamin which keeps the ciliae — tiny hair-like projections inside the fallopian tubes — healthy. The ciliae help to move the egg down the tube to the womb. Vitamin A keeps the mucous membranes healthy and is important for overall reproductive health. It is needed for sperm production, healthy testes and conversion of cholesterol to testosterone in the male, and to oestrogen in the female. A deficiency can lead to degeneration of the sex organs.

Vitamin B-complex

The other nutrient deficiencies implicated in low birthweight, problem pregnancies, possible malformation and increased chances of neonatal or perinatal death are folic acid (B_9), thiamin (B_1), riboflavin (B_2), niacinamide (B_3), pantothenic acid (B_5) pyridoxin (B_6), cobalamin (B_{12}) and biotin (which is helpful for candidiasis treatment). You need these preconceptually.

The B-complex vitamins, which occur together in nature, should always be taken as a group, as an excess of one can induce or disguise a deficiency in another. They are generally important to keep the hormonal balance, especially to ensure enough progesterone, which is essential for the early development of the embryo and the smooth progression of the pregnancy. In the male, B_5 is required for healthy testes, and B_{12} to increase sperm count and motility, but all the B vitamins are useful and will help to counteract stress reactions in either partner.

Experimental congenital malformation has been induced with 99 per cent accuracy in animals simply by withholding B vitamins from their preconceptual diet. Although the experiments performed to supply this information are to be deplored, the results certainly need heeding.

Thiamin (Vitamin B₁)

This vitamin is essential for maintaining the pregnancy and preventing abnormalities.

Riboflavin (Vitamin B₂)

If riboflavin deprivation occurs a month or so before possible conception, it can lead to infertility. If induced closer to fertilisation (12 days before), deprivation can cause malformation, and after conception there may be re-absorption of the embryo. This is because riboflavin affects oestradiol levels, which are needed to develop the follicle.

Take care if you are on a dairy-free diet as it may be deficient in riboflavin. Eat more mushrooms, broccoli and broad beans.

Pantothenic acid (Vitamin B₅)

This vitamin is important for healthy testes, and helps in the building of body cells, normal growth and the development of the central nervous system.

Pyridoxin (Vitamin B₆)

With the dosage set at the amount needed to relieve premenstrual tension, this vitamin may lead to a decrease in prolactin levels and an increase in progesterone levels (which is why it is useful for PMS). Progesterone is necessary to prepare the endometrium for implantation and pregnancy. Vitamin B₆ is also required for the metabolism of several other nutrients, has been shown to increase the chances of conception and is required to control homocysteine levels which, when raised, can lead to repeated miscarriages and neural tube defects.

Folic acid (Vitamin B₉)

This is one of the most important nutrients to take preconceptually, as the need for it in the very early stages of pregnancy is enormous. In the first 3–7 weeks of gestation, it is essential for the new tissue to differentiate into organs; protein metabolism is dependent on folic acid for tissue growth to occur.

A deficiency can also lead to infertility (through reducing the production of eggs and sperm), repeated miscarriage or neural tube defects (through a rise in homocysteine levels normally kept in check by this nutrient and vitamins B₆ and B₁₂), and chromosomal damage (which causes mutations). Therefore, *particular care should be exercised when coming off the Pill to ensure that you replenish your supplies of folic acid prior to conception.*

Cobalamin (Vitamin B₁₂)

This vitamin has been shown to enhance fertility in both sexes and is required to ensure adequate sperm count and motility. A deficiency can cause spinal cord damage in the infant and contribute to repeated miscarriage as it is required to keep homocysteine levels low. Excessive doses of folic acid (more than 1 mg) can mask a B₁₂ deficiency. *Vegetarians beware: the main source of B₁₂ is animal products.*

Inositol

Inositol is important in the male for a healthy prostate.

Ascorbic acid (Vitamin C)

Vitamin C is necessary for the production of sex hormones; a continuing pregnancy is dependent upon a rich supply. The ovaries are very rich in vitamin C, suggesting a strong need for its presence. It has been shown to start ovulation in women with anovular cycles, and can help with heavy periods and infertility. It will cut down on the chance of infections and lead to the formation of a healthier child. It is necessary to prevent non-specific sperm agglutination (the tendency to clump together), which can decrease motility and cause infertility. The effects on agglutination should be noticeable within a week. Being an antioxidant, it will help to prevent mutagenic and teratogenic activity, and assist in the elimination of toxins. Always take a preparation that contains the bioflavonoids, which will automatically be present in any food source, such as fruit and vegetables.

Vitamin D

This vitamin is necessary for the growth of bones and teeth, and for calcium and phosphorus absorption. A deficiency is a factor in many deformities. If you spend some time in the sun (not too long — beware the hole in the ozone layer!) you will form your own vitamin D.

Mixed tocopherols (Vitamin E)

This vitamin used to be called the fertility vitamin. It is necessary to ensure conception and a healthy pregnancy. A lack of it can trigger a spontaneous abortion, when the embryo is expelled very early in the pregnancy (these miscarriages can be mistaken for a heavy, possibly late, period). It is required for an adequate sperm count, and a deficiency can lead to a total lack of sperm in the semen. It is an antioxidant so will help to prevent the negative effects of toxins. It facilitates an easy delivery.

Essential fatty acids

Here we go on the essential fatty acid–saturated fats–prostaglandin roundabout again. EFAs are required for the development of your child's brain, eyes and nervous system, the walls of all cells, and can protect against SIDS. The prostaglandins control the fine-tuning of the baby's body functions. A deficiency in the EFAs can lead to a general impairment of gonadal function, chromosomal defects, spontaneous abortion and congenital malformation. Males need even more than females (and we've seen how much they need). The prostaglandins that need to be present in the seminal fluid are the PG1 and PG2 types.

Calcium

This mineral is essential for several reasons. It is required for the development of your baby's bones, for uterine muscle tone, for the formation of stretchy fertile mucus and to counteract the negative effects of manganese in the vagina, which can cause the mucus to become sticky. Male needs are not as high as female. Men can halve the dosage requirements unless there are high lead levels.

Zinc

Zinc is the most important mineral and antioxidant of all. It is used in detoxification and improves all aspects of reproductive health for both partners. It is necessary for normal production of the egg, and vital for a viable sperm count, motility. and a high percentage of normally shaped and live sperm in the semen. It is usually present in fairly large amounts in semen; excessive loss of semen through ejaculation may lose 2–5 mg of zinc a day. A deficiency can cause chromosomal abnormalities and lead to retarded development or spontaneous abortion. It is also required for an easy, on-time delivery, a healthy postnatal experience and a happy, calm and well-balanced baby. It can even help you avoid stretch marks! Take zinc daily for at least 4 months before conception and use the zinc taste test (see earlier section) to assess need.

Magnesium
This mineral is important for muscle tone and hormonal balance. A deficiency can lead to retarded development of the foetus, miscarriage and low birth weight. Magnesium is also essential to avoid toxaemia in later pregnancy and is important for healthy sperm.

Manganese
A deficiency in this mineral can lead to spontaneous abortion, bone, heart and nervous system defects in the foetus, and if the deficiency is severe, a total lack of sperm.

Iodine
This nutrient is needed for healthy thyroid function, which influences hormone balance. An iodine deficiency in pregnancy can lead to cretinism in the baby. Iodine, like copper and iron, is dangerous in excess.

Iron
Iron is required for your baby's bloodstream, brain, bone and eye development, and rate of growth. It's also necessary for your mucous membranes and general fertility (see Chapter 12 for cautions).

Copper
Too little or too much copper can lead to fertility problems. Zinc deficiency may indicate excessive levels of copper. Check this on your hair-trace mineral analysis. Most people these days, especially urban dwellers, have plenty — if not too much — as their water is delivered through copper pipes.

Boron
Boron use is restricted by legislation as it is toxic in excess, so it is not present in over-the-counter supplements. You should get all you need from your diet as long as you eat plenty of fresh fruit and vegetables.

Selenium
This nutrient is an important antioxidant which is especially useful for detoxifying heavy metals. It is present in large quantities in semen but is lost through frequent ejaculation, and a deficiency decreases sperm count, motility and the percentage of normally shaped sperm. Deficiencies in either parent have also been liked to Down syndrome, SIDS and asthmatic children.

Chromium
Chromium is an important nutrient for blood-sugar control, which can be a problem in pregnancy for both mother and child.

All minerals
All the minerals you take should be chelated and, where possible, from an organic, natural source.

Essential amino acids
These nutrients are present in complete proteins. Essential amino acids are needed for sperm production and motility, and for healthy testes. Dosage (in cases of male fertility problems):

◆ arginine — specific for sperm count, but not if there is a history of herpes — 2–4 g, 3 x daily

◆ carnitine — for count, motility and morphology (proportion of normally shaped sperm) — 600–1200mg, 3 x daily

◆ histidine — specific for motility — 300–600mg, 3 x daily.

◆ All to be taken with water between meals. A deficiency in either parent can lead to foetal malformation.

Complex carbohydrates
These are required for energy (not to be found in refined cereals). However, it's important not to have excessive amounts of carbohydrate in your diet, and to choose low glycaemic carbohydrates such as vegetables over high glycaemic carbohydrates such as sugars and refined grains.

CAUTIONS
Avoid megavitamins. Some vitamins taken in large quantities can cause adverse effects. Some examples.

◆ High levels of folic acid (more than 1 mg daily) can mask a B_{12} deficiency.

◆ Too much B_6 can be toxic and lead to numbness in the upper lip, hands and feet. (Up to 200 mg daily is very safe and symptoms are reversible.)

◆ Too much copper can decrease zinc levels and fertility.

◆ Too much vitamin A is toxic. Much more than 10 000 iu a day can lead to birth defects. Use as mixed carotenoids (or Beta-carotene) to avoid this problem.

◆ Too much iron affects zinc absorption.

◆ Too much phosphorus increases the need for calcium.

◆ Too much manganese can make your mucus sticky.

SUGGESTED DOSAGE LEVELS FOR SUPPLEMENTATION

Mixed carotenoids (or Beta-carotene) — 6 mg or vitamin A — 10 000 iu

Vitamin B-complex

folic acid — 500–1000 mcg

B_1, B_2, B_3, B_5, B_6 — 50 mg (B_6 dosage may need to be higher if progesterone levels are low, or to treat PMS)

B_{12} — 400 mcg

Biotin — 200 mcg

Choline, inositol and PABA — 25 mg

Vitamin C — 2–5 g (+ 300 mg bioflavonoids)

Vitamin D — 200 iu

Vitamin E — 500 iu (in first two pregnancy trimesters, 800 iu in last)

Omega 3 and 6 essential fatty acids (from *Evening Primrose*, flaxseed and fish oils) — 3000 mg

Calcium — 800 mg, or more (1200 mg in second trimester of pregnancy)

Magnesium — 400 mg, or more (half calcium dosage)

Manganese — 10 mg

Zinc — 20–60 mg (elemental)

Iron (only if blood test shows the need, and organic) — 15 mg with ferrum phos.

Selenium — 100–200 mcg

Chromium — 100–200mcg

Potassium — as potassium chloride (cell salt) or 15 mg

HELPFUL HINTS FOR TAKING YOUR SUPPLEMENTS

You may seem to be taking an awful lot of tablets to achieve the dosage levels recommended here. These dosages are important because you only have a short time to compensate for all those years of inadequate nutrition (even if you've been eating well, it's difficult to maintain the levels required for a conception). So here are some ideas to help make it all a bit easier:

◆ Try to find combination supplements that give you what you need in a minimum number of pills.

◆ Maybe once a week (on a Sunday evening perhaps?) make up a small container (old vitamin pots are ideal — plastic bags will suffice) for each day of the week, containing all the tablets you need to take daily, except zinc, which should be taken separately from other nutrients. This way you avoid having to count them out each morning, and, by taking your container with you, you can space them out through the day and prevent indigestion (which will cause malabsorption as well as being uncomfortable).

◆ Think daily of the positive step you are taking for the health of your pregnancy and your child.

Above all, both of you, enjoy your food. Then, well-nourished and happy, you can embark on an adventure which starts like this.

The romance of the egg and the sperm

Your healthy, well-nourished egg is released from your ovary and is caught by the waving arms of the tiny filaments (fimbriae) around the end of your fallopian tube. This tube is about as wide as a hairbrush bristle, and about 10 cm (4 inches) long. The egg itself is even smaller than the dot at the end of this exclamation mark!

You think that's incredible? Well, to the sperm the egg is a giant. Twenty-five million sperm could fit on this full stop.

As far as sperm are concerned, we always talk in millions. 'Normal' sperm count is in a range from 30–60 million per mL of seminal fluid, which will result in a healthy male depositing 280–400 million sperm in one ejaculation.

This may seem like an enormous number when only one is needed to fertilise your egg, but there are different types of sperm, and only some — the fittest — are there to fertilise the egg. The others are kamikaze sperm, whose function is to identify and kill any sperm belonging to other men. They do this by ramming (they are obviously the macho types) or poisoning them. Others block entry to sperm belonging to anyone who might subsequently have intercourse with you. This is an easy job — they just sit tight in the cervical mucus, which helps to filter out the less fit or defective sperm.

They also have to face many other hazards on their journey. Sperm move along by lashing their tails; they are enabled to do this by a substance found in your reproductive tract. It takes them several hours of vigorous tail-lashing to complete the 18 cm (7 inch) marathon from the cervix to the place in the fallopian tube, the ampulla, where, hopefully, your egg is waiting. This was succinctly put by Dr Edward Lyons, a Canadian research doctor who said, 'Sperm are not salmon. They don't swim unaided upstream.' Muscular contractions present in the uterus and tubes of fertile women produce waves which the sperm can surf to speed up their journey.

While your egg waits, a constituent of the fluid that surrounds it is sending out love letters', messages to the sperm alerting them to its presence and triggering their swim in the right direction. It's possible that these messages are selective, attracting the highly mobile and vigorous sperm rather than the very young or old, which might be less viable. The signals may also encourage the sperm on from their resting places along the way.

Sperm

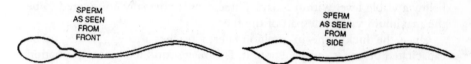

SPERM
AS SEEN
FROM
FRONT

SPERM
AS SEEN
FROM
SIDE

On this journey, many of the sperm will be immobilised by the acidity in the vagina before they reach the relative safety of the alkaline cervix. Others will be killed by the white cells produced by the woman directly after intercourse, if they haven't already been repelled by the muscular contractions of orgasm. However — it's not all hostility — at orgasm the cervix dips into the pool of semen and sucks it up.

Then many get lost in the uterus, simply swimming around and around until they die, never finding the two exits to the fallopian tubes, in one of which your egg is waiting. Also, many that do find one of the tube entrances, will choose the wrong one. An egg is normally only released by one ovary in each cycle, usually alternately. So, what starts off like the crowd at a fun run, thins out just as rapidly.

Your egg will wait for Mr Right for 12–24 hours, then, if he hasn't arrived, give up and die (broken hearted — or just tired of waiting?).

The sperm live longer, up to 3–6 days. Although they take up 116 days to be produced, once released into the vaginal tract, 6 days is the most they can survive. It is extremely unlikely that such a geriatric sperm could hobble its way to your egg and win this very competitive race.

The Progress of the Fertilized Egg

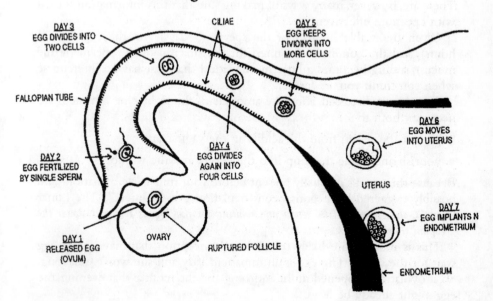

DAY 3
EGG DIVIDES INTO
TWO CELLS

CILIAE

DAY 5
EGG KEEPS
DIVIDING INTO
MORE CELLS

FALLOPIAN TUBE

DAY 6
EGG MOVES
INTO UTERUS

DAY 2
EGG FERTILIZED
BY SINGLE SPERM

DAY 4
EGG DIVIDES
AGAIN INTO
FOUR CELLS

UTERUS

DAY 7
EGG IMPLANTS IN
ENDOMETRIUM

DAY 1
RELEASED EGG
(OVUM)

OVARY

RUPTURED FOLLICLE

← ENDOMETRIUM

In fact, sperm life reduces by a third each day; 16–18 hours is an average lifespan. The number of sperm (sperm count) also lowers each day, and falls below a viable level within 3 days. Three days is normally considered to be the maximum viable lifespan of the sperm.

Once the lucky one-in-a-zillion sperm reaches the egg, it has to be capacitated before it can penetrate it. This may sound like a scary initiation rite, but in fact, hormonal secretions in the female release two enzymes from the sperm, making the way clear for the final breakthrough, by enabling the sperm to burrow through the egg's outer coatings.

Then the fertilised egg is majestically wafted down the rest of the tube, by rhythmic contractions and the little ciliae that line the tubes. It takes about a week of this slow and stately progress until the egg is in the uterus and implants in the endometrium. From that moment on, everything moves very quickly.

The moral of this story is …

Timing is critical

You have spent some months preparing for the big event and you want to be sure that you know which sexual act will result in conception, so you need to know *exactly when to do it*.

Learning when you are fertile is the same process whether you want to avoid or achieve pregnancy, so the best way to achieve it is to avoid it first.

Since you will need at least a few months to prepare yourself nutritionally, and to ensure good health (hormonal and otherwise), there will be plenty of time to learn how to apply sympto-thermal and lunar cycle methods to identify your fertile days.

Timing for conception is a bit like timing for contraception in reverse. There are, however, many ways of making sure that this information is used with optimum effectiveness.

Given the viable lifespan of the sperm (3 days) and the egg (12–24 hours), and the conditions required for the survival of the sperm (fertile mucus), timing becomes a little more critical than just having intercourse when you think you are fertile.

As we have discussed, adequate amounts of the right type of mucus are necessary both to

◆ protect the sperm from the acidity in the vagina, and

◆ nourish and guide them up into the cervix and the womb.

Because this mucus is usually present before your mid-cycle ovulation (and possibly triggered by a spontaneous ovulation; see Chapter 7, 'The Lunar Cycle'), *the sperm can be ready and waiting for the egg as it comes down the fallopian tube*.

This is much more likely to result in conception than having the egg wait for the sperm. The egg is an impatient lady and she won't wait long. So, if ovulation happened in the morning and intercourse that evening, the egg might already be dead.

Also, we aren't that good (yet) at telling precisely when ovulation occurs, so *it is vital to know in advance that ovulation is about to take place.*

Information (such as that given by your basal body temperature readings) that tells you that ovulation has already taken place will be useless if there is any chance that it happened up to or more than 12 hours ago, or if there is no opportunity for intercourse in the next 12 hours.

Recent research also suggests that the time of day may be a critical factor when planning your conception attempt. Sperm count has been found to be highest between 5.00 pm and 5.30 pm, while ovulation peaks between 3.00 pm and 7.00 pm. Late afternoon seems to be the optimum time of day for a conception attempt.

BABY SNATCHING

There is another timing factor to take into consideration to ensure a healthy conception. *Ageing sperm and ova are potentially defective.*

You need to be using your timing techniques to make sure that the romance between the egg and the sperm is a story of young love!

Two scenarios to avoid.

◆ A single sexual act several days *prior* to ovulation, likely to furnish the ovum with ageing and potentially defective sperm.

◆ A single sexual act just *after* ovulation, creating a higher risk of the sperm meeting an ageing and potentially defective egg.

Frequent intercourse throughout the peak fertile time until ovulation is over ensures that fresh sperm meet a fresh egg. Having waited until the right moment to start, you then keep going until you are sure that you have ovulated.

CONCEPTION ON THE HORMONAL CYCLE

The best way to tell that you are about to ovulate and ready to receive sperm is through the mucus observations. Hopefully, you will be getting good at this by the time you plan to conceive.

Another advantage of spending a few months learning about symptom observation is that, after the birth of your baby, you will already be an expert in natural contraception. Breastfeeding is not an easy time to practise natural birth control if you are a novice.

Once fertile mucus has been detected, there is a good chance that sperm deposited in the vagina will be ready and waiting for the egg when it is released. However, this procedure can be improved upon.

By using a combination of temperature and mucus observations over several cycles, it is possible to come to a refined understanding of your ovulation timing within your mucus pattern.

Using the day at the beginning of the temperature rise as the most likely day for ovulation to have taken place, you can learn if there is a regular mucus pattern preceding this day. There usually is.

For example, you may find that you usually ovulate on

◆ the third day of wet mucus, *or*

◆ usually the fifth, *or*

◆ the second day of *spinn*, following 3–4 days of wetness.

Personal repeating patterns are uncovered in this way; *mittelschmerz* can help to confirm this.

You cannot necessarily expect to pinpoint ovulation to the exact day, but you can expect to refine your understanding considerably. This can make a great deal of difference to how you time your conception attempt. Let's take an example.

Suppose you generally had 5 days of wet mucus, followed by 1 day of *spinn*, followed by a return to dry, sticky mucus (your BIP), and you then determine through your temperature readings that you usually ovulate on the day after the *spinn*-type mucus.

The day before ovulation is the most important day for you to have intercourse; that way, you can be sure that fresh, vigorous sperm are ready and waiting for your egg, as the front-runners are the healthiest, the less viable sperm trailing along behind and taking longer to complete the journey. Bear in mind that the peak symptom occurs in the majority of women 12–24 hours before ovulation (Mother Nature is at it again). In our example, you would avoid sexual activity for at least four of the wet days, and concentrate on the fifth day of wetness and the day of *spinn*.

Depending on how regular your mucus pattern is, and bearing in mind that you don't want to start your conception attempts after ovulation, you might even refine this further by only starting to try to conceive on the day of *spinn*.

Without this information, you might have started your attempts 5 days before ovulation, when the wet, fertile mucus started, and thus have wasted valuable sperm.

Pinpointing ovulation is especially important if sperm count is at all low. There is a Monty Python song which goes:

> *Every sperm is sacred,*
> *Every sperm is great,*
> *If a sperm gets wasted,*
> *God gets quite irate.*

While this is intended as a satire on Roman Catholic attitudes to contraception, it's a jingle that can remind you of the best way to approach your conception attempt.

Several days (3–5) of abstinence (no ejaculation) can help to build a high count of healthy sperm.

This will ensure that the sperm responsible for the conception are fresh and healthy. It also prevents the loss of large amounts of the essential nutrients zinc and selenium, which are plentiful in healthy semen. A greater period of abstinence can, however, be counterproductive as the sperm may age before ejaculation.

The best time to have intercourse is in the late afternoon, as ovulation and peak sperm count most frequently occur then. Sperm should be deposited high in the vagina, near the cervix (penetration from the rear is most successful). After ejaculation, leave the penis in the vagina until it is flaccid, to prevent pulling the semen out.

The woman should then lie down for a few minutes, to keep the semen high in the vagina. It is not necessary to put your legs up or stay prone for an extended period of time because healthy sperm will find their way into the cervix quite rapidly. Avoid lubricants as they may interfere with sperm motility; even saliva has been shown to be spermicidal. It's possible that the woman's saliva at mid-cycle, when it is ferning under the influence of increased oestrogen levels, might be more friendly to sperm, but the only substance definitely shown to be unharmful is raw egg-white. This should add a touch of humour to your conception attempt!

If your mucus pattern changes suddenly and you suspect that ovulation has happened, but you have missed it, don't try anyway — avoid the possibility of fertilising an ageing egg by waiting for the next cycle.

Temperature readings obviously do not, by themselves, give you this warning of ovulation. However, they are an essential part of the process of refining your understanding of the significance of your unique mucus pattern.

Temperature readings also confirm that ovulation is taking place and on which day of the mucus pattern this normally occurs. They also give you valuable information about the length of the pre-ovulatory (follicular) or post-ovulatory (luteal) phases. This is important information, which will help you lessen the chances of miscarriage and defective eggs.

The optimum time for ovulation is on Day 14 or earlier, when the chances of fertilisation producing healthy offspring are greater than 90 per cent. If you ovulate on Day 15 or later, your chances of a good conception drop to 43 per cent. Remember, these statistics are taken from women who are not necessarily taking care of their health. Your chances of a healthy conception if you have prepared well are considerably higher. However, they do show the relative rates.

Size of the Follicle at Different Stages of the Cycle

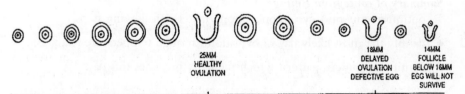

25MM
HEALTHY
OVULATION

18MM
DELAYED
OVULATION
DEFECTIVE EGG

14MM
FOLLICLE
BELOW 16MM
EGG WILL NOT
SURVIVE

1   14   22

This has to do with the size of the follicle at different times in the menstrual cycle. On the first day of the period it is about 2 mm. Over the next 14 days, it grows to 25 mm. This increase, the fastest growth observed in any human tissue during the normal human lifecycle — apart from the initial development of the embryo — is of the order of twelve times the initial diameter, and 1000 times the initial mass.

Long pre-ovulatory phases (greater than 16 days), in which ovulation occurs when the follicle is already reducing in size, have been associated with changes in the corpus luteum and the efficiency of progesterone secretion, which is necessary to maintain the pregnancy. This is because the corpus luteum is formed from the follicle after ovulation (see Chapter 3, 'Your Bodies'). If ovulation occurs very late (20–25 days), there is a higher incidence of miscarriage and abnormal eggs.

A delayed ovulation, which can be the result of hormonal imbalance, ovarian or pituitary dysfunction, smoking, alcohol excess, drug use, environmental toxins or nutrient deficiencies, may occur when the follicle is, for example, at about Day 22, only 18mm. If the follicle is below 16 mm, the egg will not survive.

Because a long pre-ovulatory phase can result in lowered progesterone levels, it may lead to a post-ovulatory phase which is too short, an additional problem. The fertilised egg takes about a week to travel down the fallopian tube, so progesterone levels need to be peaking at about this time to ensure a receptive endometrium. The progesterone peaks midway between ovulation and menstruation, and if the luteal phase is less than 12 days long, this will occur before 6 days have elapsed, which is too early for the egg's implantation. If the length of the luteal phase is 10 days or less, the peak will be reached in 5 days at the most, and the cycle will be infertile.

Reduced progesterone levels and a shortened luteal phase are termed a 'luteal defect' and may be caused by many other factors. Hormone balancing treatments described in Chapter 12 may be helpful in correcting imbalances of either phases of the cycle. If, despite your preconception health care, your temperature readings indicate that your pre-ovulatory phase is too long, or your post-ovulatory phase too short, then you should turn to your health practitioner for advice and treatment before trying to conceive.

If you find that ovulation does not occur, or only happens rarely, then therapy is also indicated.

Summary of conception timing

To optimise your mid-cycle conceptions, take the following steps.

◆ Identify the most likely day of ovulation (through temperature readings).

◆ Identify the mucus pattern which regularly precedes this day.

◆ Identify the day before ovulation according to this mucus pattern. This may be the peak symptom day and is the best day to attempt conception.

◆ Identify the day which is usually 3–5 (4) days before this (if your mucus pattern is not evident this long before ovulation, you may need to identify the day of the cycle). This is the best day to start abstinence, after an ejaculation to get rid of old sperm.

◆ Continue conception attempts at least every other day (to ensure fresh sperm are always present) until ovulation is over (temperature readings have risen and mucus has dried up), *or* you reach day 17 of your cycle, after which no more unprotected intercourse should occur until you are confident ovulation is over and conception cannot occur.

◆ If your pre-ovulatory phase is consistently greater than 16 days, or your post-ovulatory phase less than 12 days — seek help before attempting conception.

CONCEPTION ON THE LUNAR CYCLE

Most conceptions occur on the hormonal cycle, or when the two cycles synchronise. However, for some women the lunar peak seems to be a viable alternative. If this occurs separately from mid-cycle ovulation, a spontaneous ovulation will need to be triggered for conception to take place.

Much of the 4 days of possible and potential fertility on this cycle is only fertile if, after being deposited, the sperm live until the peak time when an ovulation might occur. Unless this cycle synchronises with the hormonal cycle, spontaneous ovulation will only happen if triggered by some event, the most likely being sexual activity.

Spontaneous ovulation only seems likely to occur if intercourse takes place within the 24 hours preceding the exact return of the natal angle.

If intercourse takes place 2 days before the peak, the spontaneous ovulation would be unlikely to occur and conception would only be possible, theoretically, if some other event triggered the ovulation (for example, masturbation or high levels of excitement).

So, if you want to make sure that you conceive at your lunar peak, it's best to make love within the 24-hour peak time. Intercourse is then likely to trigger the release of the egg and deposit the sperm simultaneously, ensuring fresh egg and sperm.

In order to trigger the ovulation, sexual activity can be frequent within 24-hour peak period. Then ovulation is more likely to be triggered and the timespan is within the viable life of the sperm.

To recap, a 4-day lunar fertile period looks like this.

24 Hour Peak Fertile Lunar Time

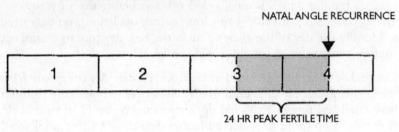

) *Remember that your lunar time remains fertile wherever it falls in your hormonal cycle.*

The most fertile situation seems to be if the mid–cycle ovulation comes at the lunar peak, with a menstruation–lunar combination also having a high rate of success (see Chapter 7, 'The Lunar Cycle').

Very often, the breakthrough in infertility cases comes when the two cycles synchronise for the first time. If your cycles do synchronise, you will be preparing for conception by anticipating ovulation, abstaining from intercourse, and creating a mood of optimism and relaxation. If the two fertile times do not coincide, then you will prepare in just the same way before your lunar peak day.

Since the lunar peak time is determined in advance, it will be easy to see which days are required for preparation and when the attempt should start. If the two fertile times come close together, you will need to use your own judgement as to whether to treat them as one continuous fertile time or separately, with renewed abstinence between.

Whenever you are anticipating an ovulation and preparing yourself for a conception attempt, abstinence is not the only important way to prepare. The days leading up to it need to be as productive as possible.

Having completed your long-term training, now is the time for the final warm-up at the starting blocks. With all your nutrients in place and a fit body, let us turn our attention to your mind.

I did think of running a competition. Count up the number of times the following words appear in this book:

'Fertility', 'moon', 'mucus', 'natural', 'herbs', 'vitamins', 'nutrition', and … 'stress'. Even if you didn't win with 'stress', you do get to read on.

Stress

It's true that stress is one of the root causes of reproductive and sexual problems. It even robs us of our nutrients. Love and marriage may not go together quite as often as they used to when the song was written, but stress and sexual activity are a far more common (and less successful) combination than ever.

Stress is endemic to our modern lifestyles, especially for urban dwellers. Of course, what we are talking about here is *too much stress*, or the inability to cope with the stress in your life. There is also such a thing as *too little stress* — it's called boredom! Some stress is necessary, and even fun. This has been termed 'eustress' ('eu' being a Greek prefix meaning 'good' as in euphemism, euphoria and eulogy).

If it weren't for eustress, conception might never occur at all. You may have noticed (and if by some strange chance you haven't, the romance writers soon bring it to your attention) that as you get sexually aroused, your pulse quickens, your heart beats a little faster, and this is probably rapidly followed by an episode of heavy breathing!

Now, if there is too much stress or you are in such bad shape that you can't handle it, then all these responses change. Either the male can't get it up, the female is too tired, or you're both feeling too cranky.

Not only that, but fertility is also affected by stress. Your regularity is the first thing that you notice is affected. Your menopause may come earlier, and long-term stress, via the pathways linking the hypothalamus, the sympathetic nervous system, the pituitary, the adrenals and the gonads (ovaries and testes) may have an extremely negative effect on your reproductive capacity. So, stress reduction needs to be part of your long-term preparation for conception, just like nutrition and exercise.

Too much stress at the moment of conception presents its own immediate problems, apart from disinclination.

In childbirth, stresses such as moving the labouring woman around and attaching her to endless gadgets are now known to delay contractions because they interfere with the action of oxytocin, the hormone that causes the contractions. The same responses can inhibit the process whereby the sperm is added to the seminal flow. If the prospective father is too stressed, he may have little or no sperm in his semen.

If the prospective mother is under stress, there may be a chemical alteration in the uterine and vaginal secretions which facilitate the motility of the incoming sperm (if there are any) and the secretions of enzymes necessary for capacitation. This is the process whereby two enzymes are released from the sperm, making the way clear for the final penetration of the egg's two outer coatings.

You can see that you need to have up your sleeve all sorts of techniques for turning your conception attempt and the few days leading up to it into as pleasurable an event as possible.

PREPARATION FOR CONCEPTION
One of the ways of reducing stress is to have sex. But we've already seen how ejaculation should be avoided in the 3–5 days before conception. Sexual contact doesn't always need to include ejaculation, of course, so you can use this time to express your love for each other in different sexual and

sensual ways. You may also find it helpful to find other means of relieving physical and mental stress while maintaining affection, good communication and contact.

Touch is a vital way of destressing and making contact; it doesn't have to be sexual to be effective and supportive.

MASSAGE

Massage is touch with an extra. As well as giving stress release for the nervous system, it can affect our minds and bodies profoundly through relaxing the muscles.

During your few days abstinence, cuddle and hug, and massage each other's neck, shoulders, head, face, hands, feet, back and tummy.

If you've never done any massage before, don't worry; almost anything you do will be welcomed. Use your fingers, thumbs, hands and even elbows to knead away the tensions. If you're worried that you might hurt your partner, extract a promise before you begin that if you cause pain, they will scream, yell, leap up — or simply tell you. Then you can put some energy into the rub, which will make it more effective.

Here are a few massage ideas.

Feet

You can't really go wrong here, except if someone is ticklish. Then you thump the bottom of the foot (all over) with your fist until it relaxes. Ticklishness is really tension.

Head, neck and shoulders

Get your partner to sit on the floor at your feet with you in a chair, or to lie down on their back with you kneeling at their head.

◆ Start with the shoulders.

◆ Move on to the neck. Dig in firmly on either side of the spine, moving the flesh away from the bone and up towards the skull, using your fingertips. Using your whole hand, stretch the muscles up towards the head in long, sweeping movements.

◆ Dig in very firmly under the base of the skull (usually lots of tension here), and move around to the ears and back to the spine. Do this several times.

◆ With your fingers firmly under this ridge, place your hands over your partner's ears, and then (when they can't hear you) say, 'Now I'm going to stretch your neck!' This is not dangerous even if you pull hard (which you should), *as long as you make no sudden movements*. Lean back to pull, and lean in towards the head as you release. Slowly. You can then pull hard (it's easiest in the lying down position), and you will gap the vertebrae, giving them a chance to realign.

◆ Now, move on to the ears. This bit is delicious, and if the massage is being done as part of your lead-up to a conception attempt, this may be as far as you get.

◆ Jaw and chin come next, with smooth, upward movements over the throat.

◆ On the face, you need to use small circular movements, to avoid stretching the skin. However, they should still be vigorous, and generally from the centre of the face out toward the sides, as tension tends to purse our faces up towards the middle.

◆ Up and over nose and cheeks, around the eyes, eyebrows and temples, and around the eyeballs (not too hard here). Then, it's very soothing to place the palms of your hands over your partner's eyes and hold them there, still and quiet, for a minute or two.

◆ Smooth away the frowns between the eyebrows and over the forehead.

◆ Finish with vigorous rubbing over the whole scalp, even grasping the hair and pulling gently to stimulate the hair follicles. This is a wonderful feeling.

◆ The whole massage can even be done while watching the television in the evenings, although it is better in peace and quiet, or with some relaxing music. You'll be hooked for life.

Back
This is the area with perhaps the most scope for a long massage. There are infinite possibilities on this large expanse of flesh, but always spend some time pulling the flesh away from the bone, digging in firmly on either side of the spine. Long, sweeping movements up and down the whole back are very soothing.

The recipient will need to lie flat on their front, on the floor or on a massage bench (beds are too soft).

Tummy
There is a particular massage which is ideal for the preconceptual time. Peristaltic massage releases abdominal and pelvic tensions, right there in the area you're targeting.

As you relax, there is one activity in your body which speeds up — peristalsis. All the others slow down — heartbeat, breathing and thoughts — but as you relax, the action of your intestines, as they pass the food along, actually increases. Because it's such a rhythmic, loose action, it is inhibited by stress.

There are whole therapies based on encouraging peristaltic motion to release negativity, tension, and emotional and physical blocks. Therapists train for years to use these body-centred methods to contact and release emotional blocks, but the techniques are easily adapted for home use.

◆ The person to be massaged should lie down on their back, legs slightly apart, arms down beside the body, preferably with palms facing up.

◆ Start breathing deeply, rhythmically and easily. Don't force it but feel yourself pull the air right down to the base of your lungs and push it out again.

◆ The masseur then strokes, gently at first, then with increasing firmness, from the diaphragm down towards the pubic bone on the out breath. (The exhalation can be recognised as the time the abdomen deflates.)

◆ This can be continued for as long as it's comfortable.

◆ The strokes can then be changed to a circular movement, in a clockwise direction, following the path of the intestines, up on the right-hand side of the body and down on the left.

As you relax with this massage, you may find that your tummy starts to gurgle. *This is good.* It means peristalsis is happening, the organs are relaxing, and you are releasing abdominal and pelvic tensions.

Peristaltic massage is especially useful as part of foreplay before your conception attempt.

AUTOSUGGESTION

As you release physical tensions, so your mind calms and clears. This is a good time for using suggestion and affirmation techniques, to increase your confidence and optimism. You can put the following ideas on tape, create them in your mind, or get a therapist to do it for you. If you order a conception kit from Natural Fertility Management (see Appendix 1), you will receive a tape which has on it a visualisation and affirmations very similar to the following text.

Just find a comfortable place to sit or to lie and follow the text in Chapter 8, 'Synchronising Cycles', up to the point where you have visualised yourself under the phase of the moon which was present at your birth. Follow on like this.

Now see clearly again your whole reproductive system, ovaries, tubes, womb, cervix and vagina, still glowing with warmth and light, full of vital, healthy energy, relaxed. (If your partner is with you he should at this point imagine testes, vas deferens, seminal vesicles, prostate and penis, and see the production of millions of motile, healthy sperm.)

See the cervix and vagina full of wet, fertile mucus and know that your body is preparing for its mid-cycle ovulation. In the wet, fertile mucus there are millions of motile, healthy sperm swimming vigorously up through the cervix and the womb and into the tubes.

See one of your ovaries release an egg, which is captured by the tiny filaments at the end of the fallopian tube. The egg passes down into the tube, swept along by the rhythmic contractions of the tube and the little ciliae that line it.

See the egg being met by many sperm, dancing around it, bombarding it, until one of the sperm penetrates the egg, burrows in to the nucleus and fertilises it.

Now see the fertilised egg, wafting slowly down the tube, entering the womb, and implanting in the endometrium.

It starts to change, to divide, to multiply and to grow.

You can see the head and limbs develop, and the cord, which attaches it to the wall of the womb, throbbing with blood.

The baby grows, perfectly, becoming fuller and rounder, filling your womb, which is stretching. Everything is growing, your belly is getting larger and larger.

The baby continues to grow, full of health and beauty, until it's ready to be born (you can visualise the baby as of a particular sex if you have a preference).

Now you can see the cervix dilate, and the uterus contract, and the baby is being pushed, down and out, in rhythmic surges.

You see the baby's head emerge, and the hands of your helpers guide the child out in to the world. The baby is perfect, beautiful, and healthy, and everyone is smiling.

You are handed the child, and you put it to your breast, and everything is good.

Return to your breathing, in and out.

Follow the rhythm of your breath.

Sink right down into your centre, deeper and deeper, further down with each breath, each movement, each word.

Come at last to your most central, private and unique place, where you are your very essence.

In this place you know exactly who you are, what your real goals are, and that you can and will accomplish them.

Say to yourself in your mind, in this central place, substituting your own phase of the moon, when your fertility peaks.

> *My reproductive system is getting healthier and healthier, and my fertility is increasing, every day. I will find it easy to do all that is necessary to achieve a healthy conception, pregnancy and birth. I will regularly ovulate at mid-cycle [n] days before (after) the new (full) moon. I will continue to do so cycle after cycle until I conceive. When we are ready, with healthy bodies, eggs and sperm, I will conceive a healthy child and give birth to it/him/her easily after a successful pregnancy. I can feel my child getting nearer and nearer.*

(Or, if this is just before the conception attempt, substitute the day on which you expect your lunar peak to fall.)

> *I will ovulate on my hormonal cycle next ... day. I will now conceive a healthy child and give birth to it/her/him easily after a successful pregnancy. I can feel my child getting nearer and nearer.*

Return to your breathing, in and out.

Feel the energy return to your mind and body with each breath.

Feel the normal body muscle tone return.

Feel the circulation speed up to normal levels.

Feel your heartbeat and breathing speed up.

Feel your mind coming back up to normal wakefulness, alert and full of energy.

Open your eyes!

Wide awake!

Have a big yawn and a huge stretch.

Remember — don't play relaxation recordings in the car or while you or anyone else within earshot is operating machinery, using sharp knives or being involved in any activity which could be dangerous if drowsy.

Now your body and mind are relaxed with massage and visualisation. It's time to celebrate.

Have a great evening, with a candlelit dinner, evening celebration, or whatever turns you on. Bring some joy to this most important occasion.

Enjoy yourselves and the conception of your child will be just as memorable as its birth.

OTHER REMEDIES FOR STRESS CONTROL

Although visualisation and massage are both wonderful ways to assist relaxation, there are many others to choose from.

Exercise, good nutrition and adequate sleep are all important; they should be part of your daily life during your preconception health care. Other remedies which can be part of your daily preparation for pregnancy and can be used on the occasion that you attempt conception, are aromatherapy, herbal nervines and Bach flower essences.

When you are decorating your bedroom with candles, flowers or whatever you feel is appropriate to this momentous occasion, use some sweet-smelling oils in a burner to create a relaxing environment. These can also be added to your massage oil. Oils for relaxation and stress include

◆ *Lavender*

◆ *Marjoram*

◆ *Neroli*

◆ *Ylang Ylang*

◆ *Rosewood*

◆ *Rose*

◆ *Myrtle*

◆ *Sandalwood*

◆ *Geranium*

◆ *Mandarin.*

Herbal nervines and Bach flower essences are wonderful for calming the nerves and changing negative states. Bach flower remedies are flower essences, in homoeopathic dilution, which unblock negative energy states by dealing with such emotions as

◆ discouragement (*Gentian*)

◆ hopelessness and despair (*Gorse*)

◆ impatience (*Impatiens*)

◆ resentment (*Willow*)

◆ sense of physical unhealthiness (*Crab Apple*)

◆ uncertainty re correct path in life (*Wild Oat*)

◆ protection from outside influences (*Walnut*)

◆ self-reproach and guilt (*Pine*)

◆ lack of confidence (*Larch*)

◆ despondency, but struggling on (*Oak*)

◆ fear of known things (*Mimulus*).

Herbal nervines work to calm the nervous system and the nerve tonics to tone it. They do not make you sleepy, although they can help you to sleep. *Chamomile* tea is especially good for this; it can be bought at a health food shop and made at home. Use the recipe in Chapter 12, 'Natural Remedies for Hormonal and Reproductive Health', to make an infusion. Or use tea bags, but leave them steeping in the water long enough for the herb's active ingredients to seep into the water. Other useful herbs are

◆ *Motherwort*

◆ *Skullcap*

◆ *Passiflora (Passionflower)*

◆ *Valerian*

◆ *Hops*

◆ *Vervain*

◆ and *Oats*, as a long-term nerve tonic (eat porridge for breakfast). This nutritious food is also indicated to build a healthy sperm count.

If you are lethargic and depressed, try *Oats* again, *Ginseng* and *Damiana*.

Dealing with daily stress may be harder if you have a fertility problem, especially if you have been trying to conceive for a while. Some infertile situations may be resolved by attending to the preconception health care program outlined in this chapter, and further explored in my book *The Natural Way to Better Babies*. The advice in Chapter 12, 'Natural Remedies for Hormonal and Reproductive Health', may also be useful, though an intractable or serious problem may need professional help. However, even though you may feel that your fertility problem is physiological in origin, coping with the fear and tension inherent in the situation is an important part of its resolution.

THE STRESS OF INFERTILITY

Ah! Here we come to a *big one*! The question is — which comes first? Infertility or stress? The catch is that the longer the infertility continues, the greater the stress on the aspiring parents, and the longer the infertility continues.

Although there is a mass of evidence showing the adverse effect of stress on fertility, most orthodox treatments for infertile couples tend to exacerbate, rather than treat, the problem.

Holistic medicine, on the other hand, treats the entire situation, so there is much more chance of success in overcoming infertility if the stresses inherent in the situation are acknowledged and dealt with.

Psychological blocks to conception are very real. In some cases, there may be a deep fear of pregnancy originating in childhood (or in another lifetime, if you believe in reincarnation). These problems may need the expert help of a therapist to uncover and release. However, it isn't always that complex an issue.

Infertility is in itself so stressful an experience that what may start out as a low level of fertility can become a psychologically based, intractable problem. Women who are infertile have been shown to have anxiety and depression levels equivalent to women with cancer, heart disease or HIV-positive status. Many report that infertility is the worst crisis of their lives, worse than divorce or the loss of a parent. High levels of stress affect ovarian, tubal and other reproductive functions, such as hormone balance. They also affect other organs and systems which can, in turn, have an indirect effect on fertility, such as the adrenals, the digestion and absorption of nutrients, and immune function.

Effective therapies include:

> psychotherapy (including counselling)
> hypnotherapy
> relaxation and breathing techniques
> meditation and prayer
> aromatherapy
> herbal, homoeopathic and Bach flower remedies
> acupuncture and acupressure
> exercise
> massage and body work

It is certainly not necessary to use all of these. Everyone will have a different preference. We've already seen how stress affects fertility. Now let's look at how infertility affects stress levels. There's a lot you can do to help yourself.

Is sex a chore?

So many infertile couples start to identify their sex lives with their conception attempts. Each sexual act becomes solely concerned with conception and often experienced as a 'probable failure' by those who've already been trying for a while. The whole sex act can then become contaminated with negativity as the personal pleasure and expression of love — that used to be such a good stress release — become obscured.

It is as important to identify the infertile times as it is to recognise the fertile. Then, you can have just-for-us sex at the times of the cycle when conception can't occur. Even if you never have a child (and some fertility problems don't get solved), you can always have each other.

Don't destroy what you have for what you want, and don't let sexual activity become associated in your mind with negative results and disappointment. Give it a breathing space. That way, you derive all the benefits from the destressing effect of sexual activity and from your loving support of each other. Express your trust in your private relationship that is to endure whether the longed-for children come or not.

In your preparation time leading to the conception attempt, don't feel that in order to raise sperm count you must lie on opposite sides of the bed! Allow your sexuality expression in kisses, cuddles and caresses. If you raise your sexual energy at this time, with no resultant ejaculation, sperm count will benefit more than if you simply abstain.

Bring the magic back into your relationship.

On the days when you know you are fertile and you are trying to conceive, let in a little joy. Energy levels are raised, relaxed and given positively through enjoyment.

Joy is the most important emotion, but often difficult to experience if conception has repeatedly failed. Just beware of having unrealistic expectations.

Too high an expectation

Do you set your sights so high each month that you come crashing down with each menstrual period? This emotional rollercoaster won't help you either to enjoy life or to conceive.

In cases where infertility is long-standing and causing depression, it's perhaps inadvisable to build your hopes too high each month. Celebrate that you have another chance to conceive, rather than any certain outcome.

Approach each attempt as a new chance and celebrate by making the evening special. Use some of the ideas we've discussed already, go out to dinner, go for a moonlit walk by the sea.

Try to shelve responsibilities at this time, farm older kids out to friends or relatives and have the evening to yourselves. Take time off work. If the home environment is too reminiscent of past failures, use another room or go away for the night.

The key is to relax, be optimistic and enjoy yourselves. Then, even if it doesn't work this time, at least you can look forward to the next.

Fear of childlessness

Do you have a great fear of childlessness? Is the prospect of becoming a parent the only possible future you can entertain? Do you constantly suppress any thoughts of failure as negative?

Well, they're not. They're not only realistic but need expression and are much more dangerous if repressed. Although many cases of infertility will respond to treatment, there will always be some that won't. For some infertile couples, there is no final breakthrough. For every couple with a fertility problem there is a chance that a solution will not be found. This is a fear that is better faced.

I must not fear. Fear is the mind killer. Fear is the little death that leads to total obliteration. I will face my fear. I will permit it to pass over me and through me, and when it is gone I will turn the inner eye to its path, and where it was there will be nothing.

So goes the litany from Frank Herbert's novel, *Dune*. Your fear of not having a child may become, in itself, such a source of stress that it ends up as part of the problem.

Just because you don't express this fear doesn't mean it isn't there, eating away at you. It may be helpful to come to terms with infertility and remove its sting. Sit down and draw up a list acknowledging the advantages of a life without children. There are many. Here are some examples.

◆ More time.

◆ More money.

◆ More flexibility.

◆ More chance to travel.

◆ More chance to advance a career.

◆ More chance to pursue your interests.

◆ More chance to relate to and spend time with each other.

◆ More chance to realise and achieve other life goals.

◆ More chance to contribute to world population control.

If your list can be seen as a real alternative and not as a failure, then some of the fear and stress may be removed (and you may have a better chance of conception). You will certainly develop a more patient attitude, and allow your therapy to take its course.

If you find this is too difficult but feel it is a real issue for you, a good therapist can help.

Fear of parenthood, childbirth and pregnancy

For some of you, it may not be the prospect of childlessness that distresses you; rather, the reverse situation may be true. You may have a deeply ingrained fear of motherhood, childbirth or pregnancy.

This may be because of a contraceptive attitude you developed when you were younger, when becoming pregnant would have been disastrous and caused great trauma.

Try to get clear what these attitudes could have been in the past and on what they were based. Then clarify how the conditions in your life have changed since then.

Fear of childbirth is often fed by having horror stories fed us when we were children. 'I nearly died having you,' says Mum to show how much she loves you. The result is that, in your mind, having children and suffering are synonymous.

These fears are further fed by ignorance. Demystify the process by reading about childbirth, talking to your doctor or, if possible, attending the birth of a friend's child. Even if the birth is not as planned, it will nearly always turn out well, the baby beautiful, the mother ecstatic, the father glowing and the whole thing over in a day at the most.

Fear of motherhood is often fed by childhood role models and ignorance. Subconsciously, you may be very afraid of repeating the mistakes you saw your parents make. Every parent makes mistakes. You will, too. We're humans, not angels, and we're people before we're parents. Forgive your parents — then you will feel free to make your own mistakes.

If you have never had much contact with children and are anxious that you won't be able to cope with them, start making time to be with them. Babysit your friends' kids (they'll love you for it). Hold and rock babies, play with the little ones, develop your nurturing self. Get the juices flowing.

If you feel any of these fears are very deep-seated, seek professional help. You'll feel much better for it.

Pressure from family and friends

♦ Do you really want a child?

♦ Does your husband/wife really want a child?

♦ Do your parents/family really want you to have a child?

♦ Do your friends really want you to have a child?

♦ Are the answers to all these questions the same? *Can you differentiate?*

Your needs and priorities are not necessarily the same as those of your family or your friends. Some women, and men, feel extraordinarily pressured to have a child and never have a chance to find out whether they truly want one or not.

Some women, and men, subconsciously sabotage their therapy simply because either

♦ they don't really want a child but feel they ought to, *or*

♦ they do really want a child but are resentful of the pressures on them to perform.

If you are unsure about your motivation, a little counselling can help you discover and own your decisions.

Femininity, masculinity and self-esteem

It is customary for 'barren' women to be, and feel, outcasts. It used to be traditional for childless wives to be replaced, and men, always mindful of their virility, seldom accepted blame. The stigma of sterility is different these days, more subtle, but still present. Motherhood is glorified (and rightly so, although often romanticised beyond belief) and old attitudes die hard.

Many women who are infertile feel bereft of their femininity and self-esteem. This is even common to those who don't want children, as it is after menopause or tubal ligation (sterilisation).

While the bearing of children is, of course, a big part of the female role, it certainly isn't the whole story. If you feel less feminine or desirable, find other ways to affirm your sexuality. Talk it over with your partner; you may be reassured.

These days, we know that the difficulties often don't lie with the woman, but that the sperm may be deficient in some way. This can be just as hard for the man. The reason women were traditionally scapegoats was because the men couldn't handle it either.

Masculinity, virility, potency — measured so often by the ability to impregnate — is a large part of male self-esteem, which needs bolstering and reassurance.

These difficulties with sexuality and self-esteem may not be the only way the stresses of infertility affect your relationship.

Poor communication

'A troubled shared is a trouble halved', should perhaps be, 'A trouble aired is a trouble halved', because the fact that someone else is in it with you is only helpful if you *talk about it.*

Sometimes in counselling, if a couple is asked (individually), 'How do you think [your partner] feels about this?', the answer is surprisingly tentative, and often denied by the other.

Don't assume you know how your partner is feeling. Talk things over. You both may discover not only how your partner feels, but also how you feel. And you will probably both feel a lot better. Loving and communicative relationships are more likely to relieve stress and produce a baby. They are also good training for family life.

There are groups that are formed expressly for the support of infertile couples, where people in similar circumstances can meet and learn of possible treatments and feel that they are not alone. These groups can help you to share your problems, gain support and learn to communicate your needs (see Appendix 2, 'Contacts and Resources').

Unresolved grief

If you have previously experienced a stillbirth or loss during pregnancy, or had a child whose health is severely affected, your grief may be so overwhelming (or repressed) that you can't move on. You may also be afraid that the problem will recur.

You need to learn to let go and create a more confident and optimistic environment for your next conception. As difficult as this may seem, it can be made a lot easier in two ways.

First, you can seek help from professional therapists or support groups which can offer a safe situation in which to express your grief and fear. Second, you can have a great deal of faith in the benefits of preconception health care. As the Foresight study shows, and as we experience at our health centre, a complete preparation before pregnancy can be enormously successful in the prevention of such problems.

So — go back to the beginning of this chapter and, as you put all the suggested measures in place, allow yourself to hope and dream.

Take a break

If you are giving conception all you have, that's great. If you've been doing that for a long time, maybe that's not so great. Repeated failure can be very dispiriting. But if you've already tried some of the changes in attitude suggested here and you still feel depressed, *take a break*.

Forget about conception for a while. Let go. You can return to it later with renewed vigour and optimism — and a greater chance of success.

Infertility

What is infertility? Well, officially, a couple is considered infertile if conception has not occurred within 1 year of trying (although if the woman is 35 years of age or more, this time frame may be shortened to 6 months). This is a statistic that covers all sorts of conditions (which may have been treated by all sorts of remedies), but the number of couples who fall into this category is growing all the time.

It is currently estimated that in the Western world, as many as 15 per cent of couples can be considered infertile, and one in six has difficulty conceiving — and the figure is growing. Infertility is big business. Millions of dollars are poured into the hi-tech treatments.

Although one can argue that on a global scale we have enough children, it remains an immense personal tragedy for those who find, on deciding to start a family, that they can't. Infertility has huge social ramifications for the individual and for the human species.

First, we have to become aware that nearly all the world's environmental problems originate with exploding population levels, and that we all have a personal responsibility not to have too many children.

Having children at all may well become a privilege, not a right, unless we solve some of the huge problems of environmental concern and population growth.

Usually, when a species reaches plague levels, which humans could well be seen to have done, Mother Nature steps in and wipes great numbers of them out. Possibly, the increasingly high levels of infertility can be regarded in this light. They are certainly a by-product of the kind of society in which we live, which is, in turn, an inevitable result of our population density, our overuse of the earth's resources and our polluting lifestyles.

Children are our future so let's give them a future with which they can live.

Even if we accept a responsibility to have limited numbers of children and, at the very most, only replace ourselves, it's essential for any species to be optimistic about its future and to feel confident that it has one. On a collective level, that means having fewer and healthier children, but on an individual level, it still means reproduction. This is what life on earth, in a physical sense at least, seems to be about — the continuation of the species.

The main causes of infertility seem to be

> stress
> poor nutrition
> environmental pollution
> radiation
> toxicity
> drugs (medical and social)
> contraception programs
> genito-urinary infections
> immune dysfunction
> greater age of parents

These can all, to some extent, be seen as lifestyle conditions. And that is how you need to start treating your fertility problem. Let's look at your chances.

The 15 per cent figure for infertility translates into

◆ 3 million couples in North America (including Canada)

◆ 400 000 couples in Britain

◆ 100 000 couples in Australia and New Zealand.

This is a great many, so if you have this problem, you're in good company.

However, not all women, or men, may wish to have children. It is estimated that about 85 per cent of both men and women do, and that of these, 60–80 per cent will have conceived within a year (thereby avoiding the label 'infertile'), and 80–85 per cent within 2 years.

The average time taken to conceive is a lot longer than most people suppose, being between 4 and 6 months.

It breaks down like this:

◆ 25 per cent of couples conceive within 1 month.

◆ 60 per cent of couples conceive after 6 months.

◆ 85 per cent of couples conceive after 12 months.

So you may be superfertile, very fertile, fertile, subfertile or infertile.

Infertility is a very doom-laden word, and one likely to make you want to give up, here and now. That's the trouble with it. It may have a ring of finality to it, but there is nearly always room for hope. In this chapter we are trying to improve the odds.

Surprisingly, up to 50 per cent of infertile situations are regarded as arising simply because the couple isn't 'doing it right'! By understanding the physical processes involved in the timing of conception, optimum use can be made of fertility (even if it's low) in either partner, which may well result in success without recourse to treatment. *Correct timing may be all you need.*

If your fertility is low, with the chances on the very few fertile days each month lower than normal, it only needs a busy lifestyle, one or other of you to be tired or have a headache, and months can go by without success.

Without precise timing, conception has the following possibilities of success.

◆ Chance of conception mid-cycle — 20 per cent.

◆ Chance of conception at any point in cycle — 2–4 per cent.

◆ Chance of conception with a single act — 0.65 per cent.

There are many natural therapies that can be effective for infertile states. These have none of the possible side-effects that may result from the more orthodox approaches, and will result in improved reproductive and general health for both parents and child.

Fertility drugs can have quite severe ill-effects on the health of both mother and child, and do not actually improve reproductive health or innate fertility. Apart from the physical implications, they can often result in far-reaching emotional changes.

The more invasive hi-tech procedures such as in vitro fertilisation also have an extreme emotional effect. Many women (and men) who go through these programs experience high levels of stress, low self-esteem and lack of control. This may well be a contributing factor to their low rate of success, generally assessed at less than 15 per cent. The Foresight study showed, on the other hand, a success rate of 81 per cent, and no side-effects (other than improved health of mother and child).

Although one can only be glad for the couples who have had success through assisted reproductive programs, there are a great many questions that are raised by these procedures.

Vast amounts of money are spent to bring success to a very small number of couples. This money might be better spent educating many more women and their partners in some of the ways they might help their reproductive health. (Diet, for example, as well as stress, is usually ignored on these programs.)

It is also questionable whether we are doing the human race a favour by helping infertile couples to get around their infertility problem rather than solve it. In many cases, infertility results from such poor levels of health, that we are merely ensuring the survival of the least fit. Indeed, studies show an approximate three-fold increase in perinatal deaths in children born through assisted reproductive programs.

There are huge ethical and moral questions that arise from the following practices.

◆ Use of embryos for research.

◆ Donor eggs and sperm.

◆ Surrogate motherhood.

◆ The rights of the embryo.

◆ Freezing of embryos.

◆ Disposal of unused embryos.

◆ The use of neomorts (newly dead women on life support systems) as surrogate wombs.

◆ The rights of frozen embryos to inherit.

◆ Custody of frozen embryos in divorce.

◆ The 'rights' of postmenopausal women to have children.

◆ Babies being born from five parents (an egg donor, a sperm donor, a surrogate and two legal parents).

◆ Eggs being fielded from aborted foetuses for donor programs.

Happily, natural therapies are generally non-invasive and non-traumatic. They offer a chance for the individual or couple to feel that they are in control, and that they are contributing to the solution of their problem.

In cases of low fertility, the problem may lie with either partner — or both. As male fertility is affected increasingly adversely by the effects we have listed (and the sperm, being smaller than the egg and produced from scratch in the offending environment, is even more vulnerable), more and more studies are showing that fertility problems are being equally shared between the sexes. Although the studies give varying figures, the causes of a couple's infertility can be approximately assessed as

◆ 30 per cent female problems

◆ 30 per cent male problems

◆ 20 per cent mutual problems

◆ 20 per cent unexplained problems.

The causes of these problems can be further broken down.

Causes of infertility in women

- ◆ 20 per cent — disorders of ovulation
- ◆ 30 per cent — disorders of fallopian tubes
- ◆ 15 per cent — endometriosis
- ◆ 10 per cent — disorders of mucus
- ◆ 5 per cent — other mechanical causes (such as fibroids).

Causes of infertility in men

- ◆ 50 per cent — disorders of sperm (quantity and quality)
- ◆ 30 per cent — disorders of sexual intercourse.

Causes unknown

20 per cent of infertility in both men and women is unexplained in medical terms, though may have a lot to do with the factors discussed above.

DIAGNOSTIC TESTS FOR INFERTILITY

If a couple presents as infertile, the man's fertility will usually be tested first once it has been established that intercourse takes place reasonably often, with ejaculation inside the vagina, and no other obvious reason for infertility is present.

This is because the tests to establish male fertility levels are easier to do, with many fewer intrusive and painful (although sometimes embarrassing) procedures, involving no surgery or possible side-effects. *Also, these tests are much more conclusive.*

The tests for female infertility can be much more complex, traumatic and less definitive.

To gauge a man's fertility, the semen is tested for volume, sperm count (the number per millilitre), sperm motility (the ability to propel themselves forward, and the number still active after a few hours) and morphology (the percentage of abnormally shaped sperm). Further diagnostic tests for the man are described later in 'Male Infertility'.

If a woman's fertility is suspect, she can also elect to have various tests. These range from simple blood tests to check hormone levels, to surgical procedures such as laparoscopy in which a telescopic lens is inserted through a small incision (usually in the navel) so an inspection of the internal organs can be made, thereby enabling a diagnosis of conditions such as endometriosis, PID, blocked fallopian tubes, ovarian cysts, or polycystic ovarian syndrome (PCOS). A general anaesthetic is required.

Many women who decide to use natural methods have already been through a whole barrage of tests and have either identified the problem or are still left with no apparent reason for their infertility.

For other women, natural remedies are their first choice. These women will usually wait to get at least some initial clues from their observations before going any further with fertility tests.

You may choose to try natural remedies before going for tests, or you may prefer to get hold of any available information first.

There is a great deal that can be done through optimising timing, nutrition, stress control, and general tonic natural remedies without even knowing what the specific problem is. This applies to both partners.

This tonic effect of many natural remedies can raise the general performance of the organs and systems. Other remedies and treatments can have specific effects.

If the general remedies don't work, they can be made more specific to your needs as information is gathered through various fertility tests. Some women prefer a more specific approach from the very beginning, and are quite prepared to have invasive tests carried out.

MUTUAL INFERTILITY

If the man's sperm count is fine, and the woman is seen to be ovulating, has no blocked tubes or diseases of the reproductive or endocrine systems, then the compatibility of the couple can be tested.

Post-coital tests are carried out to find if the sperm are surviving once they are in the female reproductive tract. It is also possible to test for sperm antibodies in the woman's blood or mucus, and the mucus can be assessed for other factors causing hostility, such as acidity, insufficient amount or lack of ferning (see section on mucus production in Chapter 12).

If the mucus contains sperm antibodies, the sperm are immobilised. This is a result of the woman's reacting to the sperm as an allergenic substance, an invading pathogen, from which it needs to protect itself. (This can happen in the man's body, too; see below). High toxin levels in the sperm may also contribute to this problem.

The medical treatment used to be with immunosuppressive or antihistamine drugs, which are, of course, the cause of many undesirable side-effects. More frequently these days, the couple is referred to an in vitro program. Unfortunately, if the woman has antibodies in her blood, these will be present in all her body fluids, so a conception is unlikely.

Natural medicine can treat the woman's immune system, and ensure that the cervical mucus is not a channel for toxic-waste elimination. Detoxification of the male is also advisable.

While a condom is used for between 3–6 months to allow the woman's immune reaction to subside, her immune system is treated with diet, supplements, and herbal or homoeopathic medicine, and a program of detoxification is followed. (Fasting may be recommended, but only do this under competent supervision.)

During this time, the signs of fertility are well learnt, so that the condom is removed *only at the moment of conception*, not giving the body time to build up any antibodies.

Sperm Antibodies

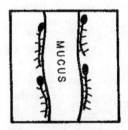 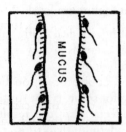 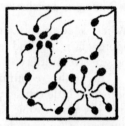

SPERM ANTIBODIES IN THE MALE CAUSE THE TAILS OF THE SPERM TO STICK TO THE CERVICAL MUCUS

SPERM ANTIBODIES IN THE FEMALE CAUSE THE HEADS OF THE SPERM TO STICK TO THE CERVICAL MUCUS

SPERM ANTIBODIES CAUSE THE SPERM TO STICK TOGETHER (AGGLUTINATION) HEAD TO HEAD, HEAD TO TAIL AND TAIL TO TAIL

This has the added benefit of starting the pregnancy with a healthy immune system, which will, of course, be necessary to prevent allergies or sensitivities to foods or environmental agents, which may also be evident in women with this problem.

MALE INFERTILITY

Sperm quantity and quality are of concern worldwide, as counts and the markers of sperm health (motility and morphology) consistently fall and the incidence of testicular disease rises. This is commonly regarded as the effect of increased pollution and toxicity in the environment, so full preconception health care is of extreme importance to ensure that there are adequate numbers of healthy sperm.

Here is a list of possible causes of male infertility.

◆ Hormonal imbalance (e.g. excessive prolactin — see female, or inadequate testosterone; high levels of FSH indicate testicular failure).

◆ Damage to testes (from drugs, radiation, glandular disease such as mumps or glandular fever, GUIs and STDs, TB and physical injury).

◆ Blocked tubes (vas deferens or epididymis).

◆ Excessive heat or pressure (beware saunas, wetsuits, tight trousers, underwear made from synthetic fabrics).

◆ Antibody production (especially after vasectomy reversal).

◆ Undescended testes.

◆ Varicoceles (varicose veins) in the testes (see below).

◆ Infection of prostate or seminal vesicles (treat as for vaginal infections — internally).

◆ Abnormal penile erection or ejaculation (usually a stress or emotional reaction).

◆ Nutrient deficiencies and high toxin levels.

When a couple is attempting to deal with infertility, the first line of approach is to find out if there is a low sperm count, low level of progressive motility or morphology.

This is the recommended course of action because the test, although perhaps a little embarrassing for some, is not surgically intrusive or painful, and has no possible side-effects. Also, the results (allowing for periodic fluctuation) are much more definite than those that can be performed on the woman (which are also generally more invasive).

It is useful to take a check on sperm count and quality reasonably often during therapy to measure progress and see which factors affect the result. Always note the conditions (such as number of days abstinence preceding each ejaculation) that apply to each individual test, so that comparisons can be made.

The guidelines for diet, exercise and supplements for male reproductive health have been discussed earlier in this chapter.

Normal Sperm

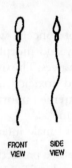

FRONT VIEW   SIDE VIEW

Sperm Abnormalities

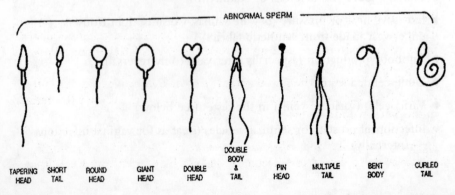

| TAPERING HEAD | SHORT TAIL | ROUND HEAD | GIANT HEAD | DOUBLE HEAD | DOUBLE BODY & TAIL | PIN HEAD | MULTIPLE TAIL | BENT BODY | CURLED TAIL |

Sperm abnormalities, as well as count and motility, seem to be greatly affected by cigarette smoking, alcohol and other mutagenic agents such as radiation, heavy metals, chemicals, drugs and environmental toxins. It's a squeaky-clean life for healthy sperm.

Another test which may be helpful is to look for varicoceles (or varicose veins in the testes) which can cause problems with the production of adequate numbers of healthy sperm. If there are obvious problems with the quantity or quality of the sperm, this test can be performed through palpation and ultrasound. An operation is frequently successful, and stress management has also been found to be effective.

Sperm antibodies in the male are more difficult to treat than in the female, as it is impossible to isolate the man from his sperm. However, herbal and nutritional treatment for autoimmune conditions is sometimes successful.

Acupuncture is helpful for treating sperm problems, as are herbs. With some additions for individual health problems, the following herbs may prove beneficial for achieving good numbers of healthy sperm.

◆ *Gotu Kola*

◆ *Sarsaparilla*

◆ *Ginkgo*

◆ *Damiana*

◆ *Oats Seed*

◆ *Astragalus*

◆ *Saw Palmetto*

◆ *Panax Ginseng*

◆ *Tribulus*

◆ *Kava*

◆ *Withania*

◆ *Schisandra*

These are best dispensed in fluid extract form (which is most potent) by an experienced herbalist, who can treat your unique situation. Encapsulated herbs work well, too. Expect an increased growth of facial hair, renewed vigour, and heightened sexual appetite.

Herbal nervines are helpful if stress is part of the problem (it very often is), and Bach flower remedies if emotions are frayed (see Other Remedies in the Stress section of this chapter, above).

Bee pollen has a reputation for being of assistance, as do the amino acids arginine, carnitine and histidine, co-enzyme Q_{10} and octocosanol, a substance that is found in wheatgerm oil (also high in vitamin E). All these remedies can be obtained from your natural health practitioner or your health food shop.

Another possible aid in the cases where the count is low is the use of the male lunar peak time (see Chapters 7 and 8 for more on this).

If normal levels are obtained through treatment and conception still does not occur, it's time to start checking out mutual problems and arranging further diagnostic tests for the woman's fertility to see if there is some specific problem that has not been discovered previously.

However, there's more you men can do. Although sperm quantity and quality is definitely raised through abstinence, which must be practised for 3–5 days before each conception attempt, it's possible to improve on this.

Lengthy abstinence (greater than 5 days) is not generally helpful, but you may find great assistance in following the advice of ancient Oriental medicine.

Oriental philosophy teaches that semen is a concentrated valuable essence of fluids and energy to be nurtured and not indiscriminately wasted. This is contrary to the Western understanding that frequency of ejaculation has no effect on the health of the individual.

One way to strengthen the sexual potency of the male is to practise sensual sex.

Sensual sex can be practised in your run-up of 3–5 days as well as at other times. It involves intimate contact, with extensive and prolonged foreplay and sensual games, *but no ejaculation.*

When the urge for orgasm becomes too strong for comfort, sexual contact is ceased until the penis is flaccid. You can try a cold shower or a run around the block or a game of Scrabble! Then, sensual contact is resumed. This should really only be attempted by those with some experience in these techniques — or the benefits of abstinence may be threatened.

The idea is that the erotic stimulation, coupled with the gaining and losing of an erection, acts over a period of time as a pump to increase sexual energy and sperm quantity and quality.

The same idea is behind the suggestion that, at the conception attempt itself, foreplay should be extensive, raising the sexual energy, and allowing for several gains and losses of erection. Sperm count is higher when the man is highly sexually aroused — so make your conception attempts exciting and stress-free!

Another useful technique (especially if the volume of semen is too great) may be the split ejaculation, where only the first gush of the ejaculate (which contains the most numerous and healthiest sperm) is deposited in the vagina, after which the penis is withdrawn. The healthy sperm may have a better chance if unhindered by their less healthy brothers.

CONTINUING INFERTILITY
Even if you are one of those who don't make the breakthrough, you, too, can still have a success story.

By working through your underlying fears of infertility and by feeling that you have done all in your power to resolve your problem (not simply handing it over to an 'expert'), you stand a much better chance of having a healthy and positive reaction to your childless state.

Feelings of resentment, guilt, blame and inadequacy can ruin your chances of changing your life's direction in a positive way. Learn to channel your nurturing qualities in other ways to lead a fulfilling, positive, successful and loving life, and leave the rest behind.

Counselling and therapy are available to help couples or individuals work through the grief and feelings of emptiness. Avail yourself of these services, treat yourself well. If these feelings are not resolved, they can harm your health, your life's direction and your relationships.

AGE

Age is undoubtedly a factor for both sexes in decreasing fertility.

◆ One in seven couples aged 30–34 is infertile.

◆ One in five aged 35–39 is infertile.

◆ One in four aged 40–44 is infertile.

Also, in women under 15 or over 45, the problems of congenital malformation increase greatly, with 25–29 being the age group least at risk.

For example, the risk of Down syndrome in the general population, according to age, is as follows:

◆ at age 24 — 1 in 1299

◆ at age 34 — 1 in 465

◆ at age 39 — 1 in 139

◆ at age 40 — 1 in 109

◆ at age 45 — 1 in 32.

Recently, it has been acknowledged that the age of the father is also an important consideration. However, it has also been found that, apart from conditions caused by chromosomal defects, age is not a factor in other abnormalities.

Levels of nutrients and toxins can affect even chromosomal defects. Radiation exposure, for example, has been linked with a higher incidence of Down syndrome, as have nutrient deficiencies. It may be that many of the congenital malformations that have previously been associated with age are, at least partly, a result of accumulated exposure to toxins and nutrient deficiencies. Good preconception health care, along the lines suggested in this chapter, has been shown to virtually eliminate these problems. You may want to bear this in mind when deciding whether to have prenatal tests, which carry a risk of causing miscarriage and often give false results.

Fertility will be lower in older prospective parents. With women being at their most fertile at about 25 years of age, there is a slight decline which accelerates at age 30, another quite significant decline at 40, until after 45 the possibility of conception is very low. Women over 50 have conceived, but generally speaking, the chances are minimal. Infertility usually precedes the menopause by about 3 years and can drop dramatically up to 10 years before. It is now known that it is the quality of the eggs that decreases with age, not the ability of the uterus to support a pregnancy.

Remember — you can reduce the effects of ageing with good nutrition, exercise and a healthy lifestyle.

Relationship Between Maternal Age and Congenital Malformations
(after Hendricks, *Obstetrics and Gynaecology 6*, p592, 1955)

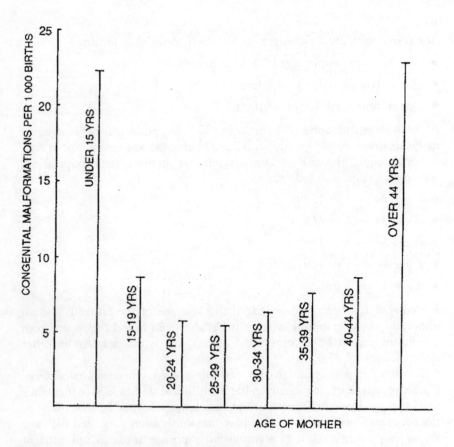

Preventing problem pregnancies
Some couples don't so much have a problem conceiving, but of conceiving well. In some personal and family histories, there is a recurring theme of miscarriages or birth defects (5 per cent of all babies born suffer some abnormality). For these couples it is especially important that both prospective parents prepare preconceptually to ensure that all possible mutagens or teratogens (substances causing congenital abnormalities), or

any conditions likely to cause miscarriage are avoided, and that all deficiencies corrected.

Earlier in this chapter, guidelines were given on preconception preparation that provided for optimum health during your pregnancy and for your child. Here is a list of substances, conditions and deficiencies which may be mutagenic, teratogenic, or cause miscarriage if ingested or experienced by either parent.

PROBLEM SUBSTANCES

Nitrosamine (formed in the stomach after ingestion of delicatessen meats)

Green potatoes

Heavy metals (mercury, aluminium, cadmium, lead; also excess copper)

Chemical and industrial pollution

Chemical cleaning agents

Paints, glues, solvents

Nicotine

Alcohol

Caffeine

Drugs (medical and social)

Environmental and ingested chemicals

Organochlorines

Spermicides, especially if they contain mercury

PROBLEM DEFICIENCIES

Vitamin A (an excess can also cause problems)

Vitamin B-complex (especially B_1, B_2, B_5, B_6, B_{12} and folic acid)

Vitamin C

Vitamin D

Vitamin E

Zinc

Magnesium

Manganese

Calcium

Selenium

Iron

Chromium

Copper

Iodine

Essential fatty acids

Protein

Amino acids

Progesterone

PROBLEM CONDITIONS

Age (for chromosomal defects only, but this can be offset by health and nutrition)

Rubella

Toxoplasmosis

Cytomegalovirus

GUIs, including mycoplasma and ureaplasma

Recent use of oral contraceptive pill (OCP)

Low birthweight

Ageing sperm or ova

Sperm abnormalities

High temperatures (e.g. saunas or fevers)

Birth-spacing interval <2 years

Pre-ovulatory phase >16 days

Post-ovulatory phase <12 days

Ionising radiation — from X-rays or flying (cosmic radiation)

Non-ionising radiation — from computer monitors, mobile phones, microwaves, TVs

Electromagnetic pollution — from waterbeds, electric blankets, kitchen gadgets

Autoimmune conditions and immune system dysfunction

Remember, some mutagenic substances, deficiencies and conditions can affect the embryo by affecting the egg or the sperm — even if you are exposed to them prior to conception.

One way to decrease their effects is to ingest antimutagenic food (see earlier in this chapter) and nutrients (especially antioxidants).

Nature has her own ways of weeding out non-viable infants; the majority of them never reach full term and most deformed embryos never reach maturity.

One in every 130 conceptions ends before the mother even realises she is pregnant, the defective zygote (fertilised egg) never attaching to the uterine wall. Twenty-five per cent of conceptions never reach an age where they can exist independently outside the womb.

Miscarriages are often the result of a defective embryo, so the list above is relevant for any woman with a history of spontaneous abortion.

Where there have been repeated miscarriages and the problem is not due to infection or a defective embryo, herbs, homoeopathic remedies or acupuncture can be used to help provide a supportive environment for the growing baby.

Treatment should be carried out under the supervision of a qualified therapist.

HEAVENLY CONCEPTIONS

As we have discussed, radiation can cause abnormalities in the egg, sperm and foetus. Especially problematic is ionising radiation, one source of which is cosmic radiation, that bombards the earth and to which you are particularly exposed when you fly at high altitudes.

Dr Jonas, when working with the lunar cycle, also came up with some findings on non-viable pregnancies (those resulting in miscarriage or abnormalities). These are the conclusions he refers to in his Rule 3 (see Chapter 7, 'The Lunar Cycle').

Although his findings are astrological in the sense that they have to do with the position of the planets in the sky at the time of conception, there is much evidence to support the idea that the effects that he noticed are related to sunspot activity and radiation.

The studies that Jonas carried out looked simply at the effects of certain aspects at the time of conception and he assumed that conception took place at the lunar peak time. Radiation effects, however, are known to affect eggs and sperm before conception, as well as the foetus, especially in the first trimester, and conceptions are more likely to occur at mid-cycle.

Despite these limitations, his studies are interesting, though I know of no systematic research carried out since.

Jonas studied cases where the children had been born deformed and concluded that there were recurring planetary aspects present at the conceptions, notably when the sun and major planets were in opposition (that is, when the angle between them, as seen from the earth, is 180°, as it is between the sun and moon at full moon).

Full moon itself he identified as being associated with particular problems if that was when the mother herself was born as well as when she conceived her child.

The nervous and, perhaps, hormonal instability experienced at full moon is well known, more births happening at this time than at any other. (Full-moon births were not found to be a problem, only conceptions.)

Full moon is a time of greater electrical potential (see Chapter 7), and the opposition of the sun and major planets is associated with solar flare activity.

Space research shows that at times of major oppositions, sunspots tend to occur, there are shifts in magnetic fields, magnetic storms, cosmic radiation and changes inside the earth. Astronauts cease taking moon trips at these times to avoid being killed by solar radiation, cyclones form over the ocean, anticyclones over land, diseases spread in epidemic proportions, the number of icebergs peaks, drought and famine occur and Burgundy wines have vintage years! With all this happening, it's not surprising one little conception gets disturbed.

As well as the known toxic effects of radiation, there also seems to be a disturbance to the electrodynamic fields that surround all living things. With the embryo, these give form to the body, so that it is this field that determines what happens — not the cells themselves. If a blob of tissue is moved from the leg position to the place where the arm should grow, an arm results.

Kirlian photography, developed by Russian scientists, reveals these electronic matrices on which the physical body is formed. Through this process it is observable how solar flares and other solar system phenomena affect the energy body.

More research from the space program shows that the subtle magnetic field changes in the earth that are caused by the sun, moon and planets, *actually alter the force field of the human body*, and thus the nervous system.

Other data show that the moon, the sun, cosmic and gamma rays, sunspot radiation and other disturbances of the earth's magnetic field had the same effect. Soviet scientists discovered an effect of magnetic field changes on the genetic substances DNA and RNA, and two American atomic scientists state that natural sources of radiation are known to cause mutations in humans. Radiation is also known to affect chromosomes and sperm, as we have already discussed.

All this adds up to a convincing argument that certain planetary configurations may have an effect on developing humans. Indeed, a well-respected British scientist is currently publishing data supporting his theory that planetary aspects present at birth can alter the personality and physical development of the child (the astrological assumption).

Jonas' theory is clearly in agreement with all this evidence, although there seems to be no particular research which backs up his claim that the moment of conception is crucial. What we do know is that the rapid changes taking place directly after conception are crucial to the healthy formation of the embryo.

Jonas' calculations have worked well enough in practice to be seriously considered by anyone who has a tendency to problem pregnancies.

If you wish to have these calculations done, you will need to consult a professional astrologer or Natural Fertility Management (see Appendix 1).

For further reading on all aspects of Dr Jonas' work and the developments since then, you can refer to my previous book, *The Lunar Cycle* (see Appendix 1).

Before attempting conception
CHECKLIST — THINGS TO BE COMPLETED BEFORE CONCEPTION IS ATTEMPTED

◆ Negative result on all tests for GUIs and other infections.

◆ Clear hair-trace mineral analysis for heavy metals.

◆ Adequate zinc status.

- Adequate nutritional status.

- Adequate ferritin levels.

- Adequate protection or detoxification from radiation and chemicals.

- Minimum of 4 months good nutrition (diet and supplementation).

- Minimum of 4 months abstinence from all drugs (including caffeine, nicotine and alcohol).

- Weight normalisation.

- Management or treatment of allergies.

- Eradication of candida.

- Adequate exercise program.

- Adequate stress-management program.

- Absence of reproductive disease.

- Regular cycles and balanced hormones.

- Adequate sperm count and healthy sperm.

- Understanding of timing techniques for conception attempt, allowing fresh sperm to meet fresh egg at the optimum time in the cycle.

Now you are pregnant

During your pregnancy, you should continue to take supplements and eat as outlined in this chapter. Zinc and ferritin levels should be regularly checked to ensure that your dosage is adequate, not excessive. Exercise, stress management and avoidance of toxins continue to be important.

Other than natural remedies to prevent miscarriage (taken under professional supervision), take no medicine at all for at least the first trimester unless taking it is unavoidable and cleared as harmless by your health practitioner. To find out all the other things that you want to know about your growing baby and its delivery, read *The Natural Way to Better Pregnancy* and *The Natural Way to Better Birth and Bonding* by myself and Janette Roberts. See Appendices 1 and 3 for these and other helpful books.

Acupuncture, reflexology, massage, osteopathy and herbal remedies can all help the various complaints of pregnancy, and hypnotherapy is a wonderful aid to an easy birth.

Once you have had your baby, reread the section on Lactation (and, if you need it, Postnatal Depression and Irregularity) in Chapter 12, 'Natural Remedies for Hormonal and Reproductive Health', and the After Childbirth section in Chapter 11, 'Times of Change', so you can practise non-invasive contraception.

It is important to space your children well. You may feel mentally and emotionally drained after pregnancy, and your body will be nutritionally depleted: it will need time to recover.

Now is the time that you become the preferred recipient of nutrients, rather than the baby, unlike during the pregnancy when the developing foetus had first pick.

The baby gets what's left over, through the breast milk, so it's still vital to consume adequate nutrients. You and your baby are both in great need. The infant has an enormous amount of growing to do, and there is a need for you to replenish your supplies. This is even more important if you are planning a second child, so that it will not be nutritionally compromised.

SPACING OUT YOUR BABIES

The *optimum spacing interval between births is between 2 and 3 years*. If babies are born within 2 years, not only does the second baby risk nutritional losses, but there is also an increased chance of miscarriage; neural tube defects (anencephalus and spina bifida) are more likely, as are the host of other problems we looked at earlier in this chapter.

There is also increasing evidence that the child needs to be the baby for at least the first 3 years of its life; the traditional spacing of 2 years between children deprives the first child of its bonding experiences and the second of its nutrients.

Give yourself a break. Use natural birth control until you're ready for your next conscious conception.

CHAPTER 14

Case Histories

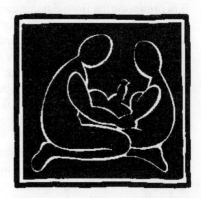

Success stories

In this chapter, I want to give you some insight into how these methods have worked in individual cases. Some of these case histories have been chosen to illustrate one particular point, while others record a whole variety of interrelating problems and solutions. Many will demonstrate how a holistic approach (one that takes care of all aspects of a case, both physical and psychological), can work so much better than a purely symptomatic treatment.

Naturally, I have not used anyone's real name, though the initials and home towns given at the end of the letters are those of the sender.

I have divided the cases into categories according to the effect that I think they demonstrate most clearly, although, as you might expect, many cases show more than one problem, treatment and result.

It was very gratifying to me while doing the research for this chapter to see how many women and couples I have been able to help. It's so good to have been a channel for benefit and assistance. My thanks go to all my patients — past, present and future — for the endless interest and satisfaction I have derived from treating and teaching them, and from seeing how wonderfully women and their partners can manage their own health, fertility and lives.

Natural fertility management — avoiding and achieving pregnancy

ANGELA

Angela hadn't experienced any particular problems with contraception, but she felt she could do better. She came to see me and used natural methods of birth control for 4 years. Then she decided it was time to start a family.

She came to see me again and we talked through her needs for the best possible conception. I gave her some nutrient supplements, organised to have tests done for GUIs and heavy metals, and made a relaxation tape with suggestions for synchronisation of her hormonal and lunar cycles, as well as for an easy and successful conception, pregnancy and birth.

Three months later, having prepared well, Angela conceived at her mid-cycle ovulation (her lunar and ovulation cycles still not quite coinciding). She had a splendid pregnancy and gave birth to a beautiful baby girl.

While breastfeeding, she kept a good watch on her mucus, avoided her lunar peak times, and came back to me when she first noticed her mucus changing. She was still using supplements, and although in excellent health, felt itchy around her vulva. She wanted to revise her contraception program and make sure that her cycles resumed as regularly as possible.

We made another tape for her, suggesting synchronisation (and no conception, this time), and put her on a short course of reproductive tonic herbs. She started sitting in the *Tea-tree* and vinegar solution twice a day.

Angela's itches went, her cycle resumed regularly, almost exactly coinciding with her lunar times. Maybe I'll hear from her again for the conscious conception of her second child.

Successful transitions to natural birth–control methods

Here are some letters that I have received from people who have attended my health centre, received postal NFM kits or read this book. I'm happy to say I get a quite a few like this.

> I am just writing to let you know how successful your program has been for me. I first came to see you a year ago, and now I am very comfortable and confident in my own ability to control my fertility and contraception. I don't even need to take my temperature any more! Since coming off the Pill, I have felt so much healthier, and have an overall feeling of well-being. I haven't had cystitis again, either.
>
> I have told other women I know about this natural method of birth control, and they are interested.
>
> Well, once again, thank you for the help.
>
> *Kerrie, New South Wales*

> It's been 12 months now since I began charting my cycle, and it's been a real voyage of discovery around myself. A very strange, but exhilarating, experience, those first few months were: unlocking a

secret code that I'd carried inside of me for about 20 years.

My cycle turned out to be so regular and straightforward that I was amazed that it hadn't always been obvious to me. But no, I'd been completely in the dark. Finding out where my ovulation regularly fell in my cycle explained such a lot about how I felt — my highs and lows and madnesses — and when. I couldn't believe that — couldn't understand why — my cycle had been a mystery to me for so long.

So, it's clear from what I've written here so far that my first, and main, impressions of the NFM program are concerned with the revelation of my cycle. Its value to me as a method of contraception has been secondary. Overall I have found the benefits of NFM to be the increased feelings of self-awareness and self-control, in terms of my fertility and my general health.

R. A., NSW

Just a short note but a hearty thank you. It has been 1 year now since meeting you and using ' the natural approach' to my contraception needs. Thank you so much again, it's a wonderful service and knowledge that you offer.

L. K, Melbourne

I have been using Natural Fertility Management for over a year now very successfully and, I may add, with much pleasure. I have learned to understand and enjoy all the aspects of my cycle. I feel more in touch with my body, more confident and empowered around my sexuality and fertility as I now know exactly when I can conceive and when I can't. I can't thank you enough.

G. M., London, England

I am so inspired by Natural Fertility Management. Thank you for opening my mind to nature where man's technology has previously ruled.

P. McL., NSW

Thank you for your instruction on the lunar cycle and for compiling my charts. I have found this new information of my fertility patterns most enlightening.

Y. D., Sydney

I am writing to thank you for the methods of Natural Fertility Management that demonstrate so clearly for women (and men) a way towards empowerment in their life, health and fertility.

K. H., Western Australia

I have had no difficulty with contraception since starting on your methods 3 years ago, and in approximately 1 year plan to use the charts for conception purposes. Thank you in advance!

D. P., Italy

I have been amazed by how easy it has been to observe my fertility cycles. I can't imagine how I never noticed before! It has made such a difference to my confidence and our sex life. Contraception was meant to be easy.

M. G., Brisbane

The rewards of using this method have extended well beyond feeling confident about contraception. It has opened up a whole new understanding of my body, and given me great peace of mind.

B. A.., Melbourne

Thank you for your pioneering work in this hugely important area of women's health. May it help other women as much as it has benefited me.

L. C., England

I congratulate you on the beautiful, simple and yet powerful methods of Natural Fertility Management. As I embark on using these methods I have a great sense of enjoyment and adventure. It has put another important piece of life's jigsaw together. Thank you.

M. S., Adelaide

I knew there had to be a better way!

M. V., California

Here is a letter from an NFM practitioner who trained with me about a couple who came to see her for birth control.

One young couple who came to me for contraception methods (after she'd briefly gone on the Pill and not been happy with the side-effects) have worked out a good system so they both have a contribution to, and awareness of, their chart each day.

He's an early riser (4.30 am to go to work), so he pops the thermometer in her mouth when he gets up and takes down the reading 5 minutes later, after showering. She fills in the other details during the day. I'm very excited and encouraged by these young people (she's 19, he's 20) taking joint responsibility for their fertility, and by the love, respect and commitment that they share.

Another young couple (she's 21, he's 22) came to see me and brought their delightful 3-month old daughter. Although she's still breastfeeding the mother was aware that that would not necessarily mean that she couldn't conceive. They'd decided to wait a couple of years to be more established in their new family before having another child.

They were a very tuned in couple: she'd noticed mucus changes around the full moon, so she wasn't surprised to find, on receiving her NFM kit, that she was born at a full moon, and she knew that they'd conceived their daughter at a full moon.

I see these couples as wonderful examples of the hope we can hold for the awareness and empowerment of future generations.

Glenda Lindsay, Melbourne

Here is another account, in her own words, of a successful transition to NFM, from a woman who is now, in her enthusiasm, teaching these methods to other women.

BLYTHE

Early in my relationship with my partner, we chose to use condoms as our contraception method. On one occasion, the condom broke. I visited my general practitioner in a state of panic, requesting the morning-after pill. He provided me with the hormones and proceeded to question me about my methods of contraception. When I informed him that my partner and I were using condoms, he responded, 'So when are you going to go on the Pill? You can't expect him to use condoms all his life.

So began my 3-year course on the Pill. Although I did not suffer any apparent side-effects, I am an extremely health-conscious person (as many of us are these days), and I detested the thought of putting synthetically constructed hormones in my body. Furthermore, I came to resent my partner for the fact he was not required to take any responsibility for birth control. Looking back, I can see the huge injustice that my general practitioner did me. Not only had he encouraged me to take a contraceptive with many unpleasant and often dangerous side-effects, but he had also contributed to my feelings of resentment towards my partner by implying that it was my duty to take the Pill for my partner's sake.

After 3 years of continuous use of the Pill, my partner and I agreed that I should have a 6-month break from the Pill to give my body a rest. Originally, I truly planned to recommence with the Pill after the 6-month period. However, I found that the longer I stayed off the Pill, the more reluctant I became to start using it again. I began my search for a natural contraceptive.

Three months after I stopped taking the Pill, I came across *The Billings Method* by Dr Evelyn Billings in a bookstore. I was so excited that I read the book immediately and attempted to put the technique into practice. I was considering becoming a Billings method instructor when a wonderful women friend advised me to learn about Francesca

Naish's combination of contraceptive techniques. I sent away for the NFM kit for contraception, and was soon promoting the methods to anyone who would listen. Initially, it was a real quantum leap for both my partner and myself to have 'unprotected' sex after having been told all our lives that sex without the use of condoms or the Pill inevitably resulted in pregnancy. In my medically oriented university course, even learned lecturers taught that condoms, the Pill and other invasive, unnatural contraceptive methods were vital for avoiding pregnancy. It took some courage to ignore these voices of authority, both for my partner and for myself. However, we came to trust the method implicitly, and I feel a glorious sense of liberation, control and a newfound sense of personal awareness.

I'm absolutely thrilled with the Natural Fertility Management methods. In addition, my partner has found that not only does the chart show him when I am fertile and when I am not, it also has space for mood, and he's able to tell to keep well out of my way!

Because I'm so enthusiastic about these methods, I recently completed the Natural Fertility Management course. It was a fabulous, informative weekend with a lovely group of people. During the course, I learnt how to recognise the signs of fertility problems. In fact, I was convinced after examining my own charts that I had not ovulated for 2 months until I learnt that my darling partner had thoughtfully washed my thermometer in hot water, rendering all of the readings meaningless! Despite these occasional hiccups, I feel that my partner and I have become a lot closer since using the natural fertility methods. Now the responsibility falls on both our shoulders.

Choosing natural contraception is one of the best things I've ever done. I would encourage any woman to try it, whether for contraception, conception or simply for self-awareness. In these times when so much in else in the world seems to be escalating out of control, it's a relief to know that through being informed about all of our fertility management options, we still do have control of our bodies.

This next story is also written by a woman who attended one of our professional training courses. It shows how the use of these methods can empower and enable women to come into their feminine, cyclical, creative birthright — before they've even thought about having children.

MELANIE

I remember my mother taking me to see a gynaecologist because I had experienced heavy menstrual bleeding since menarche (about age 16). After seeing the gynaecologist, I was prescribed the Pill (from memory, a heavy dose pill and one without cyclical distinction). Being prescribed the Pill eased my own and my mother's anxiety and in addition appeared to ease the flow of my menstruation. I remember the gynaecologist pronouncing that this was a solution that alleviated both problems — heavy bleeding and protection against my budding sexuality. I remained on the Pill for 13 years.

I don't believe I experienced any adverse reactions from taking the Pill. My focus was more on being safe. Having not been educated on my own cyclical nature, I was not focused on detecting changes. The effects were more on the positive side, i.e. decreased blood flow and pain. At this point I had no idea about my body or what negative effects could become apparent, so either I didn't notice them or I attributed them to other causes, e.g. puberty, endometriosis, etc. In hindsight, however, I am now not sure what effect oral contraception may have had on my body. I was diagnosed with endometriosis at age 25 and cervical dysplasia (CIN2) at age 33. I believe such reproductive problems have been influenced by my use of the Pill — the suppression of my natural cycle (and subsequent inability to track or detect underlying conditions) kept me in a state of fertility limbo. It wasn't until I stopped taking the Pill that I became alerted to the fact that my reproductive system needed urgent attention.

After being diagnosed with dysplasia and having a colposcopy (loop incision) and then having another recurrence of dysplasia (CIN1) 12 months later, I realised I needed to go back to a more fundamental approach. I am currently seeing a naturopath monthly and working with her on balancing my hormones and using homoeopathic medicine to continue the healing from my last diagnosis of mild dysplasia. My desire now is not to use orthodox medicine.

After being diagnosed with endometriosis, I was put on synthetic hormone tablets for 12 months, which stopped my bleeding. I cannot say that this treatment was ineffective. What I can say is that I continued to experience fertility problems. As a result of this I have chosen to look at other options to support my well-being.

I chose naturopathy because I no longer wished to override my health through the use of chemically based medicines. Through naturopathic medicine, I have also had to face other problematic factors such as diet, level of exercise, smoking and the amount of energy and stress I devote to my professional life. I doubt if this would have occurred if I had followed a more orthodox regime. Working with a natural therapist on an ongoing basis more readily allows me the right to take responsibility for my health (this could also be so with an orthodox medical doctor, though my experience to date has shown that different dialogues and language distinguish the two — the alternative practitioner being the one I am more able to now walk alongside of).

The effects of the Pill on my relationship were initially positive in that I saw its use as a way of having a relationship without fear of pregnancy. However, my ignorance was so great that I can still remember experiencing great anxiety preperiod just in case — in case

I didn't take the Pill at exactly the same time each day, etc. For me, using the Pill was a fear-based action. Not being provided with knowledge of any alternative practice I took up my duty as the one who would take responsibility for safeguarding against unwanted pregnancy. I didn't realise then how much of a trade-off this was.

It was very black and white for me then — the Pill or risk pregnancy. Now I see it as take the Pill and compromise my well-being, particularly now I have become aware of alternative methods of contraception. I'm saddened by the fact that I wasn't amid a culture that questioned the theories of orthodox medicine and so followed on in ignorance only to give my power away to a doctrine that said it was the 'easiest and best' way. This outcome was also given rise to by the distinct lack of role modelling around me. From my perspective, I didn't know any better.

Coming off the Pill was a culmination of many factors, one being the support of my partner (it was actually he who introduced the idea to me and encouraged me to make the decision). I had also been participating in many body and self-awareness programs where I became increasingly sensitive to the impact of all natural and unnatural choices I made around my physical and emotional being. None of my friends were using natural methods of contraception so I had no direct means of checking, or a place where I could alleviate some of my anxiety. When I finally made the decision I did feel a high degree of fear — more fear of the unknown. Mainly because I saw this decision as a shedding and a letting go of an element of control (though at that point I paradoxically thought I had the control over my sexuality through the use of the Pill, rather than what I later was able to see as the other way around). I did not experience any initial problems after coming off the Pill and my cycle lengths remained reasonably constant.

I believe I received enough information to get me going on the Pill, i.e. how to take it. I know that in my youth I didn't ask the questions that I would ask now of any doctor, seeing him/her for whatever reason. I find that now, after coming off the Pill, I am much more inclined to go armed with questions to the doctor, whether they may be medical or alternative. I have also found that the recent questions that I asked of my gynaecologist were not answered to the degree that I felt satisfied.

It has been my experience with the general practitioners I have visited that they will use my appointment time available to represcribe existing treatments. It was only when I went to a female GP and asked her what my contraceptive options were, that I was provided with such information. I believe the current medical system is set up to find immediate and expedient solutions to people's concerns. To me it is a sign of our times that indepth enquiry and dialogue are luxuries and not rights. This exposure has shown me how necessary it is for me to take charge of my own health and to be the one who is the questioner. Gone is the time that we should be looking for, and holding responsibility against, a doctor who will take charge of our lives.

I am using a natural method of contraception because it is not my desire to conceive. By natural, I mean that I continue to chart my cycle through mucus and temperature observations. At times of hormonal and lunar fertility, my partner and I use condoms. Yes, I am more than happy — relieved — to be using a more natural form of contraception. It has allowed me to relate to my womanhood in ways that previously were not open to me. I have also become more attuned, as a rediscovered cyclical being to the cyclical nature of this planet and feel blessed to be walking through this doorway. I have also become more accepting of my own and others' sustainable right to ebb and flow rather than feel restrained and disciplined by a more linear way of being (as mirrored by the use of a non-cyclically based pill).

My current thoughts around my identification as a woman and all that this entails have changed dramatically over the years. I see my own self-education as a necessary path to my own freedom. I am thankful for the knowledge I have sought out and that which has been made available to me, particularly NFM. This particularly relates to my position as a working woman — the hours and responsibility I manage as a general manager for an international business consultancy while maintaining a home, relationship and operating my own small business as an artist constantly challenges my sense of balance.

My cycle and that of this land has also played an important part in my developing art work. I am more likely to paint at the times of ovulation or menstruation. This is because at these times I am more directed by inner changes and movements. Creativity for me is a way in which I can transfer internal experiences into tangible form. This has developed within me an interest in how my own cycle relates to the cycle of life. Studying lunar activity has led me to appreciate the changes brought by the seasons and how this is represented and respected within a spiritual framework. The elements of fire, earth, air and wind and how they are manifested throughout the year along with the observation of sacred festivals has opened my awareness of the beauty around me. Being a woman with her own internal seasons allows me to pay homage to nature — and to the nature of life.

A point of reflection for me as an artist is that in pursuit of this experience I feel closest to what I would term as 'source' — bringing into form that which has been conceptualised by my own being. It is a magical endeavour, one which I believe has helped me manage a deep need to be a creator and through which I am given endless opportunity to express my inner most self. Particularly as many of my paintings express the feminine essence and what it means to me to be a woman (there have also been a lot more crescent moons appearing in my work, their shape representing my own lunar angle). I have found solace in my artwork as increasingly I use it as a vehicle from which I draw clarity around my feelings as a woman and potential mother.

I have a woman friend who is very close to me with whom I openly share details of my menstrual cycle. She ovulates when I menstruate and vice versa. We both use natural cotton pads and speak endlessly on the influence of ritual and the Goddess in our lives. Our communion is a haven for me, a place where I feel truly able to share my joys and sorrows in being a woman. The value of blood honouring is something I consider missing in the mainstream of today's rights of passage. Educating our young to respect their own and others' sexuality needs to go hand in hand with revolutionising our lack of respect for the earth's cyclical nature and its continuing environmental neglect. It is of no wonder to me that limited passion in these areas are providing stilted results in a world that desperately requires an increased open maturity in how we all relate to each other and ourselves.

MEGAN

Megan had been on the Pill for 7 years, had suffered from weight gain, headaches, depression and a host of so-called minor problems. Then she tried an IUD and it perforated her uterus. In despair, she turned to the diaphragm, and suffered toxic shock syndrome, with 24 hours of extreme symptoms for which she was hospitalised.

The only time she had felt comfortable about her contraception method was during 18 months of mucus testing. But she had taught herself, was not fully confident, and this had resulted in a pregnancy, which had itself been problematic. The child was 2 months premature, and this after a full month of haemorrhaging.

Megan suffered quite a lot with her periods, experiencing bad pain, PMT, hypoglycaemia (low blood-sugar leading to depressed energy states) and lumpy breasts.

Herbal and vitamin and mineral therapy cleared up the dysmenorrhoea and PMS, and renewed her hormonal health. She embarked on a new contraceptive program of mucus and temperature testing, and observance of the lunar cycle. She felt symptom-free and confident, and has used the method successfully ever since.

GILLIAN

Because of painful periods, Gillian's doctor put her on the Pill at 18. Later, she became unhappy with this solution and started to use a diaphragm. She was not shown how to use it properly or how to check that it was correctly inserted and consequently became pregnant three times in 1 year; she had a termination each time. After this experience, Gillian went back on the Pill, seeing it as the only possibility. However, it led to raging thrush (vaginal candida) which drove her to distraction.

After seeing me, she came off the Pill, took herbal remedies and nutrients, used the Tea-tree oil and vinegar douche, and the thrush abated.

She learnt to use her diaphragm properly, and uses it as infrequently as possible, preferring to abstain at her fertile times. She feels physically 'terrific' and confidently in control of her own fertility.

ALISON

For 15 years, Alison was on and off the Pill. She felt 'bad' when on it, a vague feeling she could define no more clearly than that. Like Gillian, Alison also stopped taking the Pill, and although she felt much better, she used her diaphragm incorrectly and conceived twice.

Each time she bled during the pregnancy and terminated it. She then bled almost continuously *for a whole year*, and so went back on the Pill. She was very worried about coming off it, in case the bleeding started again.

I put her on a herbal mix designed to both eliminate the Pill from her system and prevent atypical bleeding. It worked. She feels, 'So much better and in control of my life — it's wonderful!'

JUDY

Judy had used an IUD for years without any problems and enjoyed the sexual freedom it gave her. However, she had started bleeding very heavily and was experiencing bad pain at her periods. Her doctor had suggested she find another form of contraception.

She couldn't go on the Pill because of her tendency to high blood pressure, and she didn't fancy using a condom or a diaphragm. Since she also felt it was important to be able to make love without restraint, her solution was not clear.

After some counselling, she decided she could cope with a diaphragm occasionally, but felt that she must try to ensure that this was as infrequent as possible. She was impressed by the literature on the lunar cycle, but felt that needing to use a mechanical contraception twice a month would be unworkable.

We did weekly hypnotherapy to influence her hormonal cycle to synchronise with her lunar peak, and gave her herbs and nutrients for the bleeding and dysmenorrhoea. Her periods became much less problematic, but she became concerned that her cycle was getting longer.

I reassured her that it was probably a result of the suggestions, and sure enough, within three cycles, her mid-cycle ovulation was coinciding with her lunar fertile time, upon which the cycle reverted to a 29 day interval. She became confident in her identification of her fertile signs, and even in her use of the diaphragm.

ANTHEA

Anthea was also anxious to avoid two fertile times in 1 month, but felt uneasy about staying on the Pill. I started giving her herbal sand nutrient supplements to offset the effects of the Pill as quickly as possible, and hoped that her cycle would resume regularly straight away.

Assuming that this would be so, we calculated when her first ovulation would need to come in order to synchronise with her lunar peak. She stopped taking the Pill so that her withdrawal bleeding would start 15 days before this.

Everything worked to plan, her cycles resumed normally and continued on an average 29-day interval.

VALERIE

Valerie didn't come to me for contraception advice. She came because she'd had an abnormal Pap smear, which was thought to be related to the genital wart virus. She wondered if there was anything she could do about it using natural remedies.

This was the second time this result had come up; the first time she had received laser treatment and a curette. This time the virus was more widespread, on the vaginal wall and the cervix. I advised her to come off the Pill and said that condoms and diaphragms could possibly aggravate the condition, especially if she used chemical spermicides.

We treated the wart condition and the cervix became healthy within 3 months. Her PMS also cleared up. She learnt successfully to control her own fertility and came back within a year to see about conceiving a child.

MAGGIE

Maggie had tried an IUD and had suffered from infections which, luckily, were diagnosed and treated early; there had been no resultant scarring to the tubes. Then, having been scared by the possible threat to her fertility, she had decided to have a child. Everything had gone fine; her son James was now 3 years old.

Not being game to try another IUD, Maggie had gone on the Pill after his birth and had experienced recurring and debilitating bouts of vaginal candida (thrush). As she was enjoying a partial return to her career, she didn't want another child yet, but this time she wanted to use natural birth control methods.

There was, however, a problem. Until we brought the candida under control, it would be difficult for her to have enough discharge-free time to learn her mucus changes.

She stopped taking the Pill, started using condoms and began douching with *Tea-tree* oil and vinegar. She got some relief, but found that the itching and discharge returned every time she stopped douching. She was also feeling very tired and disoriented, and had eczema on her hands.

I convinced her that there was a good chance that the candida had become systemic, that it would go on recurring vaginally until it was eliminated from her gut and that her other problems would probably also then clear up.

Maggie went on the very strict anticandida diet and took other remedies that I prepared for her. Three months later, her health was greatly improved, her mucus observations were coming along fine, and she was using condoms less and less.

Other effects of the Pill

HELEN

After taking the Pill for many years, Helen decided to start a family. She was horrified when her periods did not resume. She came to me after 8 months of amenorrhoea. With the help of herbs and nutrients, we got her periods flowing.

Then it became apparent that she was not ovulating. We fixed that. Then her mucus production seemed almost non-existent and we cured that. Finally, she conceived, by using the lunar and hormonal cycles for timing. She was unsure on which cycle she conceived — but she didn't mind!

LEIGH

Leigh also had problems after she came off the Pill. There was a delay in her cycle returning. When it did, insufficient mucus was being generated around ovulation. This may have been partly an after-effect of the Pill usage but also partly due to the cauterisation of the cervix carried out when she had suffered from cervical erosion (another side effect of the Pill).

After treatment and learning to time her hormonal and lunar cycle, she promptly conceived. She then came back to me to help successfully plan her second child.

Other successful conceptions

Here are a few quotes from letters sent to me by couples who found various benefits in using a natural approach to solve their fertility problems.

> After 3 years of trying unsuccessfully to conceive we experienced two failed attempts at the GIFT/IVF program in 1993, and a miscarriage later in the same year. We decided that this program was not for us and set about obtaining a more natural approach to our problem.
>
> Early in 1994 we met Francesca Naish. After our first meeting we felt very positive while enjoying the feeling of being more in control of our situation. We made changes to our lifestyle immediately through a healthy, nutritious diet, exercise and nutrient supplements. We also listened to a relaxation tape prepared by Francesca, which helped us to visualise conception and the birth of a baby actually happening for us.
>
> Francesca advised us to take a break from trying to conceive. In June 1994, we were given the 'go-ahead' to begin trying again. We were elated to discover that we were successful on our second attempt. After enjoying a strong, healthy pregnancy, our beautiful baby boy was born on the 5th April 1995. Thanks to Francesca, our most treasured dream has come true.
>
> *D & D. M., Sydney*

Our conception occurred as soon as the lunar and hormonal cycles coincided. We are ecstatic!

J & M. D. Darwin

I am now nearly 3 months into your diet and treatments, and am feeling much better. I've also lost over 14 pounds in weight. To top it all off — I'm pregnant! Eight weeks today, and the scan showed the baby in the uterus (not an ectopic!). So, all in all, a wonderful success story! I plan to stay on the diet, and feel much better for it!

W. K. Box Hill, Australia

At last! An approach that offers me hope in my quest to have a child. I now feel confident that I can achieve a conception without having to continue suffering the horrors of the medical approach.

T.N., New Zealand

Many thanks for the natural fertility methods. I was on the verge of IVF which cuts across my commitment to Nature's strength. (In the face of advice from my gynaecologist.)

J. N. Sydney

Thank you so much for all that you have given us. We are 16 weeks and all is well for the future! We are so happy!

R & T. H. Sydney

I have a new confidence and feel empowered to achieve a pregnancy. I am feeling positive that I will become pregnant and have a healthy child — You are no idea how much this means to me.

F.M. France

I write to thank you for your help — with affirmations, visualisations, knowledge of menstrual cycles and vitamins for good measure! They helped me conceive the most beautiful embodiment of joy I've ever met. Myles is now 13 months old, a little shaky on the legs, but big and strong.

T.D., Sydney

We have been using your methods of conception for 3 months now, and have just conceived. What a wonderful help Natural Fertility Management has been! I wouldn't be without it now and will use the methods for contraception after the birth of my child. I recommend it to all my friends and clients.

A. B., Shepparton, Australia

We have used your methods to have a healthy girl, then a boy, and are now thinking our family is complete. Luckily we can now use the methods for contraception with no worries (about health or effectiveness). We are also glad we discovered your methods.

R & F. C. Sydney

ANNE

Endometriosis had blighted Anne's hopes of a pregnancy. She had a severe case with a long history. I was able to treat her successfully, although, since the treatment involved use of herbs contra-indicated during pregnancy, she used a condom while she learnt to isolate her fertile times and prepared for pregnancy.

Anne conceived at her mid-cycle ovulation within 2 months of ceasing treatment.

MARSHA

Marsha came to me after several unsuccessful attempts at in vitro fertilisation. There was no apparent reason why she did not conceive, and the quantity and quality of her husband's sperm were fine. Then we got to the part of the consultation where I took down details of her diet.

'Breakfast?' I enquired innocently.

'Two shortbread biscuits and a cup of black coffee,' she replied.

'Well,' I said, 'the coffee will have to go, and so really will the biscuits. Perhaps we could substitute something a bit more nutritious, such as porridge, or wholemeal bread.'

She said she had recently bought a nutrient-enriched white bread for her daughter. Cursing the bread manufacturers (under my breath) I explained that wholegrain bread didn't need enriching as it still had everything in it in its natural form.

'However,' I said in good faith, 'let's move on to lunch.'

'Chips.'

'Often?'

'Every day.'

'Oh dear. What with?'

'Nothing else, just chips.'

Well, I was beginning to get the hang of this, but still I remained optimistic. Perhaps something nutritious for dinner? A plate of fish and vegetables, or a salad?

'Steak.'

'Steak and what?'

'Steak and pasta.'

'White, or wholemeal?'

'White.'

There wasn't really very much nutrition in a diet like that. Did she ever eat fruit or vegetables at all? No, and neither did her husband, who was glaring at me, obviously aware that I was going to suggest something outrageous such as brown rice and vegetables.

I toned down my suggestions as much as I could. Wholegrain cereal or bread for breakfast, a salad and wholegrain bread sandwich for lunch, and fish, free-range, organically fed chicken or meat for dinner with vegetables. Fruit and nuts for snacks in between.

There was great resistance at first, but she soon got the hang of it. Her husband did, too. I expect her first child (who was 8) benefited as well. When they had built up a sufficient store of nutrients, she conceived. It was much cheaper than IVF.

ROSEMARY

Rosemary simply couldn't cope with not being a mother. Her fear that her infertility was a permanent state was causing her such stress that she couldn't sleep and was rapidly becoming extremely run down. There was no obvious physical reason for her infertility; previously irregular cycles had come good.

Hypnotherapy and counselling changed her attitude and her ability to conceive. By doing regular relaxation and visualisation, Rosemary achieved a pregnancy within 4 months.

JUDITH

For 18 months, Judith had been trying to conceive. After 7 months she had a laparoscopy, and dye was used to test the patency of her fallopian tubes.

This showed enormous fibroids on her uterus, adhesions to her left fallopian tube (which was not yet blocked, although the flow of dye was minimal), and a cyst on her right ovary. She also suffered quite distressing dysmenorrhoea.

Despite these problems, which affected the whole of her reproductive system, she conceived a month later, but miscarried almost immediately. Eight months later, she started taking a fertility drug, as she had no mucus production. Still no conception occurred and 2 months further on, her quest led her to me.

On a very strict diet and with the help of nutrient supplements and herbal remedies, we cleared up the fibroids in 4 months. The left tube was clear, the cyst was gone, and she had plentiful mucus production and no more painful periods. A miracle. But, one more stage to go.

Two more months, 2 years down the track from the beginning of her journey, Judith conceived and didn't miscarry. The miracle was topped!

FIONA

Fiona felt herself to be very fit and was extremely puzzled and a little resentful that her cycles had stopped just when she wanted to conceive. She was athletically active and ate mostly a raw vegetarian diet. She didn't know that both of these conditions could cause amenorrhoea.

When Fiona cut back on her training, introduced more protein into her diet, such as cooked fish, her cycle returned and she conceived.

STACEY

This was an unusual case. There was nothing wrong with Stacey at all. She wanted a child, as she was in a stable relationship and felt the time was right. However, since her relationship was with another woman, she had a problem.

She had found a willing father, but, as she preferred not to use a syringe to inject the sperm, and because of her sexual preference, she wanted to isolate the fertile time and cut down on the number of attempts. I never heard what the outcome was, but wished her well.

NICOLA

At 39, with a history of no conceptions, and with adhesions to the tubes and ovarian cysts, Nicola's chances looked slim. She had no idea why she had developed adhesions; there had been no history of infection or trauma in the abdomen.

The adhesions and the cysts had been removed when they were discovered at the time the laparoscopy was performed, and the tubes were apparently clear. Conception had still not occurred and this, combined with her job as a teacher, was contributing to her highly stressed state.

After changing her teaching job to one at a Steiner school, where the pace and ambience suited her much better, learning timing techniques and using natural remedies, she conceived within 5 months.

MICHELLE

Having had no problems conceiving her first two children, Michelle was distressed at having tried for 2 years with no success for her third. Although she had no history of PID, her tubes were partially blocked. No dye was detected when she underwent a hysterosalpingogram, but minimal dye passage was seen through a laparoscope.

The probable reason for this seemed to be the emergency caesarean section she'd had at the delivery of her second child because of placenta praevia. However, she was ovulating, with regular, symptom-free periods, and her husband's sperm count was good.

Michelle realised that her treatment could take some months. She was very conscientious with her herbs, diet and supplements, and listened regularly to a motivational tape I prepared for her.

Each cycle, she was meticulous in her timing of conception, and 6 months later it paid off — she conceived.

DIANE

Having terminated her first and only pregnancy 10 years previously, at a time when she and her now husband had only just met, Diane ended up 8 weeks later in hospital, haemorrhaging.

She had no conscious regrets about what she saw as an appropriate action at the time, but was now suffering from endometriosis on one ovary and a cyst on the other. She was bleeding very heavily on the first 2 days of each period, and suffered a lot of pain.

During the phase we were treating the endometriosis and the cyst, she and her husband used condoms so she could take the more physiologically active herbs required. Although she was a vegetarian, Diane started to include fish in her diet, as she felt her protein levels were low; she also took supplements. She spent the next few cycles learning timing techniques.

After 3 months, her bleeding pattern was so improved that we decided to give conception a try. It worked. I knew it had when she came through the door of the clinic with a huge bunch of flowers and an even bigger grin.

PENNY

Penny had trouble recording her temperatures. It wasn't a lack of motivation, but her temperatures were so low that they didn't fit on the graph.

I suspected from this that she might have an underactive thyroid (hypothyroidism), which would be affecting her fertility. The appropriate natural remedies resolved the problem.

Success after previous problematic pregnancies

URSULA AND JEREMY

Ursula and Jeremy had experienced multiple problems in their quest for a baby — Ursula had experienced several miscarriages and Jeremy had been diagnosed with inadequate numbers of sperm, and those that he had were not very healthy. However, after testing both Ursula and Jeremy for the full range of genito-urinary infections that can cause miscarriage, it became apparent that Jeremy was not the only one with the problems: each of them tested positive to several infections, even though there had been no symptoms. Ursula's charting also showed a tendency, in some cycles, for ovulation to occur after Day 17.

Antibiotic treatment was prescribed, and given full support from natural remedies; a complete program of preconception health care was undertaken. Newly confident, they embarked on a well-timed conception attempt and are now proud parents of a gorgeous little girl.

ROBERTA AND CARLOS

Roberta was an older mother who had recently had a 'therapeutic' termination of a baby diagnosed as having Down syndrome. When she came to me she was very frightened of a repeat experience. Because she was also concerned about her fertility declining as she grew older, it took a lot of counselling to persuade her that the advantages of completing her preconception health care were of prominent importance and that as far as her fertility was concerned, she would be 'younger' at the end of her preparation.

Her husband Carlos was supportive. Together they undertook a comprehensive program of detoxification, nutritional supplementation, herbal treatment and stress management. We also investigated both of them for the full range of GUIs, which were, happily, absent. Carlos had previously been exposed to a high degree of radiation through X-rays he'd required after a knee injury. At the time of the X-rays, no protection had been given to his genitalia, so we focused — for him especially — on remedies that also assisted recovery from the effects of radiation.

I'm happy to say that photos of their happy, healthy children now grace my baby wall at the Jocelyn Centre.

In vitro

Some women and couples come to me before they try an in vitro conception, wanting to avoid it if possible. Some come to tone up their reproductive and hormonal systems so there is more chance of success on the in vitro program. Some come because they find in vitro such a traumatic experience that they feel they can't continue, while others come because in vitro has failed them.

Despite the enormous amount of money spent on and publicity that surrounds in vitro fertilisation programs, their success rate is still, on average, only about 10–15 per cent, although related procedures, such as gamete intrafallopian transfer (GIFT), which can be performed on women with patent tubes, are more successful.

Although I am very happy for the few for whom it is a success, I feel that the money could perhaps be spent better on teaching women how to take care of their hormonal, reproductive and general health. This would reach far greater numbers and, on the whole, does so. This approach seems to be a more successful, with the added advantage of improved foetal health.

HEATHER

Heather's blocked tubes were caused by adhesions that were so bad that neither surgery nor natural medicines would have been of any use. She'd had three attempts at in vitro conception. One time, the egg didn't fertilise; the other times the egg didn't attach in the womb. Heather wanted to optimise her chances for the next try; she had found the program somewhat traumatic and felt this was her last attempt.

Heather and I worked together to synchronise her lunar and hormonal cycles and tone her reproductive system through the use of herbs, vitamins, minerals and exercise. Her partner also practised preconception health care, though there was no obvious fertility problem. The next attempt at in vitro fertilisation took place when her cycles coincided and was successful.

GINA

By the time Gina came to see me she and her partner had been on the infertility treadmill for 6 years, during which time she had conceived several times. One pregnancy was from a natural conception after 2 years of trying; she miscarried at 7 weeks. The others were through assisted reproductive programs. Two of these miscarried early, one at 6 weeks, the other pregnancy, with twins, she carried to 6 months. A further attempt at in vitro fertilisation in the recent past had been unsuccessful.

Gina had been treated for endometriosis, although her tubes were patent and her serum hormone levels adequate. I continued the treatment for endometriosis naturopathical, and concentrated on detoxifying her system from the many (medical) drugs she had taken.

After 3 months, during which time she learnt timing techniques and used condoms as she and her partner prepared their bodies and minds for conception, we changed to a fertility boosting treatment. Within a further 3 months Gina had conceived naturally; she carried the pregnancy to a successful birth of a healthy child.

STELLA

With Stella, the initial diagnosis had been of multiple cysts on the ends of her fallopian tubes, which she had successfully treated with herbs before she came to see me. After she still had not conceived a year later, she started taking clomiphene citrate, a fertility drug.

While taking the drug, Stella was experiencing little or no mucus and her temperature did not rise mid-cycle. Interestingly enough, her serum LH levels surged at her lunar fertile time. As well as suffering other congestive mucus symptoms in her respiratory system, Stella also had dysmenorrhoea and her post-ovulatory phase was too short (less than 10 days).

She felt insecure about going off the fertility drugs, so I treated her for the effects of the drug as well as to boost fertility and, apart from assisting elimination through the liver, gave mucous membrane tonic and hormone balancing herbs and nutrients.

Stella's period and mucus production problems resolved and her luteal phase extended, but a post-coital test showed very few sperm surviving, even though there appeared to be no antibodies in the mucus. Her partner's sperm count seemed to be fine, so that wasn't the problem; besides, he was practising preconception health care anyway, to optimise their chances.

We put Stella on an anti-acidity diet and alkalising herbs. As a side benefit, her respiratory congestion cleared. We continued to include preventative treatment for cysts.

The stage seemed to be set for conception, but she felt insecure about a natural conception and was stressed about the prospect of assisted reproductive technology.

To help her make clear decisions, Stella did some hypnotherapy sessions, which resulted in an in vitro attempt during which she was supported by anti-stress herbs, a relaxation/positivity tape and weekly hypnotherapy sessions.

This was a case where treatment had to be changed many times as the situation progressed, and where patience paid off. It took us a year from the time Stella first came to see me before we got results.

WENDY

Assisted reproductive technology had not been successful for Wendy, although she was very determined to conceive. Time was not on her side as she was in her early forties, but she already had adopted one absolutely charming Korean child, who graced our consultations with his smile.

Her health was not good and she was rapidly developing an asthmatic response. The main fertility problem was one of sperm antibodies in her mucus, although her cycle was also erratic.

Wendy, like Stella, was patient and determined. Over the months that she and her partner practised preconception health care, we successfully treated all sorts of health problems. As well as seeing me, she was having acupuncture and taking homoeopathic medicine.

Since Wendy had developed an allergy-based asthma, we focused on rebuilding and detoxifying her immune system. At the same time, she used condoms to give her body a rest from the invading sperm.

Not only did Wendy's immune system respond favourably, but her general health and state of mind also became such that a conception was at last possible.

MARION

Marion had tried to conceive on an assisted reproductive program because her mucus was so deficient that her partner's sperm simply couldn't survive in her cervix. She had been given oestrogen treatment for this, but it wasn't successful.

I talked to Marion about her diet because I felt that this might be the clue we needed. As well as cutting all dairy products out of her diet and taking reasonable doses of nutrient supplements, she took high doses of calcium and magnesium. She included oestrogen-rich foods in her diet and took hormone-balancing herbs so she could produce more oestrogen herself.

Soon her mucus was wet and stretchy and profuse — conception occurred without any interference at all.

DAWN

Dawn had twice attempted an artificially assisted conception. Neither time had been successful. The second had been after she and her partner had some treatment with me, although, as she was impatient, they didn't wait as long as I recommended for treatment to take effect before attempting conception (herbal tonics work slowly over a few months). She was also very stressed about the whole situation; she found the in vitro program very upsetting and impersonal.

I felt that Dawn needed to empower herself so we started ongoing hypnotherapy while completing the herbal and nutrient preparations for conception. She overcame her impatience and allowed her therapy to run its full course.

We then made a special relaxation and suggestion tape for her to use during the next in vitro attempt and she continued to see me for the first 2 weeks of that cycle.

Dawn said she felt 'in complete control' and much more confident. The attempt was successful.

Other successes from feeling in control
GERALDINE

Geraldine's first pregnancy had come in her early twenties while she was on the Pill, and she had terminated it. Another, when she was 28, was also terminated. Then she had a couple of haemorrhages between periods and went on the Pill as treatment.

She then discovered lumps in her breast and groin which had been present for 3 months by the time she came to see me, wanting to conceive.

With the use of herbs, nutritional supplements and a healthy diet, we cleared up the lumps in 3 months . Geraldine's first attempt at conception after this was successful. Her attitude to her treatment was extremely positive, whereas before, she had felt hopelessly 'out of control'. She felt that she had been abusing her body and her health, which was an enormous source of worry to her.

As soon as Geraldine felt she was dealing with her health problems herself, in a way that suited her nature and left her feeling good about herself, her health problems cleared up. She then conceived right away.

CAMILLA

When Camilla came to see me, she was obviously very nervous. At first I thought that it was because she, a fairly conservative person, was anxious about entrusting herself to an 'alternative' health practitioner.

It turned out to be because she had not told her husband (who'd had children by a previous marriage and was not interested in having any more) that she was seeing me, or even that she was trying to conceive.

Camilla had had a myomectomy (reconstruction of the uterus and removal of fibroids), but the surgery had been in a part of the womb that was unlikely to affect a pregnancy. Other than that, she seemed to be in good reproductive health. Even so, she was very stressed, and suffered from asthma and recurrent headaches.

Her job — and the unresolved situation with her husband — were both causing her strain. Her treatment included relaxation and suggestion tapes, Bach flower remedies, herbal nervines and counselling.

I never found out whether she conceived or not because she moved away, but by the time she moved, I felt her chances were good because she had created a whole new career for herself.

Whether she conceived or not, Camilla's was already a success story, because once again she felt good about her life. She successfully resolved the issue of children with her husband and felt so good about that, as well as feeling good about her new work, that she felt she was back in control of her life.

PAMELA

I didn't help Pamela at all. All she did was phone me and ask about how she could embark on a program of natural and self-help remedies to resolve her long-standing infertility.

She never kept our appointment because, within a few weeks of the call, she had conceived. All Pamela had needed was to feel that she was tackling the problem in a way she felt good about and that involved her own efforts.

There are quite a lot of Pamelas in my files (and gaps in my appointment book)!

SALLY

Sally's endometriosis had cleared up 6 years before she saw me, but it had left one blocked tube. She had been on the Pill for 7 years but, for the last 9, had used no contraception. However, she had not conceived, despite five attempts at in vitro conceptions in the previous 3 years. She also suffered from intense PMS and dysmenorrhoea, although her cycles were regular and she appeared to be ovulating.

After 3 months on herbal treatment and through paying attention to her nutrient status, these problems had cleared up, although she was still feeling depressed about her infertility. She was so impressed with the improvement in her hormonal health, we continued to use natural medicines with hypnotherapy and counselling for her state of mind.

Sally still hasn't conceived, but feels so much better physically and emotionally that she doesn't mind so much any more. She would still love to have children, but has learned to accept that this way may not be for her.

By feeling that she has done all in her power to resolve her infertility and not simply handed the problem over to an 'expert', Sally has lost her feelings of resentment, guilt and inadequacy.

She has always been involved with the local children and has scores of them in her house every weekend. So Sally's is a kind of success story after all.

Conceptions on the lunar cycle
TANYA

Tanya was a doctor with an interest in herbs and nutrition, who ran a 'holistic' practice. She was sufficiently interested in Natural Fertility Management to attend one of my courses, intending to use the methods for both herself and her patients, mainly for contraception.

Tanya started to apply the methods with enthusiasm, but remained sceptical about the possibility of conceiving at a lunar peak time that fell outside of the middle of the hormonal cycle.

One (very gorgeous) baby and several months maternity leave later, Tanya is now a full convert!

ANNABELLE

Annabelle, who was 23 years old when she came to see me, had gone 9 months since coming off the Pill without a regular cycle. At the request of her gynaecologist, she had prepared temperature charts, and from these it appeared as if ovulation was not occurring. The mucus symptoms that she did have, although very scant, occurred only 7 days before her (occasional) period.

After I had treated Annabelle with herbal and nutritional supplements for 2 months, and she had made some changes in her diet and exercise routine, she had a regular cycle, with normal mucus production at ovulation and a subsequent period after 15 days.

She abstained during this ovulation and the next, but made love during the next lunar fertile time, which came in the second half of her cycle, after mid-cycle ovulation had already come and gone (as shown by a temperature rise).

Annabelle conceived, carried the child to term, and successfully gave birth. She came back to me when her baby was 18 months old. She was still breastfeeding and had not had any periods yet, but was experiencing pain and congestion in her ovaries. I treated her again with herbs, her cycle resumed and she continued to use the method for contraception.

JOAN

When Joan came to see me, she had been trying unsuccessfully for 18 months to conceive. During that time, she had suffered two miscarriages, one 13 months before, and the other, which was diagnosed as resulting from a blighted ovum (when there is no embryo, though an apparent pregnancy commences) 5 months after that. She had no conceptions in the 8 months prior to seeing me.

Her history was of a late menarche at 18 years, and then a vastly irregular cycle over the next few years. Although she was now only 25, Joan was despairing of having a child and quite highly stressed by the whole experience.

She had had experience of identifying her mid-cycle ovulation through checking her mucus symptoms and her temperature; her diet and exercise routines were adequate.

I treated Joan and her partner with herbal medicine and supplements, gave them additional dietary and exercise advice, made a tape for her to use for relaxation and to create positive visualisations of the outcome, and drew up charts showing her lunar fertile times.

Within 3 months, she had conceived — on the lunar cycle, which she had used in preference to her mid-cycle ovulation (which she was adept at identifying as a result of long-term practice of it, but which had not been successful for her). She carried the baby to term and gave birth to a beautiful girl.

Conception when lunar phase and ovulation coincide

JOANNA

Joanna came to see me after trying to conceive for only 2 months. She was impatient. I drew up lunar charts and instructed her in timing and preparation techniques. We made a tape for her to ease stress, create positive visualisations, and bring the lunar and hormonal cycles together. I also gave her tonic herbs.

Joanna continued to try for conception for another 6 months, using both the ovulation and lunar times, which occurred separately. During that time, by using the tape and autosuggestions for synchronising the cycles, her lunar and hormonal fertile times crept closer and closer together. On the first occasion they coincided, Joanna conceived.

LUCY

Lucy had a very bad experience before she came to see me. She was 35 and had just miscarried when 5 months pregnant, the baby having been dead in the womb since 4 months.

When she was 21, Lucy had aborted at 6 months and, although that child had been healthy in the womb, it did not live. No reasons had been given to her for these events, although she had suffered a perforated uterus before her first pregnancy when an IUD lodged in her womb. She had used four IUDs altogether, and one had been 'lost' inside her.

Lucy and her partner were tested for heavy metals, infections and antibodies that can cause miscarriage; all were absent. They learnt timing techniques on the lunar and hormonal cycles and started doing regular exercise, changed their diet along the guidelines that I gave them, and took nutrient supplements and tonic herbs for her womb, ovaries and circulation.

We did some relaxation and visualisation sessions, which techniques she used to bring positivity and synchronise her cycles. Within 3 months, her cycles were coinciding and she had conceived. The child was successfully carried to term.

CHRISTINE

Christine also had a traumatic history. When she was 24, she'd had a termination, which led to continual heavy bleeding and pain in her left side. To solve this, she was put on the Pill, which resulted in her becoming very depressed, with headaches and atypical bleeding patterns. However, she continued to take the Pill until she was 26, then stopped and became pregnant.

Then there was another termination and the insertion of an IUD, which should never have been considered, given her history of bleeding. Her body totally rejected it and she had very bad, profuse bleeding.

When the bleeding settled, an ovarian cyst was found, which was operated on. The operation led to a ruptured bowel and adhesions on the tubes. From this point on she used a diaphragm and her cycle was regular, but with very painful 6–7-day periods.

When Christine was 29, she started bleeding again and was taken to hospital. The adhesions from the previous operation had led to a haemorrhage and the ovary and tube were removed.

For the next year after this, she had a great deal of hormonal instability, with bleeding every 2 weeks but no ovulation. Her doctor put her on the fertility drug clomiphene citrate. She began to ovulate but became severely hypoglycaemic. She came off the drug 3 months later and subsequently had a 'normal' period. Then the next period came a week early; she bled for 7 days, and again 4 days later, for 2 weeks.

Christine came to me after the bleeding had stopped for 1 week. She wanted not only to 'regulate' her menstrual experiences, but also to conceive. She felt that this might be impossible, given her history.

I treated her with herbs to balance the hormonal state and to reduce pain and bleeding, and instructed her in timing. She corrected her nutrient status with supplements and diet, and exercised more to regulate her circulation.

She used autosuggestion techniques from a tape I prepared for her to help control bleeding and make her cycle regular and synchronised with her lunar return. This happened within a few months, by which time her hormonal cycle was behaving itself. Christine conceived as soon as the two cycles coincided.

Conception when lunar return and menstruation coincide

RACHEL

Rachel was a Jewish woman who, for religious reasons, avoided sex during her period. She wanted to conceive but had had no success. When I calculated her lunar cycle, it became apparent that it was coinciding with her menstruation. She decided the baby was more important to her than the taboo, and promptly conceived.

Dr Jonas also had cases such as this. One concerned a couple who had been unable to conceive a child for 7 or 8 years. Jonas found that the lunar cycle was coinciding with menstruation, which the couple had avoided, thinking it infertile. Although Jonas gave no specific advice, the couple tried conception during the period anyway and the woman conceived immediately.

This was reported by Dr Farsky, who practises Jonas' methods in Switzerland, to Margaret Lewis, a patient of mine who was doing further research on the lunar cycle. Dr Farsky experienced many such cases.

JENNY

Jenny, one of my patients, corroborated these findings by accident. She was using the method for contraception and made love during her period, not really believing she could conceive. She did, and had a termination. Since then her lunar return has coincided with her ovulation and all is going well.

The lunar cycle, pregnancy and birth

The lunar cycle also seems to influence the timing of birth. The following story beautifully illustrates this ancient connection between the moon, women and fertility.

This delightful study is from a student of Natural Fertility Management, a woman who had previously used mucus and temperature charting but was learning about the lunar cycle for the first time. She had kept extensive and accurate records of all her many children's conceptions and births, and I calculated a retrospective lunar chart for her, giving her personal lunar peak times relating to her own biorhythm over these years. There was a tendency to twins in her family, so it may be that she was particularly susceptible to the influence of the lunar cycle: this additional potentially fertile time has been found to be responsible for the conception of non-identical twins.

The following is this woman's fascinating story, which may be interesting to those of you who have previously had arguments with your doctor about conception and due dates.

During a recent Natural Fertility Management course, I was interested to learn of the effect of the lunar cycle on fertility. This was perhaps an explanation for the otherwise unexpected arrival of my two youngest children, who were conceived while we were using the Billings method. Our daughter, now 9, was conceived 9–10 days after I believed I had ovulated (*spinn*, or fertile, mucus followed by a clear sustained temperature rise lasting over 1 week). Our son, now nearly 4, was conceived 18 days after I had recorded ovulation symptoms and a rise in basal temperature. In addition to avoiding all sexual contact near ovulation, we were using a barrier method at all other times.

Throughout the pregnancies, I had experienced long-running problems convincing health professionals that my babies were due later than the dates assumed from the date of my last period (and that I was not stupid, vague, lying or having an extramarital relationship!). Interestingly, both babies arrived well past their official due dates: our daughter, 4300g, '10 days late' but with no signs of postmaturity; and our son was induced, '18 days overdue' weighing 4600g but with no signs of postmaturity.

Francesca kindly provided me with some retrospective lunar cycle charts so that I could see if there was a link. I was also interested in seeing if the lunar angle return was connected to the onset of labour.

The results? Quite amazing! I was able to remember these children's conception dates (a bit hard to forget when there had been so much debate about it during the pregnancies) and both correlated beautifully with the lunar cycle. It solved a mystery for us. Awareness of the lunar cycle may have prevented these pregnancies — though I would hasten to add that we all love these two 'lunar children' dearly and would not change anything about them or their births at all. We believe that they are special people who were really meant to be here. It may be interesting to add that both these children were conceived while we were both shell-shocked by the deaths of close family members. While I do not have any firm opinions on reincarnation, our daughter has many strong similarities in personality, talents and interests to her grandmother who died so close to her conception.

At the time, I wondered if a second ovulation was possible in some cycles. This idea was dismissed as ludicrous by an obstetrician, but I do wonder, especially in light of my strong family history of non-identical twins who have been born with significant gaps in birthweight and maturity.

The conception dates of our two older sons also tallied well with the lunar cycle — I was able to remember these easily as they coincided with easily remembered dates such as our wedding anniversary and Easter. In both cases, this was probably lunar cycle and mid-cycle ovulation being synchronised.

Of these four children mentioned, spontaneous onset of labour coincided with the lunar cycle in two cases. In the other two, it didn't. I did, however, experience false labour significantly enough to spend the night at the birth centre. I could remember the date too — it was my niece's birthday and she was disappointed that her cousin missed her birthday by a week. It would be interesting to see if other parents or midwives have noticed the effect of the lunar cycle on uterine irritability.

Other unwanted conceptions
RUTH

Ruth came to me after having conceived while using the sympto-thermal method. She was adept at observing both mucus and temperature changes so felt confused and let down that she had conceived, despite being scrupulous in her attendance to detail in following the method.

I calculated back to the cycle in which Ruth had conceived and, as she kept comprehensive records of her sexual activity, found that her lunar return had coincided with the only time she had unprotected intercourse that month (believing herself to be safe).

This has occurred quite often in my experience.

SAMANTHA

Samantha had also been using the mucus method and conceived against her wishes. She felt conception had occurred during her period, as this was the only time that she had not used a barrier technique. She wondered if her lunar cycle had fallen then. I calculated, and no, it hadn't.

However, while asking about her cycle history, it became apparent that Samantha often had short cycles. It seemed likely that she had ovulated very soon after her period and the sperm had lived through, fertile mucus being observed as soon as the bleeding ceased.

Samantha had a termination and is wiser now.

KIM

Kim had repeatedly conceived while using every contraception technique in the book. She conceived twice using a diaphragm, once when a condom burst, once on the Pill and once when relying on an IUD, as well as twice more when using nothing but withdrawal and a rough rhythm calculation.

All of these pregnancies had miscarried or been aborted. Kim felt that she was superfertile and that nothing would work for her. I explained that however high her levels of fertility, she was still only fertile for a few days each month.

While we were discussing whether she could possibly trust natural methods of birth control, it became apparent that she was, at the least, unsure of her decision to remain childless (she was certainly very attached to the idea of her superfertility).

On further questioning, it appeared that these ambivalent feelings had perhaps been the cause of her being a little less than rigorous in applying her contraception techniques. We used hypnotherapy to bring her subconscious desires to awareness so she could deal with them and make a conscious choice to which she could stay committed. Kim has used natural methods successfully ever since.

BELINDA

Belinda was *most* disillusioned, as she had conceived while on the Pill. As she was unhappy about the circumstances and the possible effects of the Pill on a pregnancy, this contributed to her reluctance to have a child so she had a termination, which caused her to became very insecure: she felt that if the Pill didn't work, there was no safe way for her to avoid conception.

When we calculated backwards, the conception seemed to have occurred at a lunar peak fertile time. Feeling better with at least a possible explanation, Belinda found the confidence to start using natural birth control methods and has been doing so from that time on.

Failure to conceive due to subconscious blocks

Subconscious psychological blocks to conception can be very real, and often much more complex than the understandable and natural stress reaction experienced by so many infertile couples. The blocks in the following cases come from very different causes, but I have little doubt that, in each case, were the main reason for the woman's infertility.

SANDRA

Earlier on in her life, Sandra had had two terminations, followed by the premature birth of a child with a congenital brain disorder. She felt very guilty about this, believing that the terminations had caused an incompetent cervix (which may well have been the case), resulting in the premature birth and ensuing disorder.

She was suffering from extremely bad dysmenorrhoea, accompanied by vomiting, diarrhoea, very heavy bleeding and pain, but she wanted to conceive again.

In Sandra's case, I feel sure that with psychotherapy her guilt and doubts could have been allayed, and her dysmenorrhoea and infertility healed. However, she did not continue treatment with me.

Many people who catch a glimpse of their psychological blocks are alarmed at having to confront them and choose not to do so. That is up to them. However, many use the help of a therapist to bring them to awareness and come to a successful resolution.

VICKY

Vicky was very anxious to conceive. She had married late in life and was impatient to start a family. When she was much younger, she'd had two terminations, an IUD had become 'jammed' and rejected, and she had been on and off the Pill for some years.

Her husband's sperm count was lowish (we soon fixed that) and she had bad dysmenorrhoea (we fixed that, too). She was eating well and had a healthy lifestyle except for smoking cigarettes, which she gave up very easily when we used hypnotherapy, despite enormous initial resistance (her husband also gave up as part of his treatment).

When Vicky came to me she had been trying to conceive for 18 months. She achieved conception 6 months later but miscarried. Then she admitted to me that she had experienced sexual fantasies involving children for some time and felt extremely guilty about them.

When we worked on her acceptance of these fantasies, not only did they disappear (sexual feelings feed off guilt) but she also conceived quite easily and carried the baby to term.

MARIA

At the same time as Maria began trying to conceive, her mother became terminally ill. She was ill for a year before she died, and during this time Maria did not become pregnant. She was experienced with mucus and temperature checking, and tests showed that her hormone levels were fine, and that her husband's sperm, which survived well in her reproductive tract, were also fine.

Two months after her mother died, Maria developed bad dysmenorrhoea; she was also diagnosed as having endometriosis. It wasn't extensive, and was treated and eliminated, except on one tube.

Six months later her periods were coming every 2 weeks. Hormone therapy was started, her cycle went to 28 days, and she was put on the clomiphene citrate as well as a program for in vitro conception.

She conceived, but miscarried at 12 weeks and bled for 2 months, with clotting and bad pain. Her cycle resumed on a 6-week interval. An ultrasound showed that her ovary had enlarged as a result of the hormonal medication.

When Maria came to see me, she had been trying to conceive for 3 years altogether and was very depressed, particularly since her best friend had just conceived with ease. She was not experiencing much mid-cycle mucus and her period was still coming every 6 weeks, with discomfort.

I gave her herbs to regulate her hormones and eliminate the drugs from her system, as ovulation must come before Day 20 for conception to be viable. She started taking nutrients to prepare for a healthy pregnancy and we did considerable work over a few weeks on her emotional state.

It came up through counselling that Maria had felt very guilty at trying to conceive during her mother's terminal illness, and had never really allowed herself to grieve. Processing this grief seemed to overcome the final hurdle to a successful conception.

It was certainly a very speedy cure, because within 2 months, her cycle was normal and she had conceived a healthy child, who, when I saw her at the age of 4 months, was being fully breastfed.

MONICA

Monica's history was one of a very secure childhood with a father who adored her. There was no apparent physical reason for her infertility and she could see no possible cause in her very happy childhood memories of her parents as role models. As far as she could see, her attitude to parenting was based on the extremely successful relationship she'd had with her own parents, especially her father.

What emerged as she did therapy was a fear that her own husband would form such a strong bond with her daughter (she was sure it would be a girl) that she would be neglected. Once these fears were addressed and her husband reassured her successfully. Monica conceived.

VICTORIA

Victoria had mother-in-law problems. She was not a very assertive woman and had married into a close-knit, emotionally intense family dominated by an eccentric woman whose favourite child was Victoria's husband, Edward.

Edward was reasonably assertive himself, but instead of standing up to his mother, he conspired with her to influence Victoria, who felt totally overwhelmed.

Victoria's mother-in-law chose the furniture, bought the house she and Edward lived in and generally ran their lives. Victoria was becoming unable to make her own decisions or assessments, except out of irritation and resentment. She continually asked for my opinion of her chances of conceiving, although I had endlessly repeated the same information.

I thought her chances were quite good, but I could see that there was some deep work needed first. Her desire to have a child, although strong, was so confused with her mother-in-law's determination for a grandchild and her own resistance to that pressure that she had 'given herself' endometriosis and an imbalance in her hormones to avoid the whole issue.

Her reproductive conditions were not severe at all, and the physical problems could quite easily be overcome with a little dedication. And dedication Victoria had, but it was mostly channelled into thwarting her mother-in-law, about whom she could not stop complaining.

We spent most of our sessions in counselling until she had come to see that she had to reclaim her life, her possessions, her home and her need to conceive — and do it for herself.

Then we introduced some hypnotherapy to firm her resolve. Slowly, she made changes in her life that were based on her own decisions, without giving in to hate and spite. She even came to feel that she could be happy to let her mother-in-law love and take pride in her grandchild and still keep her own relationship with her child intact.

She made changes in the home, to make it hers, and grew to like it enough to plan the nursery. Once she had made a space in her life for her child, it came.

JEANETTE

Jeanette was a therapist so spent her life sorting out other people's problems. This was a source of resentment for her husband, who felt she was abandoning him. Their relationship, although potentially good, suffered from a certain lack of commitment.

When Jeanette first came to me, she felt unsure if she was ready for a child. She had been trying for a conception for a while, but was not surprised that it hadn't happened, given her ambivalence.

During the course of therapy with me, she came to feel that she was ready to conceive but something was still holding her back. Everything physical had come good, although there had been problems previously, and what came up next was that she wasn't sure if she wanted to conceive in that relationship.

Jeanette determined to take some time out from her practice and spend some of her very nurturing energy on herself and her relationship. She's doing that right now, and I'm sure we'll get some good results soon.

NATASHA

Having recently experienced the stillbirth of her baby, Natasha was understandably devastated. In her life, however, there was little room to express this since, as a very high-profile person in the entertainment business, her every mood was public property.

There was no reason to suppose another child would be stillborn, as the cause had been a very high temperature in the last few days of the pregnancy, a result of an exotic virus contracted from a traveller.

Natasha's problems were that she hadn't had the opportunity to grieve and was still very fearful of a repeat experience.

Her therapy was to take time out from work and public life, and involve herself preparing for an optimum conception, taking time and responsibility to create a new chance and thereby work through her grief and fear of the old.

ZOE

In this case, the block wasn't subconscious — or even Zoe's. It was her husband's, and although it may have been subconscious on his part — I never got to see him — I didn't get to form an opinion. The result of the problem, however, was absolutely clear. Zoe's husband would not make love to her and hadn't since they married.

There wasn't really a lot I could do to help. Zoe learnt how to time conception very precisely and we made sure her reproductive health was up to scratch so that if there was a breakthrough, it wouldn't be wasted.

Zoe then had three options: to continue to have faith that she could engineer a change of heart in her husband, to find another father and risk her relationship, or to choose motherhood over marriage and leave in search of a more obliging partner.

I don't know what she did, but I know I'll never get a harder case!

Many of the women who come to see me have husbands or partners who are not interested in having children. Some are even definitely opposed to it. Sometimes, although less often, it's the other way around. We saw how Camilla worked through this to a happy resolution, but the situations are not always amenable to negotiation.

These situations are becoming more and more common as people move on from one relationship to the next. One partner may have children from a previous relationship and feel that they have passed that period of their lives.

For these situations to be resolved, both partners need to be sensitive to each other's needs. There aren't always easy answers. Unfortunately, the sensitivity is often lacking, as we shall see in this next case.

Relationship problems
AMANDA AND COLIN

Amanda wanted children, Colin didn't. Amanda came to see me, Colin didn't. Amanda wanted to talk about it, Colin didn't. Amanda was very clear about her desires and needs, Colin wasn't. Amanda was childless, Colin wasn't. Amanda was prepared to go through surgical procedures to find out if there was anything wrong with her fertility. Colin wasn't prepared to ejaculate into a pot to see if there was anything wrong with his. Amanda was saddened but not threatened by the thought of infertility. Colin was threatened but not sad. Amanda began to think of Colin as an insensitive pig. Colin began to think of Amanda as a demanding harridan. Amanda got divorced. Colin did, too.

PHILIPPA AND TED

Philippa and Ted both wanted children and were both willing to do anything to solve their long-standing infertility. However, Ted found it more difficult than he expected to give up smoking, and Philippa became more and more impatient with him, refusing to start her conception attempts until he had uncontaminated sperm.

Having spent many months persuading Ted of the importance of that very approach, I now found it necessary to emphasise to both of them the very real effort Ted had made in other areas. It was that or become a marriage guidance counsellor.

Often, when a preconception health care program has been enthusiastically undertaken but not completed, I need to remind a couple that, although it is indeed important to try to achieve all the preconception goals, they are still well ahead of the majority of couples and what they have achieved is well worthwhile.

Hormonal and reproductive health

Although most of the problems of hormonal health we deal with at the Jocelyn Centre are part of a fertility or contraception consultation, we also help women who have no need of help in either of these areas.

Most of these women have problems that we have looked at already, such as PID, endometriosis or PMS. Some women who come to us are reaching the end of their fertile lives and need to understand what is happening to their bodies so they can avoid conception during the fluctuations of menopause, as well as reduce the discomfort they are experiencing during this time.

In Chapter 12, 'Natural Remedies for Hormonal and Reproductive Health', we looked at some ways of dealing with commonly experienced hormonal ill-health. Here are a few case histories to illustrate them.

BEVERLY

Continuous and horrendous PMS was debilitating Beverley to the point that she was almost suicidal. It was getting worse as time went on, particularly since the birth of her last child by caesarean section.

Beverley was already taking a multivitamin and mineral tablet formulated for the relief of PMS, as well as some iron tablets, which she found gave her some relief. But, as well as her cyclic symptoms, which included heavy bleeding, pain and nausea, she was chronically constipated, and suffered from digestive problems and very low sexual energy.

I took her off the iron tablets and substituted *Bladderwrack* (seaweed), which I mixed with other herbs such as *Chastetree* for hormonal balancing, nervines, sexual tonics and liver herbs.

The *Bladderwrack* was much easier for her to metabolise than the iron, and the constipation cleared. As we changed her diet to eliminate fats (particularly in the second half of her cycle), increased the sources of vitamin B$_6$, calcium, magnesium and zinc, and gave her *Evening Primrose* oil capsules, she became a completely renewed person.

'For the first time in so many years, I feel like a human being again. The water retention and other symptoms have gone, and I am so much less depressed and anxious. I even feel interested in sex!'

BARBARA

Barbara thought she had her PMS licked. She was doing all the things I had recommended and it was getting better all the time. Then, along came a demanding and stressful week or two when she gave in to the desire for a little piece of chocolate, 'Just to help her through'.

Her one piece of chocolate became several, and came to be accompanied by a drink or two. Before she had time to take stock, she was cramming in sugar and alcohol in an effort to keep afloat and the PMS symptoms all came rushing back.

When Barbara came in for her next appointment and had made her confession, I asked her to read a book on systemic candida problems and see if she could relate to the descriptions therein. She did, and she could. So we started her on an anticandida diet with appropriate medication. Now her PMS stands a chance of being permanently cured.

ELIZABETH

Elizabeth also suffered from candida. Having got that almost under control, she now found herself entering into an early menopause. The hot flushes, low energy, weight gain and general feeling of malaise were sufficiently similar to her previous candida symptoms for her to guess they might be related.

Indeed they were. While she kept her candida under control and ate well — avoided all sugar, alcohol and refined carbohydrates, fermented foods and fungi — the menopause treatments worked, her cycle resumed fairly normally and her symptoms abated.

If she lapsed with her diet and allowed herself to respond to stress by craving and eating stimulants such as caffeine and sugar, then the oestrogenic herbs, the hormonal balancers, the essential fatty acids and the absence of saturated fats from her diet didn't hold the menopausal symptoms at bay.

Elizabeth didn't want to conceive by mistake at this point in her life, so she had another reason to keep herself in good hormonal health. She found it easy to identify her fertile times, even in the slightly changed patterns she was experiencing.

Enough of the ladies; let's give the blokes a turn!

Sperm count problems

MAX

Max's story was one of *very* low sperm count. His partner, Mia, had never been pregnant; nor had any of his previous partners conceived. Mia had normal cycles; tests indicated no fertility problems.

Even so, we put Mia on herbs as well as Max, just to be sure; each of them also took supplements and paid much greater attention to their diet and health.

Max achieved his higher sperm count through using these treatments and the lunar cycle peak times, as the results from tests done at these times were considerably better than those done at other times. Mia synchronised her ovulation (which she identified through mucus and temperature observations) to his lunar peak with the help of autosuggestions and a tape I prepared for her.

FRANK

Frank's sperm count was *very, very* low. He and Eunice had been on a program of assisted conception with no success; donor sperm, which neither of them felt good about, was the next step. In Frank's case, hormonal drugs had had no effect, but herbal remedies combined with vitamins and minerals brought his sperm count up so much — from 'very, very low' to 'more than adequate' — that it was hardly necessary to use the lunar chart.

He did anyway, to make sure. His wife had her own fertility problem, which made a natural conception impossible, but with the help of the in vitro program, Frank's plentiful sperm was used and conception achieved within 4 months of seeing me.

GEORGE

George has been mentioned before, in Chapter 13. He's the one who wore the wetsuit. It took us some time to work out why he was not responding to the remedies that he had been receiving, but in the end it was unnecessary to give him treatment. He just gave up surfing in cold weather! Wetsuits keep the testicles hot and under pressure, and so kill sperm.

ANDREW

Andrew was a farmer who had major deficiencies in all three sperm factors — count, motility and morphology. He was committed to a natural lifestyle and had converted his farm to organic methods some years before.

When his zinc levels refused to come good, I suggested a hair-trace mineral analysis. The results showed an excessively high level of many toxic heavy metals. Andrew was dismayed that, despite his new, healthy farm practices, the legacy from his earlier exposure was still affecting him so adversely.

As well as the normal program of preconception care for both he and his wife, Andrew undertook intravenous chelation therapy to eliminate the heavy metals.

His semen analysis, 6 months later after new, healthy sperm had had a chance to develop, was sufficiently good to achieve a healthy conception.

STEWART

In Stewart's case of very low sperm count and motility, we combined all the approaches. He also used some Tantric yoga techniques, similar to the erection gain and loss routine described in Chapter 13.

His count went up from 1 800 000 (which is low, believe it or not), to 52 million (which is more than adequate). These readings were taken at trough and peak lunar times with treatment in between.

DANIEL

Daniel's main problem was the poor motility of his sperm and their tendency to clump together. As well as the usual herbal remedies and supplements, I gave him high doses of vitamin C. His wife Joanne still didn't conceive. Daniel became very distressed, taking the blame upon himself.

It turned out that Joanne, who had initially refused to come with Daniel to see me (thereby increasing his feelings of responsibility and guilt), was getting very little fertile mucus. Once she agreed to treatment, this problem righted itself. But, by then, Daniel was so stressed, his sperm count was down. The final solution was joint counselling.

CRAIG

Craig's difficulty was not sperm count or motility problems, but a high proportion of abnormal sperm — far too many of the sperm he produced were not healthy.

First, we cleaned up his diet and put him on herbs and supplements. This gave us a better result, but not good enough. Craig resisted and resisted giving up smoking. Finally, he agreed to do hypnotherapy, which was successful. Two months later, the greater proportion of his sperm was normal. Conception followed in a few months.

HARRY

Harry also had abnormality problems. He didn't have to give up smoking, because he already had. Harry had to give up his job. Handling chemicals all day long probably didn't do much for his overall health anyway.

We used a homoeopathic chemical detoxification remedy and liver herbs, as well as reproductive tonics and increased nutrients. The treatment was a success.

KATE AND TERRY

Kate and Terry were superfit, and the only real problem was a slightly low sperm count. After that had been boosted, and they both had stayed on the preconception diet, raised their nutrient levels and learnt exact timing techniques, we expected conception to follow easily. It didn't.

A post-coital test was done. It showed no sperm *at all* alive in Kate's mucus after intercourse. No antibodies could be found, the mucus wasn't acidic, and it ferned beautifully. The test was carried out again, in case a mistake had been made: the same result came back.

Terry's sperm was tested in donor mucus, and donor sperm in Kate's mucus. The results were not helpful. Only one thing remained — they both had to give up smoking.

Hypnotherapy came to the rescue again; within 2 months, Kate conceived.

Although, because of her small size and her baby's disinclination to turn around and face the right way, a caesarean section had to be performed, the following letter shows that this really didn't matter.

We are absolutely delighted, ecstatic and in a state of bliss over the safe, happy, healthy birth of our 'heaven on earth', a daughter, Tara, born 7th June!

Thanks for your advice and support. Will call in sometime and introduce you to the third member of our family!

Although many natural therapies can be successful in cases of infertility and for some, one approach is better than another, my own love is for herbs — perhaps I was a witch in another lifetime or I may have learnt it all in this one. Herbal remedies have not only fascinated me, but they have also brought great success to many of my patients, as well as to my family and myself.

That is not to say that the results achieved in many of these cases could not have been accomplished equally well with homoeopathy or acupuncture, for example. Other psychotherapeutic techniques could have been substituted for hypnotherapy.

These stories illustrate many of the points I have tried to make in this book — there are so many others for which there is not room. My thanks to all my patients, included here or not, and to you, the reader, for your time and attention.

The moral of these stories is that natural, non-invasive and holistic therapies and techniques can work. Whatever the outcome, they will leave you better off than you were when you started treatment. I hope this book has helped you to see how they can work for you, and that they will help you achieve

◆ confident contraception

◆ conscious conception

◆ functional fertility

◆ hormonal health

◆ preparation for pregnancy, and —

◆ greater joy and satisfaction in your life.

Available Services

Francesca and Natural Fertility Management also offer the following services that can augment and update the information in this book.

The Books

These books by Francesca Naish and Janette Roberts (the Australian representative of the Foresight Association) are available through all good bookshops by mail order or through the Internet. All prices are quoted in Australian dollars and include GST.

The Natural Way to Better Babies: Preconception Health Care for Prospective Parents, Francesca Naish and Janette Roberts, Random House, Sydney, 1996, $27.50.

The Natural Way to a Better Pregnancy, Francesca Naish and Janette Roberts, Doubleday, Sydney, 1999, $25.00.

The Natural Way to Better Birth and Bonding, Francesca Naish and Janette Roberts, Doubleday, Sydney, 2000, $27.50.

The Lunar Cycle, by Francesca Naish, Nature and Health Books, Sydney, 1989, $13.00.

For the above books, send cheque, money order or credit card details (Visa/Mastercard/Bankcard) to

> Natural Fertility Management
>
> P O Box 786
>
> Castlemaine Victoria 3450
>
> Australia
>
> Phone (61-3) 5472 4922 Fax (61-3) 5470 5766

or order through our website: **www.fertility.com.au**. Please include postage costs: $10.00 for up to four books (within Australia); $25.00 for up to two books (overseas economy air).

Natural Fertility Management

Francesca is the director of Natural Fertility Management (NFM), which offers programs for

◆ natural contraception

◆ conscious conception and preconception health care

◆ overcoming fertility problems (male and female)

as well as holistic health care for

◆ reproductive health (male and female)

◆ pregnancy and preparation for birth

◆ threatened miscarriage

◆ breastfeeding

◆ menopause.

You can find out more about NFM on our website **www.fertility.com.au.**

PERSONAL CONSULTATIONS

The Natural Fertility Management clinic offers all of the above programs and treatments at

> The Jocelyn Centre
>
> 46 Grosvenor Street
>
> Woollahra NSW 2025
>
> Australia
>
> Phone (61 2) 9369 2047 Fax (61 2) 9369 5179

where a comprehensive range of holistic medical and natural treatment is provided by highly qualified practitioners, using natural and non-invasive therapies.

HOW TO FIND A LOCAL NFM PRACTITIONER

NFM provides a referral service to NFM accredited counsellors throughout Australia, as well as in New Zealand, the USA and the UK.

Send a stamped, self-addressed envelope to

> Jane Bennett
>
> NFM Network Coordinator
>
> P O Box 786
>
> Castlemaine Victoria 3450
>
> Australia
>
> Phone (61 3) 5472 4922, Fax (61 3) 5470 5766

or you can contact her through our website at **www.fertility.com.au.**
Email **enquiries@fertility.com.au.**

POSTAL AND INTERNET SERVICES

For those unable to attend personally, contraception and conception kits
are also available by mail order or through the Internet. See above for postal
and website addresses (all enquiries to the network coordinator).

The NFM kits for contraception or conception include the following
items.

◆ A copy of the book Natural Fertility: A Complete Guide to Avoiding
   or Achieving Conception (or rebate on proof of purchase).

◆ A copy of the book The Natural Way to Better Babies: Preconception
   Health Care for Prospective Parents (for conception kits only — rebate
   on proof of purchase).

◆ An audio cassette with

   − side 1: instructions for contraception or conception and use of lunar
     cycle charts, and

   − side 2: relaxation techniques, visualisations and suggestions to assist
     the synchronisation of cycles, increase confidence and motivation,
     promote reproductive health and general well-being, and deal with
     stress. In the conception kit there are also suggestions for a healthy
     conception, pregnancy and birth.

◆ Blank sympto-thermal charts for recording mucus and temperature and
   other observations for each menstrual cycle.

◆ Individual computer-calculated lunar charts showing the potentially
   fertile times on your personal biorhythmic fertility cycle for the next
   10 years.

◆ Current year moon calendar, showing moon phase present on each day
   of the year.

◆ Time zone calculator, to adjust times given on your personal lunar
   chart for different time zones.

◆ Attractively bound printed notes for conception or contraception,
   taking you through the first few months, cycle by cycle.

◆ Options

   − for conscious conception — sex selection calculations and advice

   − for male fertility problems — male lunar chart, male relaxation and
     suggestion tape

   − naturopathic advice for your personal situations from Francesca
     Naish and her Associates.

Orders can be placed through the website or by mail. Contact Jane Bennett, NFM Network Coordinator, as above.

NFM COUNSELLOR TRAINING
Residential seminars are conducted by Francesca Naish and her associates to train health professionals in NFM techniques and the *Better Babies* program of preconception health care and fertility treatments. All accredited counsellors have access to NFM kits for their patients and professional support. You can find out more about the training through the website, or by contacting the NFM Network Coordinator (see above).

NFM AND BETTER BABIES HELPLINE
Francesca Naish and her associates are also available for advice on all reproductive health issues, as well as those associated with fertility and contraception. Phone consultations for simple enquiries are charged by the minute. More complex problems can be addressed by mail or email. For enquiries, contact the NFM Network Coordinator.

Payment for online, postal or telephone consultations can be made by Visa, Mastercard or Bankcard, as well as by cheque or postal order.

Individual advice for preconception health care, fertility problems or contraception can be included with the kits available through our postal or Internet service. See above for details.

Contacts and Resources

Wherever possible, I have given national contacts. NSW contacts, when given, can usually supply you with appropriate addresses in your own state or territory. Natural health journals contain service directories that will give many more names and addresses than I have been able to list here. All addresses and phone numbers are up to date at time of publication.

To find a doctor trained in nutritional and environmental medicine, contact

Australian College of Nutritional and Environmental Medicine (ACNEM)

13 Hilton Street, Beaumaris, Vic 3193.

Phone (03) 9589 6088, Fax (03) 9589 5158.

For names of appropriate natural health practitioners, contact

Acupuncture Ethics and Standards Organisation (AESO) and Australian Acupuncture Association (AACA)

P O Box 5142, West End, Qld 4101.

Phone (07) 3846 5866.

Association of Massage Therapists (NSW)

P O Box 1248, Bondi Junction, NSW 2022.

Phone (02) 9300 9405.

Association of Remedial Masseurs

1/120 Blaxland Road, Ryde, NSW 2112.

Phone (02) 9807 4769.

Australian Association of Reflexology

2 Stewart Avenue, Matraville, NSW 2036.

Phone (02) 9311 2322.

Australian Council for Experiential Therapies and College of Experiential Psychotherapy

141 Beattie Street, Balmain, NSW 2041.

Phone (02) 9818 4188.

Australian Hypnotherapists Association
Phone 1800 067 557 (free call).

Australian Natural Therapists Association (for a comprehensive listing of a wide range of natural therapists)
P O Box A964, Sydney, NSW 2000.
Phone (02) 9283 2234. Country and interstate callers phone 1800 817 577 (free call).

Australian Osteopathic Association
P O Box 699, Turramurra, NSW 2074.
Phone (02) 9449 4799.

Australian Psychological Society
30 Atchison Street, St Leonards, NSW 2065.
Phone (02) 9906 6504.

Australian School of Reflexology
15 Kedumba Crescent, Turramurra, NSW 2074.
Phone (02) 9988 3881.

Australian Society of Clinical Hypnotherapists
30 Denistone Road, Eastwood, NSW 2122.
Phone (02) 9874 2776.

Australian Society of Hypnosis (members are doctors, dentists, psychiatrists, psychologists) and Academy of Applied Hypnosis
300 George Street, Sydney, NSW 2000.
Phone (02) 9231 4877.

Australian Traditional Medicine Society (for a comprehensive listing of a wide range of natural therapists)
P O Box 1027, Meadowbank, NSW 2114.
Phone (02) 9809 6800.

BKS Iyengar (Yoga) Association of Australia Inc.
P O Box 159, Mosman, NSW 2088.
Phone (02) 9948 2366.

Chiropractors Association of Australia
Phone 1800 803 665 (free call).

Homoeopathic Association of NSW
90 Pitt Street, Sydney, NSW 2000.
Phone (02) 9231 3322.

International Federation of Aromatherapists
P O Box 107, Burwood, NSW 2134, and
P O Box 400, Balwyn, Vic 3103.
Phone 1902 24 0125 (National Information Line).

International Yoga Teachers Association Inc.
P O Box 207, St Ives, NSW 2075.
Phone (02) 9484 2256.

Natural Health Society
Suite 28/541 High Street, Penrith, NSW 2750.
Phone (02) 4721 5068.

National Herbalists Association of Australia
P O Box 61, Broadway, NSW 2007.
Phone (02) 9211 6437.

Reflexology Association of Australia
22 Lagoon Street, Narrabeen, NSW 2101.
Phone (02) 9970 6155.

Reiki Network
187a Avenue Road, Mosman, NSW 2088.
Phone (02) 9969 1623 or 1800 804 529 (free call).

Shiatsu Therapy Association of Australia
332 Carlisle Street, Balaclava, Vic 3183.
Phone (03) 9530 0067
or
P O Box 47, Waverley, NSW 2024.
Phone (02) 9314 5248.

T'ai Chi Australian Academy
P O Box 1020, Burwood North, NSW 2134
Phone (02) 9797 9355.

To receive an organic products directory, contact

Heaven and Earth Systems Pty Ltd
Phone (02) 9365 7668.

To find a supplier of organically grown produce near you, contact

The National Association for Sustainable Agriculture, Australia (NASAA)
Head Office
P O Box 768, Stirling, SA 5152.
Phone (08) 8370 8455, Fax (08) 8370 8381.

New South Wales and ACT
P O Box 770, North Sydney, NSW 2060.

Queensland
P O Box 733, Emerald, Qld 4720.

South Australia
P O Box 207, Stirling, SA 5152.

Western Australia
P O Box 8387, Stirling Street, WA 6849.

Tasmania
Post Office, Lower Longley, Tas 7109.

Victoria
RMB 1299, Blampied, Vic 3363.

For information about water filters and water deliveries, contact

All Clear Water Aust.
Phone (08) 9257 2241.

Aqua One Water Filters
Phone (07) 3890 2900.

Crystal Clear Purification Systems
Phone (08) 8331 3376.

Crystal Flow
Phone (03) 9866 8222.

Culligan
Phone (02) 9316 4142.

Neverfail Spring Water Co.
Phone (02) 9712 1022.

Raindance Water Purifiers
Phone (07) 3849 1577.

The Freshly Squeezed Water Co.
Phone (02) 9712 1022 or (07) 3856 0988.

The Pure Water Shop
Phone (08) 8373 2096.

The Water People
Phone (03) 9885 0222.

The Water Shop
Phone (02) 9956 5677.

Unicorn — The Water Filter Advisory Centre
Phone (08) 9242 1066.

Water One
Phone (02) 9181 2983

For Bach flower remedies and Australian bush flower essences, contact

Australian Bush Flower Essences
45 Booralie Road, Terrey Hills, NSW 2084.
Phone (02) 9319 0847 or 015 432 288.

Martin and Pleasance
135 Swan Street, Richmond, Vic 3121.
Phone (03) 427 7422.

For meditation and yoga classes, contact

Siddha Yoga Foundation
50 Garnet Street, Dulwich Hill, NSW 2203.
Phone (02) 9559 5666.

Yoga in pregnancy

The Yoga Place
Level 1, 374 Darling Street, Balmain, NSW 2041.
Phone Dr Alex Sharland, (02) 9555 7544.

Other prenatal yoga classes in Sydney
Bondi Junction — (02) 9389 4694.
Gladesville — (02) 9879 5240.
Northern Beaches, Ann Watts — (02) 9799 6510.
Manly — (02) 9977 4725.
South, Yona Griffin — (02) 9522 4363.
Surry Hills — (02) 9212 4177.

For ambient music and relaxation tapes, contact

Natural Symphonies
P O Box 25,
Camden, NSW 2570.
Phone (02) 4655 1800, Fax (02) 4655 9434.

Phoenix Music
P O Box 9,
Bondi, NSW 2026.
Phone (02) 9211 5891.

For DIY acupressure machines, contact

ELF Cocoon Australia, Health and Environment Services
P O Box 40,
Merimbula, NSW 2548.

SHP International Pty Ltd.
5/212 Glen Osmond Road,
Fullarton, SA 5068.
Phone (08) 8379 0700.

For cloth (re-useable) menstrual pads, contact

Rad-pads
P O Box 78,
Castlemaine, Victoria 3450.
Phone (03) 5472 4922, Fax (03) 5470 5766.

Moonphase Pads
P O Box 101,
Bondi Junction, NSW 2022.

For more information on menstrual well-being, contact

Menstrual Well-being Network
Phone (03) 9752 0045, Fax, (03) 9752 0045.

To be fitted for a diaphragm, contact your local women's health centre or Family Planning Association (FPA)

Family Planning Association of NSW
328 Liverpool Road,
Ashfield, NSW 2131.
Phone (02) 9716 6099.

To find kits that help pinpoint the day of ovulation, look in your local pharmacy for

Clear Plan, The Right Day, and First Response.

For more information on hair-trace mineral analysis, contact

Interclinical Laboratories
P O Box 630, Gladesville, NSW 2111.
Phone (02) 9211 2200, Fax (02) 9211 4409.

For more information about Foresight or to subscribe to its newsletter, contact

Foresight Association
Mail Box 16
133 Rowntree Street, Birchgrove, NSW 2041.
Phone and fax (02) 9818 3734.

Foresight also has a range of brochures for health practitioners, and a video, *Preparing for the Healthier Baby*. For a full price list, and details of subscription costs, contact the above address.

For information about support groups for infertile couples, contact

Access
P O Box 959, Parramatta, NSW 2124.
Phone (02) 9670 2380 or 9670 2608 (all states).

To order a colourful moon chart or calendar for your wall, contact

Moon Charts
Reply Paid 20
P O Box 40, Ainslie, ACT 2602.
Phone (02) 6248 7225.

Wombmoon Calendar
P O Box 206, Manly, NSW 2095.
Fax (02) 9983 9440.

Recommended Reading

Natural fertility awareness methods

Books are listed by title, author, publisher, city of publication and year of publication.

The Natural Birth Control Book, Art Rosenblum, Aquarian Research Foundation, Philadelphia, 1976.

A Cooperative Method of Natural Birth Control, Margaret Nofziger, The Book Publishing Co., Tennessee, 1976.

The Fertility Question, Margaret Nofziger, The Book Publishing Co., Tennessee, 1982.

The Fertility Awareness Workbook, Barbara Kass-Annese and Dr Hal Danzer, Thorsons, London, 1984.

Natural Birth Control, Katia and Jonathon Drake, Thorsons, London, 1984.

The Billings Method, Controlling Fertility Without Drugs or Devices, Dr Evelyn Billings and Anne Westmore, Anne O'Donovan, Melbourne, 1980.

The Personal Fertility Guide, Terry Guay, Harbor Publishing, California, 1980.

Taking Charge of Your Fertility, Toni Weschler, Harper Perennial, New York, 1995.

The New Birth Control Program, Christine Garfink and Hank Pizer, Bantam, New York, 1979.

Natural Sex, Mary Shivanandan, Paul Hamlyn, London, 1979.

Natural Birth Control, Frank Richards, Spectrum, Melbourne, 1982.

Natural Family Planning, Anna M. Flynn and Melissa Brooks, George Allen & Unwin, London, 1984.

Mental Birth Control, Mildred Jackson and Terri Teague, Lawton-Teague Publications, California, 1978.

Fertility Awareness — How to become pregnant when you want to, and avoid pregnancy when you don't, Regina Pfeiffer and Katherine Whitlock, Prentice Hall, New Jersey, 1984.

Diamond Method, pamphlet available from Golden Glow Publishers, 2210 Wilshire Blvd, Santa Monica CA 90403.

LUNAR INFLUENCES

The Lunar Cycle, Francesca Naish, Nature and Health Books, Australia and NZ, Prism Press, UK, 1989.

Astrological Birth Control, Sheila Ostrander and Lynn Schroeder, Prentice Hall, New Jersey, 1972.

PSI, Psychic Discoveries Behind the Iron Curtain, Sheila Ostrander and Lynn Shroeder, Abacus, London, 1978.

Women's Mysteries, Ancient and Modern, M. Esther Harding, Harper & Row, New York, 1976.

The Wise Wound, Menstruation and Everywoman, Penelope Shettle and Peter Redgrave, Paladin, London, 1986.

The Mothers, Robert Briffault, Macmillan, New York, 1927.

Lunaception, Louise Lacey, Coward, McCann & Geoghegan, New York, [n.d.].

Body Time, Gay Lear Luce, Temple Smith, London, 1972.

Health & Light, John Ott, Pocket Books, New York, 1976.

Supernature, Lyall Watson, Hodder & Stoughton, New York.

Moon Madness, Paul Katzeff, Citadel Press, New Jersey, [n.d.]

The Cosmic Clocks, Michel Gauquelin, Avon Books, New York, 1969.

WOMEN'S HEALTH

The Women's Guide to Herbal Medicine, Carol Rogers, Hamish Hamilton, London, 1995.

Herbal Remedies for Women, Amanda McQuade Crawford, Prima Publishing, California, 1997.

Hygieia, A Women's Herbal, Jeanine Parvati, Freestone, California, 1978.

Women's Trouble, Natural and Medical Solutions, Ruth Trickey and Kaz Cooke, Allen & Unwin, Sydney, 1998.

Women, Hormones and the Menstrual Cycle, Ruth Trickey, Allen & Unwin, Sydney, 1998.

Natural Healing for Women, S. Curtis and R. Fraser, Pandora, UK, 1991.

Nutrition for Women, The Complete Guide, Elizabeth Somer MARD, Henry Holt, New York, 1993.

Essential Supplements for Women, Carolyn Reuben and Dr Joan Priestley, Thorsons, London, 1991.

Homoeopathic Remedies for Women's Ailments, P. Speight, Health Science Press, UK, 1985.

Homoeopathy for Women, Dr Barry Rose and Dr Christina Scott-Moncrieff, Harper Collins, UK, 1998.

Aromatherapy for Women, M Tisserand, Thorsons, London, 1985.

Natural Hormone Health, Arabella Melville, Thorsons, London, 1970.

Women's Health, Dr Sandra Cabot, Pan Books, Sydney, 1987.

Every Woman's Book, Paavo Airola, Health Plus Publishers, Phoenix, Arizona, 1979.

Body Talk, Jules Black, Angus & Robertson, Sydney, 1988.

The New Women's Health Handbook, Virago, London, 1978.

Everywoman, Derek Llewellyn-Jones, Faber & Faber, London, 1971.

The New Our Bodies, Ourselves, Boston Women's Health Collective, Simon & Schuster, New York, 1992.

How to Stay Out of the Gynaecologist's Office, Federation of Feminist Women's Health Centres, Peace Press, California, 1981.

The Holistic Health Handbook, Berkeley Holistic Health Centre, And/Or Press, Berkeley, 1978.

The Good Health Guide for Women, Jill Turner and Wendy Savage, Paul Hamlyn, London, 1981.

Alternative Health Care for Women, Patsy Westcott, Thorsons, London, 1981.

In Our Own Hands, Bon Hull, Hyland House, Melbourne, 1980.

How to Cope with Menstrual Problems, A Wholistic Approach, Nikki Goldbeck, Keats Publishing, Connecticut, 1983.

No More Menstrual Cramps, Penny Wise Budoff, Angus & Robertson, Sydney, 1984.

The Premenstrual Syndrome, C. Shreeve, Thorsons, UK, 1983.

Once a Month, Katherine Dalton, Fontana/Collins, UK, 1978.

Beat PMS Through Diet, Maryon Stewart, Ebury Press, UK, 1981.

Choice Guide to Birth Control, Penny Lane and John Porter, Thomas Nelson, Melbourne, 1984.

The Bitter Pill, E. Grant, Corgi, UK, 1992.

Breast Cancer? Breast Health!, Susun S. Weed, Ashtree Publishing, New York, 1997.

Childbearing Year Herbal, Susun S. Weed, Ashtree Publishing, New York, 1986.

The Menopausal Years, Susun S. Weed, Ash Tree Publishing, New York, 1992.

The Herbal Menopause Book, Amanda McQuade Crawford, The Crossing Press, California, 1997.

Menopause, A Positive Approach Using Natural Therapies, Nancy Beckham, Penguin, Ringwood, 1995.

Menopause Without Medicine, Linda Ojeda, Thorsons, London, 1990.

The Wise Woman, Judy Hall with Dr Robert Jacobs, Element, UK/USA, 1992.

Ourselves, Growing Older, Paula Brown Doress and Diana Laskin Siegal, Simon & Schuster, New York, 1987; Fontana, UK, 1989.

NUTRITION, HERBS AND NATURAL REMEDIES

A Modern Herbal, M Grieve, Penguin, Harmondsworth, 1977.

Dictionary of Modern Herbalism, Simon Mills, Thorsons, London, 1985.

Encyclopedia of Herbs and Herbalism, Malcolm Stuart, Orbis, London, 1979.

Botanical Influences on Illness, M. R. Werbach, Third Line Press, California, 1994.

The Flower Essence Repertory, P. Kaminski and R. Katz, The Flower Essence Society, California, 1994.

Orthomolecular Nutrition, Abram Hoffer and Morton Walker, Keats Publishing, Connecticut, 1978.

Nutrition and Your Body, Benjamin Colimore and Sarah Stewart Colimore, Light Wave Press, California, 1974.

Mental and Elemental Nutrients, C. Pfeiffer, Keats, Connecticut, 1975.

Nutrition and Physical Degeneration, Dr Weston Price, Price Pottenger Nutrition Foundation, California, 1945.

Nutrition Against Disease, R. Williams, Bantam, New York, 1971.

Nutritional Medicine, S. Davies and A. Stewart, Pan Books, London. 1987.

Do-It-Yourself Shiatsu, Wataru Ohashi, George Allen & Unwin, UK, 1979.

Stories the Feet Have Told Through Reflexology, E. D. Ingham, Ingham Publishing, Florida, 1951.

Reflexology, M. Segal, Wilshire Book Co., California, 1976.

It Might Be Allergies, It Can Be Cured, Phillip Alexander, Davont, Sydney, 1990.

Relief from Candida, Allergies and Ill Health, Greta and Michael Sichel, Sally Milner Publishing, Sydney, 1990.

Candida Can Be Beaten, Richard Turner and Elizabeth Simonsen, Oidium Books, Geelong, 1985.

Hypoglycaemia, A Better Approach, Paavo Airola, Health Plus Publishers, Phoenix, Arizona, 1977.

PRECONCEPTION HEALTH CARE

A Natural Way to Better Babies, Preconception Health Care for Prospective Parents, Francesca Naish and Janette Roberts, Random House, Sydney, 1996.

Planning for a Healthy Baby, Belinda Barnes and Suzanne Gail Bradley, Foresight, Ebury Press, London, 1990.

Preparation for Pregnancy, Suzanne Gail Bradley and Nicholas Bennett, Argyll, Scotland, 1995.

INFERTILITY

Stair Step Approach to Fertility, M. Edwards (ed.), Well Women Series, The Crossing Press, California, 1989.

Getting Pregnant, Derek Llewellyn Jones, Ashwood House Medical, Melbourne, 1990.

Living Laboratories, Robyn Rowland, Sun Books, Sydney, 1992.

Women as Wombs, J. G. Raymond, Harper, California, 1993.

The Experience of Infertility, Naomi Pfeffer and Anne Woollett, Virago, London, 1983.

Getting Pregnant, R. Winston, Anaya, London. 1989.

Success Rates of Contraception Methods

Ranges indicate varied results from different surveys.

Method	Theoretical success rate (%)	User success rate (%)
Pill		
Combined	99.5	95–99
Mini–pill	97–99	93–99
IUD	94–99	93–98
Condoms	95–99	80–93
Diaphragm/cap (+ spermicide)	92–98	80–97
Vaginal ring	96	96
Spermicide (chemical)	85–95	70–85
Spermicide (vitamin C)	96	96
Withdrawal	90	70–85
Injections (Depo-Provera)	99	99
Skin implants (Norplant)	99	99
Sterilisation (male and female)	99.5–99.9	93–99.9
Sympto-thermal method	97–99	70–98
Mucus method	97–98.5	70–98
Temperature method*	93–99	70–98
Rhythm method (regular cycles)	98	60–85
Rhythm method (irregular cycles)	55	30–55
Lunar cycle (with rhythm)	98.5	97.5–98.5

* Temperature method implies abstinence in pre-ovulatory phase.

Both mucus and sympto-thermal methods have been found to have user success rates as high as 99.8 per cent in groups that are both well-taught and well-motivated.

Note: Theoretical success rate means that rate attainable if the method is used correctly 100 per cent of the time, in other words, only accounting for method failures.

User success rate means that rate actually recorded from users, who tend to 'forget' dates, 'lose' their diaphragm, 'run out' of condoms, or just have a misplaced faith that 'It won't happen this time', all of which may have conscious or subconscious motivation.

These user 'failures' can be divided into

◆ teaching-related (a failure in the learning process)

◆ informed choice (couple took a known risk), and

◆ unexplained.

Index